NUTRITION AND DIET RESEARCH PROGRESS

QUERCETIN

DIETARY SOURCES, FUNCTIONS AND HEALTH BENEFITS

NUTRITION AND DIET RESEARCH PROGRESS

NUTRITION AND DIET RESEARCH PROGRESS

QUERCETIN

DIETARY SOURCES, FUNCTIONS AND HEALTH BENEFITS

TAIKI CHIKAMATSU
AND
YUUDAI HIDA
EDITORS

Nova Science Publishers, Inc.
New York

For permission to use material from this book please contact us:
Telephone 631-231-7269; Fax 631-231-8175
Web Site: http://www.novapublishers.com

Additional color graphics may be available in the e-book version of this book.

LIBRARY OF CONGRESS CATALOGING-IN-PUBLICATION DATA

Quercetin: dietary sources, functions, and health benefits / editors, Taiki Chikamatsu and Yuudai Hida.
p. ; cm.
Includes bibliographical references and index.
ISBN 978-1-61942-057-1 (hardcover)
I. Chikamatsu, Taiki. II. Hida, Yuudai.
[DNLM: 1. Quercetin--pharmacology. 2. Quercetin--physiology. QV 325]

615.1--dc23

2011042422

Published by Nova Science Publishers, Inc. ✝ New York

CONTENTS

PREFACE

Quercetin, the most common member of the flavonoids family, is a group of chemical compounds that can be found in the plant kingdom. Fruits and vegetables, particularly citrus fruits, apples, onions, parsley, tea, and red wine, are the primary dietary sources of quercetin. In this book, the authors present topical research in the study of the dietary sources, functions and health benefits of quercetin. Topics discussed include the formulations for pharmaceutical administration of quercetin; the action of quercetin on oxygen uptake by uncoupled mitochondria oxidizing various substrates; the oral health benefits of quercetin; in vitro antibacterial activities and murine studies of novel quercetin diacylglycosyde analogues and the suppressive effect of quercetin on intestinal tight junction permeability.

Chapter 1- Flavonoids are a large group of plant metabolites that are commonly present in fruits, vegetables, cereals and beverages, where they contribute to the bitterness, astrigency, colour, flavour, odour and antioxidant stability of the plant. Epidemiological data suggest that long term consumption of diets rich in flavonoids could provide some health benefits such as lowering arterial pressure, decreasing plasma concentration of lipids and buffering plasma glucose, together with some protection against the development of certain cancers or cardiovascular diseases. Among them, quercetin that belongs to the flavonols components is being investigated for its widespread health benefits. The plant source of quercetin is relatively inexpensive to grow and harvest, and its purification is straightforward. Quercetin is abundant in onion and has been related to diminished mortality from coronary heart disease; it has also shown to exert anticancer properties against benzo(a) pyrene induced lung carcinogenesis in mice and possesses virucidal activity against enveloped viruses such as herpes, simplex type I or parainfluenza type 3. Most of the beneficial effects of quercetin are related to its free radical scavenging activity that supports its antioxidant capability. The antioxidant nature of quercetin is defined mainly by the presence of a catechol group in the B-ring capable of readily donating hydrogen (electron) to stabilise a radical specie. Other features important for the antioxidant nature include the presence of 2,3 unsaturation in conjugation with a 4-oxo-function in the C-ring. In addition, quercetin has proved to be effective and safe for humans at low dosages (500-1000 mg/day).

Thus, available data leads to consider the possible relevance of quercetin benefits on various chronic diseases like cardiovascular, metabolic and neurodegenerative diseases associated with oxidative stress.

Chapter 2- Quercetin, the most common member of the flavonoids family, is a group of chemical compounds that can be found in the plant kingdom. Fruits and vegetables -

particularly citrus fruits, apples, onions, parsley, tea, and red wine - are the primary dietary sources of quercetin. The flavonol is present in plants in many different glycosidic forms, and the highest concentrations are found in onion where quercetin is bound to 1 or 2 glucose molecules (quercetin-3'-glucoside and quercetin-4'-glucoside). Other important sources of quercetin glycosides are apples (quercetin galactosides) and berries (quercetin arabinoses). In addition to the chemical form of the flavonol, the applied vehicule or the composition of the diet seems to have a substantial effect on quercetin bioavailability. In general, flavonoids have been described as health-promoting, disease-preventing dietary supplements, and have activity as cancer preventive agents. Specifically, quercetin, one of the most prominent dietary antioxidants, is combating the destructive "free radical" molecules that play a part in many diseases. Moreover, quercetin has healthful anti-inflammatory and anti-allergy effects, it can also improve the health of capillaries and it has shown to have anti-cancer effects.

Chapter 3- Quercetin (3,3',4',5,7-pentahydroxyflavone, Quer) is the most abundant of the flavonoids found in nature and has a long history of consumption by humans. The main source of Quer is green tea (*Camellia sinensis*), red onion, grapes, apples, berries, cherries, broccoli, citrus fruits, caper, lovage among others. In plants, Quer exhibits strong antioxidant properties, possibly protecting against harmful ultraviolet rays. Research concerning the health benefits of Quer has shown that this compound is cardioprotective and neuroprotective, mainly by acting as antioxidant, antiinflamatory, vasodilating, antihypertensive and antithrombotic. In addition, Quer is considered a potential anti-cancer agent, although some recent data suggest that it can also increase cancer growth. The mechanism by which Quer can exert its effects is not completely elucidated. Some *in vitro* and *in vivo* works showed that Quer can interact with proteins involved in cell signaling, cell cycle and apoptosis. Owing to the large number of potential health beneficial effects of Quer, its consumption has increased, and the addition of this compound to various traditional food products has grown. However, prior to the use of Quer as food supplementation or medicine a better understanding of the real health benefits, the pharmacokinetics (i.e. bioavailability, metabolism and toxicity), pharmacodynamics and the safety of this compound is fundamental. This chapter will focus in the sources, bioavailability and potential antitumoral effect of Quer, discussing data from different cell systems, animal models, and human studies.

Chapter 4- Quercetin, a plant-based secondary metabolite widely present in fruits and vegetables, is a polyphenol belonging to the class of flavonoids. Studies for the past several decades have identified the great potential of this bioflavonoid in the prevention and treatment of a wide range of diseases. The biological effects of quercetin includes antimicrobial properties; antioxidative capacity; anti-allergic and anti-inflammatory activities; blood vessel protection; antitumor properties; antidiabetic and antiaging effects, anticataract and antineurodegenerative capacity; and protection against hypertension and cardiovascular diseases. Quercetin exerts this wide spectrum of effects by targeting several proteins/enzymes that are implicated in disease progression. Because of its outstanding safety profile and its availability in highly purified forms, the clinical implications for quercetin are growing rapidly. Even though quercetin is the major bioflavonoid in the human diet, its bioavailability has been debated. Recent studies to improve its bioavailability by combining it with vitamins or encapsulating it as nanoparticles are promising. This review mainly focuses on the molecular targets of quercetin and the mechanisms by which quercetin exerts its biological effects in the prevention and treatment of cancer, metabolic diseases and aging.

Chapter 5- Quercetin, a major bioflavonoid, is one of the most prominent antioxidants in the human diet. It is ubiquitously present in fruits, vegetables, teas and wines as well as dietary supplements. Although some research has reported quercetin acting as potentially carcinogenic agent, many studies have documented the chemopreventive, cardioprotective, and neuroprotective effects of quercetin. Beyond antioxidant, antiproliferative, and antiinflammatory activities, quercetin possesses antibacterial, antiatherogenic, antihypertensive, antifibrotic, and anticoagulative properties. Even though the precise mechanisms by which quercetin exert their beneficial remain unclear, it may be involved in reducing capacities through its possible influences on intracellular redox status, modulating the gene expression of enzymes associated with biotransformation such as phase I and phase II metabolism, suppressing cell proliferation by interacting with type II estrogen binding sites, inhibiting chromosomal alterations and tyrosine kinase, modulating several signal transduction pathways through actions at MEK/ERK and Nrf2/keap1, and stabilizing p53 at both the mRNA and protein levels to reactivate p53-dependent cell cycle arrest and apoptosis. The target of this Chapter is to examine potential mechanisms of action in order to elucidate the possible health-beneficial effects of quercetin.

Chapter 6- A large quantity of quercetin was characterized from a local dish, known as maniçoba in Pará, Brazil. The fresh leaf of *Manihot esculenta* Crantz (Euphorbiaceae), a principal ingredient for maniçoba, was found to contain a large amount of rutin or quercetin 3-*O*-rutinoside which was completely hydrolyzed to quercetin during cooking processes. Antioxidant activity of quercetin and its microfloral metabolites was examined. Quercetin inhibited the oxidation of linoleic acid catalyzed by soybean lipoxygenase-1 (EC 1.13.11.12, Type 1) with an IC_{50} of 4.5 μM, while rutin did not inhibit this oxidation up to 200 μM. The progress curves for the enzyme reaction indicate that quercetin shows slow binding kinetics. In the pseudoperoxidase activity, hydroperoxides slowly oxidize quercetin to a rather stable intermediate, 2-(3,4-dihydroxybenzoyl)-2,4,6-trihydroxy-3(2*H*)-benzofuranone. A microfloral metabolite of quercetin and rutin after ingestion, 3,4-dihydroxyphenylacetic acid, also scavenged superoxide anion generated by xanthine oxidase and inhibited uric acid formation. The antioxidant activity observed with the methanol extract of maniçoba is due mainly to multifunctional quercetin's response.

Chapter 7- Quercetin (3, 5, 7, 3′, 4′-pentahydroxy flavon), is the major flavonoid in the human diet, its daily intake in foods is estimated to be 50–500 mg and it is one of the main dietary antioxidants. It is ubiquitously present in foods including onions, apples, green and black tea, in smaller amounts in leafy green vegetables and beans as well as countless food supplements. Quercetin is typically found in plants as glycone or carbohydrate conjugates. Olive oil, grapes, dark cherries, and dark berries, such as blueberries, blackberries, and bilberries are also high in flavonoids including quercetin. It is being studied for apparent benefical effects including cardiovascular protection, anti-cancer activity, anti-ulcer effects, anti-allergy activity, cataract prevention, antiviral activity, and anti-inflammatory effects. In the body, quercetin has potent antioxidant and anti-inflammatory activity, where it can protect cellular structures and blood vessels from the damaging effects of free radicals. The biological activity of this flavonol is attributed to the presence of two antioxidants in their chemical structure, the catechol group in ring B and the OH group in position 3 of ring C.

Chapter 8- Quercetin (3, 3', 4', 5, 7-pentahydroxylflavone) is a typical flavonoid presented in various fruits and vegetables. More evidences have demonstrated that quercetin exhibits anti-oxidation, anti-cancer, anti-inflammation, anti-atherosclerosis, anti-bacteria, anti-virus, anti-diabetes, anti-aging, anti-hyperuricemia and so on. Quercetin is suggested to be a candidate for preventing various body disorders such as osteoporosis, certain forms of cancer, obesity-related disorder, pulmonary and cardiovascular diseases, neurodegenerative diseases, hyperuricemia and diabetes. Therefore, we reviewed the researching achievements of quercetin principally including its dietary sources, bioavailability and functions to health promotion and disease prevention as well as the related basic molecular mechanisms. Other aspects such as the metabolism of quercetin were covered briefly.

Chapter 9- Quercetin is a polyphenolic compound synthesized by many food plants and is an abundant micronutrient in human diet. It is attracting a large interest by virtue of its numerous beneficial biological effects: in fact, it has demonstrated anti-oxidative, free-radical scavenging and anticancer activities, protective effects towards cardiovascular disease, antiviral action, etc. Nevertheless, its bioavailability and bioefficacy is generally low due to its very poor aqueous solubility and scant stability in some environments and biological fluids. Several research efforts have been recently devoted to overcome these limitations by designing and testing appropriate formulations able to improve the quercetin bioavailability, to modulate the release kinetic and to target the release to specific tissue. This review presents the most interesting quercetin delivery systems till now developed.

Chapter 10- The action of quercetin on oxygen uptake by uncoupled rat liver mitochondria was measured. Quercetin clearly inhibited oxygen uptake with several substrates. With 300 μM quercetin the inhibition degrees with the following substrates were: citrate, 73%; β-hydroxybutyrate, 68%; α-ketoglutarate, 67%; isocitrate, 41%, α-glycerophosphate, 38%. With fumarate, oxaloacetate and succinate no significant inhibition was found. Quercetin also inhibited oxygen uptake during the oxidation of various activated fatty acids with well-defined concentration dependencies.

The degrees of inhibition with 300 μM quercetin were: octanoyl-carnitine, 83%; octanoyl-CoA, 82%; palmitoyl-CoA, 74%; oleoyl-CoA, 74%; palmitoyl-carnitine, 70%; and stearoyl-CoA, 67%. An action of quercetin on the fatty acyl-carnitine transferases is unlikely because octanoyl-CoA permeates the inner mitochondrial membrane as easily as octanoyl-carnitine or long-chain fatty acyl-carnitines and oxygen uptake with octanoyl-CoA was equally inhibited.

Although direct action on dehydrogenases cannot be ruled out, the inhibition of NADH-oxidase activity suggests inhibitory effects on electron flow probably by acting on the respiratory chain complex I. This assumption was corroborated by experiments with disrupted mitochondria in which the effects of quercetin on membrane-bound enzymatic activities were measured. Quercetin did not affect succinate-oxidase activity, but inhibited NADH-oxidase activity in a dose dependent manner. There is also the possibility of generation of prooxidant metabolites in the respiratory chain by quercetin which could lead to a competition for NADH between the respiratory chain and the quercetin metabolites, anticipating NADH oxidation.

Chapter 11- Herbs are naturally occurring gifts of nature. Flavonoids are present in fruits, vegetables and beverages derived from plants (tea, red wine), and in many dietary supplements or herbal remedies including Ginkgo Biloba, Soy Isoflavones, and Milk Thistle. Flavonoids have been described as health-promoting, disease-preventing dietary supplements, and have activity as cancer preventive agents. Additionally, they are extremely safe and associated with low toxicity, making them excellent candidates for chemopreventive agents.

Quercetin, one of the most common natural flavonoids, has been reported to possess various excellent activities both in vitro and in vivo. This chapter gives brief survey of current study on quercetin that is commonly used in cosmetic and therapeutic application in oral health care. For cosmetic application it may temporarily control or reduce malodor. For cosmetic application it may reduce plaque, caries, gingivitis, periodontal disease, oral mucosal ulceration or oral cancer. The etiology of malodor involves many factors such as gingivitis, periodontitis, nasal inflammation, chronic sinusitis and diabetes. Plaque is the major etiology of dental caries, gingivitis and periodontal diseases. Antibacterial activities of quercetin could explain how it can help to prevent these diseases. The oral mucosal ulceration or oral cancer is related both on the internal factors, immunological, microbiological, saliva, with digestive, lubricating and other protective properties, and external factors such as nutrition, habits and lifestyle, including stress and coping. Quercetin may be useful in accelerating the healing process of minor aphthous ulcers and inhibiting the cellular grow of human oral cancer cells. Quercetin may be a better candidate material for maintaining perfect oral health at home.

Chapter 12- After ingestion of foods that contain quercetin glycosides, some of them are hydrolyzed to quercetin in the oral cavity, and quercetin can stay in the cavity for several hours. During its stay in the oral cavity, quercetin can suppress the nitration induced by salivary peroxidase/H_2O_2/nitrite systems by competing with nitrite for peroxidase and/or by scavenging reactive nitrogen oxide species. Accompanying the suppression, quercetin is oxidized and one of the oxidation products is 2-(3,4-dihydroxybenzoyl)-2,4,6-trihydroxy-3(*2H*)-benzofuranone. In the stomach, quercetin and its glycosides can reduce salivary nitrite to nitric oxide (NO), which has various functions. If quercetin functions as the reductant, quercetin is transformed to the benzofuranone described above, and if a quercetin glycoside such as rutin functions as the reductant, *o*-quinone of rutin is formed, which reacts with salivary component SCN^- to produce an oxathiolone derivative of rutin. In the small intestine, quercetin and rutin may be able to slow down starch digestion by binding to starch. In this chapter, various functions of quercetin and its glycoside in the digestive tract are described, especially from the points of scavenging of reactive nitrogen oxide species and inhibition of its formation.

Chapter 13- Flavonols including quercetin, kaempferol, myricetin, and fatty acids in plants have many useful health attributes including antioxidants, cholesterol lowering effects, and cancer prevention. Six accessions of roselle, *Hibiscus sabdariffa* calyces were evaluated for quercetin, kaempferol, and myricetin content, while 11 accessions were evaluated for fatty acid content as calyces matured in a greenhouse from late 2009 - early 2010. Variations for all chemical traits were found among the roselle calyces between accessions. The accession, PI 265319 produced the most quercetin (1.134 mg/g) and myricetin (0.972 mg/g). However, PI 286316 produced the most kaempferol (1.882 mg/g). Quercetin, myricetin, and kaempferol declined insignificantly as plants matured. Several fatty acids differed significantly in content among the roselle accessions. The accession, PI 286319 produced the most mono-unsaturated fatty acid, palmitoleic acid (0.046 %) and gadoleic acid (0.213 %), however PI 468409 produced the most oleic acid (5.091 %). The accession, PI 286319 also produced the most omega-6 fatty acid, linoleic acid (6.218 %) while PI 268097 produced the most γ-linolenic acid (0.093 %). The accession, PI 286316 produced the most omega-3 fatty acid, eicosapentaenoic acid (0.038 %), however PI 265319 produced significantly more docsahexaenoic acid (5.296 %) than all other roselle accessions. Stearic, behenic, and docosahexaenoic fatty acids declined significantly over time as roselle plants matured, however gadoleic and arachidonic fatty acid content increased significantly as the calyces matured. Interestingly, the red calyces produced significantly higher amounts of fatty acids overall. Significant correlations were found for many of the flavonol and fatty acid traits tested. Based on these results, sufficient variability exists in these *Hibiscus* accessions for quercetin, kaempferol, myricetin, and fatty acid breeding projects and for use as nutraceutical or functional food plants.

Chapter 14- Quercetin is a unique bioflavonoid that has been extensively studied by researchers over past 30 years. Reports of activity in the field of antibacterial flavanoid research are widely conflicting, probably owing to inter- and intra-assay variation in susceptibility testing. However, several high quality investigations have examined the relationship between flavanoid structure and antibacterial activity and these are in close agreement. In addition, numerous research groups have sought to elucidate the antibacterial mechanisms of action of selected flavanoid. The activity of quercetin, for example, has been at least partially attributed to inhibition of bacterial DNA gyrase. In addition, quercetin is one of suitable ligand among flavanoid to fit inside the ATP binding site of DNA gyrase B and Topoisomerase IV ParE. Nevertheless, quercetin can't inhibit the growth of Gram-positive bacterial strains even at high concentrations though it can inhibit the growth of Gram-negative bacterial strains at high concentration.

Chapter 15- One of the most important functions of gastrointestinal epithelial cells is to provide a physical barrier to the diffusion of pathogens, toxins, and allergens from the external environment into the tissues. Defects in the barrier function play a crucial role in the pathogenesis of various intestinal diseases, such as inflammatory bowel disease, irritative bowel disease, and food allergies. The intestinal barrier function is organized by interactions among several barrier components, including the adhesive mucous gel layer, the mucosal immune system, and intercellular tight junctions (TJ). The TJ is a multi-protein complex, which locates around the apical end of the lateral membrane of polarized epithelial cells, and selectively regulates the paracellular passage of ions, molecules and water. The TJ complex is composed of transmembrane proteins that interact with the perijunctional actin cytoskeleton through intracellular plaque proteins. TJ permeability and assembly are dynamically regulated by various intracellular signaling molecules, such as protein kinase C, mitogen-activated protein kinases, and protein phosphatases. Quercetin is one of the most abundant flavonoids in the human diet and exhibits various biological effects, such as anti-inflammatory and anti-cancer activities. Recent studies have demonstrated that quercetin participates in the regulation of intestinal TJ barrier function. This chapter presents the recent advances in our understanding of the quercetin-mediated suppressive effect on intestinal TJ permeability with a particular focus on intracellular molecular mechanisms.

Chapter 16- Quercetin is the major representative of the flavonoid subclass of flavonols which mostly present as its glycoside form in onions, olives, tea, beer and red wine. It has a broad range of biological, pharmacological and medical applications which benefit to human health. In present paper, the dietary source, function and health benefits such as antioxidant properties, anticancer properties, anti-inflammatory, anti-aggregatory, vasodilating effects, reverse multidrug resistance and other bioactivity of quercetin and its glycoside form are reviewed.

In: Quercetin
Editors: Taiki Chikamatsu and Yuudai Hida

ISBN: 978-1 61942- 057-1

Chapter 1

QUERCETIN: NATURAL SOURCES AND HEALTH BENEFITS

M. P. Gómez-Serranillos* and O. M. Palomino†

Department of Pharmacology, Faculty of Pharmacy,
Universidad Complutense de Madrid, Madrid, Spain

ABSTRACT

Flavonoids are a large group of plant metabolites that are commonly present in fruits, vegetables, cereals and beverages, where they contribute to the bitterness, astrigency, colour, flavour, odour and antioxidant stability of the plant. Epidemiological data suggest that long term consumption of diets rich in flavonoids could provide some health benefits such as lowering arterial pressure, decreasing plasma concentration of lipids and buffering plasma glucose, together with some protection against the development of certain cancers or cardiovascular diseases. Among them, quercetin that belongs to the flavonols components is being investigated for its widespread health benefits. The plant source of quercetin is relatively inexpensive to grow and harvest, and its purification is straightforward. Quercetin is abundant in onion and has been related to diminished mortality from coronary heart disease; it has also shown to exert anticancer properties against benzo(a) pyrene induced lung carcinogenesis in mice and possesses virucidal activity against enveloped viruses such as herpes, simplex type I or parainfluenza type 3. Most of the beneficial effects of quercetin are related to its free radical scavenging activity that supports its antioxidant capability. The antioxidant nature of quercetin is defined mainly by the presence of a catechol group in the B-ring capable of readily donating hydrogen (electron) to stabilise a radical specie. Other features important for the antioxidant nature include the presence of 2,3 unsaturation in conjugation with a 4-oxo-function in the C-ring. In addition, quercetin has proved to be effective and safe for humans at low dosages (500-1000 mg/day).

---

* Full Professor, Department of Pharmacology, Faculty of Pharmacy. Universidad Complutense de Madrid (UCM), Madrid, Spain. E-mail: pserra@farm.ucm.es. Tfno: + 34. 91.394.17.67. FAX: + 34. 91.394.17.26.

† Full Professor, Department of Pharmacology, Faculty of Pharmacy. Universidad Complutense de Madrid (UCM), Madrid, Spain. E-mail: olgapalomino@farm.ucm.es. Tfno: + 34. 91.394.17.67. FAX: + 34. 91.394.17.26.

Thus, available data leads to consider the possible relevance of quercetin benefits on various chronic diseases like cardiovascular, metabolic and neurodegenerative diseases associated with oxidative stress.

INTRODUCTION

Polyphenols are one of the main groups of secondary metabolites of plants; they are ubiquitously found in edible plants, fruits, vegetables, cereals and beverages. Polyphenolic compounds are generally involved in defence against ultraviolet radiation or aggression by pathogens, whereas they contribute to the bitterness, astringency, colour, flavour, odour and oxidative stability of foods.

Phenolic compounds demonstrated a potent antioxidant activity mainly due to their redox properties which allow them to act as hydrogen donators, chelating agents of metal ions or reducing agents. Epidemiological data suggested that long term consumption of polyphenols rich diet was associated with lower risks of certain cancers and coronary heart diseases, a decrease in arterial pressure and plasma concentration of lipids, as well as a protection against development of diabetes, osteoporosis and neurodegenerative diseases. These data led to a greater scientific interest in this group of compounds because of their possible beneficial effects on human health.

More than 8,000 polyphenolic compounds have been identified in various plant species; they all arise from phenylalanine or shikimic acid, primarily in conjugated forms, with one or more sugar residues linked to hydroxyl groups or to an aromatic carbon. It is also common the association with other compounds such as carboxylic or organic acids, amines, lipids and other phenols.

Polyphenolic compounds may be classified into several groups as a function of the number of phenol rings that they content and the structural elements that bind these rings to one another. The main four classes are phenolic acids, flavonoids, stilbenes and lignanes (Figure 1).

Flavonoids consist of a basic structure consisting of two aromatic rings bound together by three carbon atoms that form an oxygenated heterocycle (C_6-C_3-C_6) (Pandey and Rizvi, 2009). They share a benzene ring A condensed with a heterocyclic six-membered ring C which carries a phenyl ring B at the 2-position for flavonoids and at the 3-position for isoflavonoids (Figure 2). They are subdivided into subclasses according to the variations in the C ring: flavones, flavonols (3-hydroxyflavones), flavanones (dihydroxyflavones), flavanonols (dihydroxyflavonols), isoflavones and isoflavanones (dihydroisoflavones). More than 4000 varieties of flavonoids have been identified in plants, many of them being responsible for the attractive colors of flowers, fruits and leaves and for the protection against oxidative damage, and insects and microbes attacks (Prassain et al., 2010). Their distribution at the tissue, cellular and subcellular levels is different: insoluble molecules are found in cell walls, while soluble ones are present within the plant cell vacuoles. Higher levels of phenolics are found in the outer layers than in the inner parts of the plant; this content is affected by several factors such as degree of ripeness at the time of harvest, environmental or edaphic factors (soil type, sun exposure, rainfall etc), processing and storage conditions. The latter is relevant to protect the vegetal product from oxidation that leads to the formation of polymerized substances which induce changes in food quality.

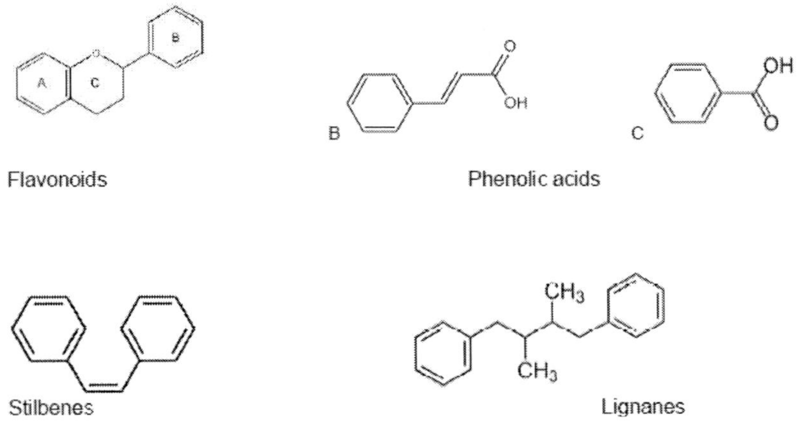

Figure 1. Basic structures of flavonoids, phenolic acids (B-cinnamic acid, C-benzoic acid), stilbenes and lignanes

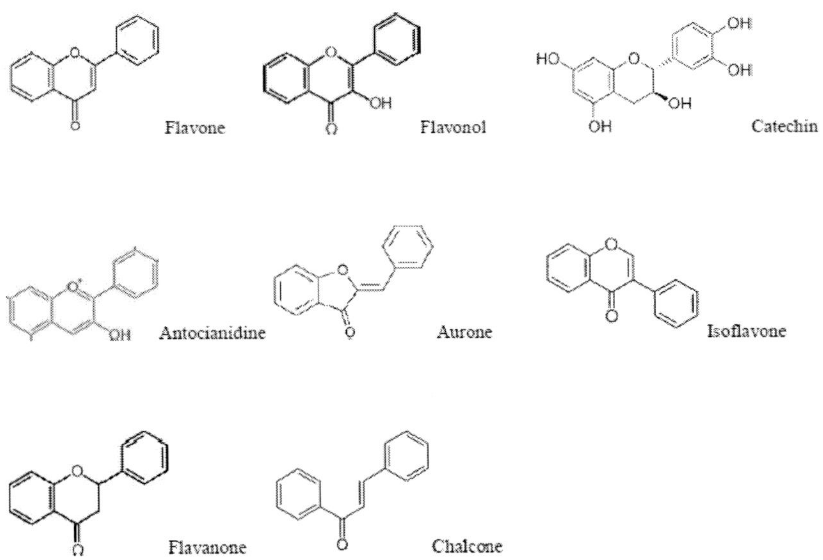

Figure 2. Chemical structures of the main flavonoids subclasses.

Recent findings show that flavonoids exert broad pharmacological effects such as antiproliferative, antitumour, antimicrobial, antithrombotic, antinflammatory, antiallergic, apoptosis-inducing and antioxidant activity that provide important health benefits related to metabolic syndrome, cancer, brain health and immune system. Great focuses of attention are their use in the inhibition of tumour development and lipid peroxidation.

The relatively low toxicity and potential efficacy of most of these compounds make them attractive to scientific as well as a large sector of the population. The effects of flavonoids are derived from their binding to or interference with enzymes, receptors, transporters and signal transduction systems; such events frequently occur in lipid membrane environments, so the bioactivity of flavonoids may be attributed to their action on the membrane as modification of any of its physicochemical properties, like fluidity by interaction with membrane lipid bilayers.

Quercetin (3,3',4',5-7-pentahydroxy flavone - Figure 3) is a natural polyphenolic compound that belongs to the flavonols subclass and is prevalent in a wide variety of food plants, including red onions, tomatoes, lettuce and celery, fruits such as apples and berries, and tea, fruit and vegetable juices, mainly in a glycosylated form. It is also found as a component of nutraceuticals or food supplements.

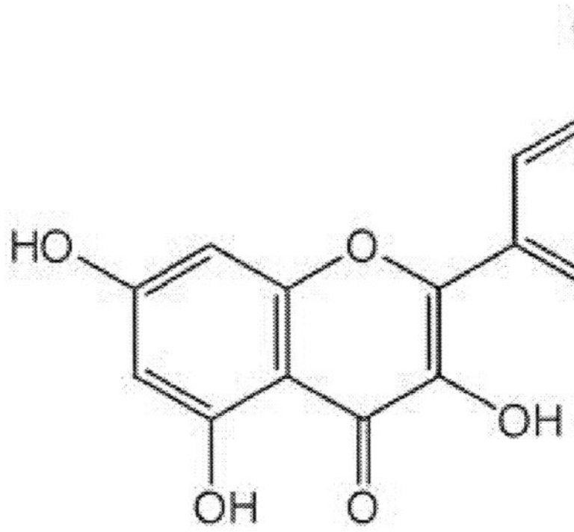

Figure 3. Chemical structure of quercetin.

Quercetin shows a strong anti-oxidant effect and also modulates the activity of many enzymes, which leads to the influence of this flavonol on a huge number of biochemical signalling pathways and, therefore, physiological and pathological processes. So nowadays, quercetin is being investigated for its widespread health benefits with great potential to address diseases and risk-factors associated with aging. The plant source of quercetin is relatively inexpensive to grow and harvest, and its purification is straightforward.

This review takes in consideration the most recent scientific data on the possible relevance of quercetin health benefits and dietary sources of this flavonol.

Dietary Sources and Bioavailability

The most important food sources of quercetin and other polyphenolic compounds are fruit and vegetables, green tea, black tea, red wine, coffee, chocolate, olives, and extra virgin olive oil. Herbs and spices, nuts and algae are also potentially significant for supplying certain polyphenols (Crozier et al., 2009). Some polyphenols are specific to particular food (flavanones in citrus fruit, isoflavones in soya, phloridzin in apples); whereas others, such as quercetin, are found in all plant products such as fruit, vegetables, cereals, leguminous plants, tea, and wine (D'Archivio et al., 2010).

Foods usually contain complex mixtures of polyphenols. Apples, for example, contain flavanol monomers or oligomers, chlorogenic acid and small quantities of other hydroxycinnamic acids, several quercetin glycosides, and 2 glycosides of phloretin and anthocyanins (Manach et al., 2004). Their concentration ranges from 0.1g total polyphenols/kg fresh weight to 10 g/kg in certain varieties of cider apples (Sanoner et al., 1999; Guyot et al., 2003). Wine also contains a complex mixture of polyphenols, most of which originate in the grape berry. They include flavonol, flavanol, proanthocyanidins, anthocyanins, phenolic acids, hydroxycinnamates and stilbenes (Forester and Waterhouse

2009; Waterhouse, 2002). The daily intake of flavonols has been estimated as 20-35 mg, of which more than 65% is quercetin and its glycosides (Pérez-Vizcaíno and Duarte, 2010). Therefore, the main source of quercetin are the daily portions of fruit and vegetables; it is present as a glycoside in all plant products: fruits like grapes, apples, pears, cherries and berries, vegetables (onions, tomatoes, lettuce, celery), cereals, fruit juices, tea, wine, infusions etc. Current dietary advice is to consume at least five portions of these products every day, each portion of at least 8.0 grams.

The beneficial activities observed *in vitro* or in animal models for quercetin and other polyphenols are not always directly related to the observed effects *in vivo*, due to the fact that some of the compounds are not able to get to the target tissue and that concentrations used are much higher than those generally contained in the human diet. Moreover, the most abundant polyphenols in our diet are not necessarily those that have the best bioavailability profile. Thus it is more important to know the bioavailability of one compound than the quantity of this compound that is present in specific food. The term "bioavailability" is used to define the concept of the "rate and extent to which a drug reaches its site of action" (Porrini and Riso, 2008); in the case of nutrition, the most appropriate definition seems to be as that fraction of an ingested nutrient or compound that reaches the systemic circulation and the specific sites where it can exert its biological action (Porrini and Riso, 2008). In other words, it simply means how much of the ingested quantity of the polyphenols is able to exert its beneficial effects in target tissues.

Bioavailability studies are not easy to carry out, since several factors may affect bioavailability directly or by decreasing polyphenol content in food. The intake of one portion of food containing the tested polyphenol should increase the blood concentration of the same compounds, but it is transitional and reflects mainly the ability of the organism to take up the polyphenol from the food matrix. Therefore, the observed increase can have only a minor implication for tissue uptake and bioactivity. When conditions of regular intake are used, even low amounts of polyphenols can be "repeatedly" absorbed and can significantly increase the concentrations both at plasma and cellular level (Scalbert and Williamson, 2000). Also the synergistic effects of the mixture of polyphenols contained in each food matrix may difficult to obtain definitive conclusions on the bioavailability and bioactivity of a single phenolic compound. This situation may improve in the future, for example, with the use of isogenic lines of onions that differ only in their quercetin contents (Femia et al., 2003), allowing comparisons between groups consuming the same food but with different polyphenol contents (Williamson and Manach, 2005).

The bioavailability of quercetin is proved to depend on the nature of its attached sugars and components of the food matrix that may affect its solubility (ethanol, fat) (Pérez-Vizcaíno and Duarte, 2010). For example, onion bulbs (*Allium cepa* L.) are one of the richest sources of dietary flavonoids and contribute to the overall intake of flavonoids (Slimestad et al, 2007). While yellow onions contain 270-1187 mg of flavonols per kilogram of fresh weight, red onions contain 415-1917 mg of flavonols per kilogram of fresh weight, quercetin derivatives being the most important ones in all onion cultivars. Their glycosyl moieties are almost exclusively glucose, which is mainly attached to the 4', 3, and/or 7-positions of the aglycones. Quercetin 4'-glucoside and quercetin 3,4'-diglucoside are reported as the main flavonols. Analogous derivatives of kaempferol and isorhamnetin have been identified as minor pigments. The outer dry layers of onion bulbs contain oligomeric structures of quercetin together with condensation products of quercetin and protocatechuic acid. Glucosides from onions show a better bioavailability than other dietary sources (Davalos et al., 2006) and even than the aglycone given as pure compound (Hollman et al., 1995).

The main factors affecting the bioavailability of dietary polyphenols in humans may be classified into External factors such as environmental factors (*i.e.*, sun exposure, degree of ripeness); Food processing related factors (thermal treatments; homogenization; liophylization; cooking and methods of culinary preparation); Food related factors (food matrix; presence of positive or negative effectors of absorption (*i.e.*, fat, fiber); Interaction with other compounds (bonds with proteins, *i.e.*, albumin) or with polyphenols with similar mechanism of absorption; Polyphenols related factors (chemical structure; concentration in food); Host related factors (Intestinal factors (*i.e.*, enzyme activity; intestinal transit time; colonic microflora); Systemic factors (*i.e.*, gender and age; disorders and/or pathologies; genetics; physiological condition).

Thermal treatment causes significant reduction in total phenolic content and their antioxidant activities in beans (Xu and Chang, 2009a) and legumes (Xu and Chang, 2009b). In general, cooking and the methods of culinary preparations influence the polyphenol content (Ferracane et al., 2008; Miglio et al., 2008; van der Sluis et al., 2001; DuPont et al., 2000; Baiano et al., 2009; Brenes et al., 2002; Xu et al., 2009), affecting also their bioavailability and bioactivity. Carrots completely lose their polyphenols after boiling, while steaming and frying has a less negative effect (−43% and −31%, respectively). For broccoli and courgettes, boiling and frying determine a higher loss of total phenolics than steaming. These results suggest that for each vegetable, a preferential cooking method could be selected to preserve or improve its nutritional qualities; *i.e.,* onions and tomatoes lose between 75% and 80% of their initial quercetin content after boiling for fifteen minutes, 65% after cooking in a microwave oven, and 30% after frying (Crozier et al., 1997).

The degree of ripeness affects the phenolic acid concentration as it decreases during ripening, whereas anthocyanins concentrations increase (Macheix et al., 1990). Although consumption of raw vegetables is widely advocated, the bioavailability of many compounds is enhanced when the vegetables are cooked: a significant increase in plasma levels of naringenin and chlorogenic acid was found after the intake of cooked tomatoes compared to the fresh product (Bugianesi et al., 2004). The steam-cooking of broccoli results in an increase in the content of polyphenols and in their antioxidant activity (Gliszczynska-Swiglo et al., 2006).

Storage affects the content of polyphenols; the storage of apple juices for 11 months resulted in a decrease in phenolic acids from 5% to 21% (Gliszczynska-Swiglo and Tyrakowska, 2003). Polyphenol content during storage over seven months in the dark was studied in red wines: the anthocyanins content decreased 88%, while no significant variations occurred in the total flavonol contents (Zafrilla et al., 2003). On the other hand, apples (Annurca variety) showed a marked increase in chlorogenic acid after four months storage: from 101 to 144 mg/kg fresh weight (Napolitano et al., 2004); and also the content of phenolic acids increased when carrots were stored under aerobic conditions (Klaiber et al., 2005).

Also technological processes, such as homogenization of vegetables, could increase the bioavailability of polyphenols by the alteration of the food matrix (Porrini et al., 1998). The study of the food matrix influence on the bioavailability of phenolic compounds reveals that the direct interaction between polyphenols and food components, such as proteins, carbohydrates, fiber, fat, alcohol, can affect their absorption (Azuma et al, 2002; Lesser et al.,

2004; Visioli et al., 2003; Donovan et al., 1999; Donovan et al., 2002). Nonetheless, the absorption of quercetin in humans is equivalent when administered in three different matrices: white wine, grape juice, and vegetable juice (Goldeberg et al., 2003). On the other hand, there may be a physiological interaction between flavonoids and fats that slows small bowel transit time (Rao et al., 1996), which would delay the absorption of flavonoids. The influence of dietary fiber on quercetin bioavailability (Tamura et al., 2007) proved that pectin might enhance the bioavailability of quercetin from rutin by altering the metabolic activity of the intestinal flora and/or gut physiological function. Recently it has also been shown that the polyphenols associated with dietary fiber are at least partially bioavailable in humans, although dietary fiber appears to delay the absorption (Perez-Jimenez et al., 2009). Other factor affecting the bioavailability is represented by the interaction with other compounds. It has been reported the existence of intermolecular bonds between serum albumin and quercetin metabolites, which supports its slow elimination from the body (Manach et al., 2004).

All the above data indicate that the real concentration of the active compound that is reached in blood must be taken in account. Most of the polyphenols present in food exist as polymers or in glycosylated forms: the sugar group is known as the glycone and the non-sugar group (the polyphenol) is known as the aglycone. In these forms the polyphenols cannot be absorbed and must suffer hydrolysis by intestinal enzymes or colonic microflora before absorption.

During absorption, polyphenols are conjugated in the intestinal cells and later in the liver by methylation, sulfation and/or glucuronidation. As a consequence of this, the forms that are found in blood and tissues are different from those present in food; this makes difficult to identify all the metabolites and to establish their biological activity. Quercetin is rapidly conjugated with glucuronic acid and/or sulphate during first-pass metabolism (intestine-liver) and a portion of the metabolites are also mehylated; therefore, the main metabolites of quercetin in human plasma are quercetin-3-glucuronide, quercetin-3-sulfate and isorhamnetin-3-glucuronide, for which limited information about their *in vitro* effects exist.

Intestinal factors and systemic factors are host related factors that influence the polyphenols bioavailability. Following the ingestion of dietary polyphenols, the absorption of some but not all components occurs in the small intestine. There are two possible mechanisms by which the glycosides could be hydrolysed: the first mechanism involves the action of lactase phloridizin hydrolase (LPH) that is present in the brush-border of the small intestine epithelial cells. LPH has two catalytic sites (Semenza, 1987): one to hydrolyse lactose (LH) and the other involved in the deglycosylation of more hydrophobic substrates. The inhibition of the LH site of the LPH complex markedly reduces deglycosylation of polyphenols (Wilkinson et al., 2003), showing that the majority of the activity is from the LH domain. The released aglycones may then enter the epithelial cell by passive diffusion as a result of their increased lipophilicity (Day et al., 2000a). The second mechanism involves cytosolic β-glucosidase (CBG) that is present within the epithelial cells, where the polar glucosides are transported through the active sodium-dependent glucose transporter SGLT1 (Gee et al., 2000).

The polyphenols that are not absorbed in the small intestine reach the colon where they undergo substantial structural modifications. In fact, the colonic microflora hydrolyzes glycosides into aglycones and degrades them to simple phenolic acids (Aura et al., 2005;

Kuhnau, 1976). This activity is of great importance for the biological action of polyphenols, since active metabolites are produced by the colonic microflora.

Prior to passage into the blood stream, the polyphenols, that now are simple aglycones, undergo to other structural modifications due to the conjugation process (Felgines et al., 2005) that takes place in the small intestine and, mostly, in the liver. The conjugation, that includes methylation, sulfation, and glucuronidation, represents a metabolic detoxication process common to many xenobiotic compounds that restricts their potential toxic effects and facilitates their biliary and urinary elimination by an increased solubility and a higher molecular weight. Glucuronidation is particularly important for increasing molecular weight, necessary for the excretion in the bile (Day et al., 2000).

Catechol-O-methyltransferase (COMT) catalyzes the transfer of a methyl group from adenosylmethionine to polyphenols that contain a diphenolic moiety, such as quercetin. This enzyme is present in a wide range of tissues, but its activity is highest in the liver and the kidneys (Piskula and Terao, 1998; Tilgmann and Ulmanen, 1996). Sulfotransferases (SULT) catalyze the transfer of a sulfate moiety from phosphoadenosine-phosphosulfate to a hydroxyl group on various substrates, among which polyphenols. Sulfation occurs mainly in the liver (Piskula and Terao, 1998; Falany, 1997). Uridine-5'-diphosphate glucuronosyltransferases (UGTs) are membrane-bound enzymes that are located in the endoplasmic reticulum in many tissues and that catalyze the transfer of a glucuronic acid from UDP-glucuronic acid to polyphenols. Glucuronidation of polyphenols first occurs in the enterocytes before further conjugation in the liver (Spencer et al., 1999; Crespy et al., 2001; Boersma et al., 2002). Although the process of conjugation on one hand produces active metabolites from some dietary polyphenols, on the other it reduces the total amount of polyphenols in the blood stream, increasing their excretion. The relative importance of the three types of conjugation may vary according to the nature of the substrate and the dose ingested. The balance between sulfation and glucuronidation of polyphenols also seems to be affected by species and sex. It is important to underline that the conjugation mechanisms are highly efficient, and free aglycones are generally either absent or present in low concentrations in plasma after consumption of nutritional doses.

Therefore, it is clear that the polyphenols are extensively modified (Porrini and Riso, 2008), not only in the small intestine and in the colon as it has been discussed above, but also in the liver, where most of the conjugation takes place. Therefore, any single polyphenol generates several metabolites, as many as 20 in the case of quercetin glycosides, although two or three usually dominate (Mullen et al., 2006). All these modifications deeply affect the biological activity of polyphenols (Day et al., 2000b; Zhang et al., 1999; Wen and Walle, 2006a, 2006b; Landis-Piwowar et al., 2008; Del Rio et al., 2010). Consequently, the compounds that reach cells and tissues are chemically, biologically and, in many instances, functionally different from the original dietary form. In general, these metabolites are less active than the parent compounds and sometimes totally inactive. However, conjugated metabolites can be deconjugated by beta-glucuronidase and lead to accumulation of flavonol aglycones in tissues (Bieger et al., 2008).

As explained above, quercetin is prevalent in fruits and vegetables in a glycosylated form but is hydrolyzed before absorption by beta-glucosidase and other similar enzymes at the point of absorption across the small intestine. As much as 93% of quercetin found in the blood is modified to quercetin 3-sulfate, quercetin 3-glucuronide, and 3- methylquercetin 3-

glucuronide (Gomez-Rico et al., 2006). Importantly no glycosylated or free quercetin is observed in blood serum.

Quercetin molecule show an amphipatic behavior (Srinivas et al., 2010): the phenyl rings from the hydrophobic part and the hydroxyl groups constitute the polar portion. This structure affects their aqueous solubility and therefore its antioxidant capacity which depends on the charge density of the hydrophilic and hydrophobic components. Following this theory, the antioxidant capacity of quercetin in a water-soluble phase has proved to be eight times greater than in a lipid-soluble phase.

After absorption, glucosides could be transported into enterocytes by the sodium dependent glucose transporter SGLT1 and then hydrolyzed by a cytosolic beta-glucosidase. Those molecules that hadn't been absorbed in gastrointestinal tract and intestine reach the colon, where microflora hydrolyzes them into various aromatic acids. After absorption, polyphenols go to several conjugation processes that include methylation, sulfation and glucuronidation to increase their hydrophilicity and facilitate their biliary and urinary elimination (Pandey and Rizvi, 2009).

Table 1. Beneficial effects of quercetin on human health

Health benefit	Effect		Reference
	In vitro	*In vivo*	
Cardiovascular system		Acute vasodilator activity	Pérez-Vizcaíno and Duarte, 2010
	Enhancing plasma NO level		Appeldoorn et al., 2009 Pérez-Vizcaíno and Duarte, 2010
	Inhibition of ET-1 release		Kahn et al., 2002 Zhao et al, 1999
	Inhibitory effect on PI3-K		Yoshizumi et al., 2002
		Extension in the lifespan of *Saccharomyces cerevisiae* and *Caenorhabditis elegans*	Belinha et al., 2007 Pietsch et al., 2009
	Cells migration through endothelia		Zhang et al, 2009
		Reduction on left ventricular hypertrophy in SHR	Pérez-Vizcaíno and Duarte, 2010
		Reduction in systolic, diastolic and mean arterial pressures after quercetin treatment	Edwards et al., 2007
		Decrease in systolic blood pressure in the apoE3 group	Conquer et al., 1998
		Reduced progression of atherosclerotic lesion in apoE deficient mouse	Hayek et al., 1997 Loke et al., 2010
	Inhibition of TNF-α production, iNOS expression and NO production in LPS-activated macrophages		Pérez-Vizcaíno and Duarte, 2010
		Increased permeability of endothelial cells	Ishizawa et al., 2011
		Reduction in HDL cholesterol and apoA1 in apo epsilon4 carriers	Egert et al., 2010

Table 1. (Continued)

Health benefit	Effect		Reference
		Protection of lipid peroxidation and the antioxidant system in diabetic patients	Pandey and Rizvi, 2009
		Decrease in mortality from coronary heart disease and to myocardial infarction with a borderline significance. Inhibition of metalloproteinase 1 (MMP1) and the disruption of the atherosclerotic plaques	Hertog et al., 1993 García-Lafuente et al., 2009
		Inverse association with stroke	Pérez-Vizcaíno and Duarte, 2010
		Decrease in lower limb volume	Rabe et al., 2011
Energy		Enhance mitochondrial biogenesis in muscle and brain	Davis et al., 2009
		Increase in peak oxygen uptake along with a substantial increase in ride time to fatigue	Davis et al., 2010
Cancer	Anticancer		Naasani et al., 2003 Norato et al., 2009
		Cohort and case-control studies: reduced risk of lung cancer	Neuhouser, 2004
		Protection of lung cancer (mice)	Pandey and Rizvi, 2009
Antioxidant		Inhibition of the FROP activity, raise in the ADS potential in the recipient organism and promoting of IRD severity reduction and acceleration of its function restoration	Zohrab'ian, 2010
Topical use		aphthous ulcers	Hamdy et al., 2010
Antimicrobial	Antibacterial		Rodríguez Vaquero et al., 2007

Methylation occurs in the C3 or C4’ positions; sulfation occurs mainly in the liver, the position of sulfation not being identified yet. Glucuronidation is observed in the C3 position and it occurs at the intestine and liver levels. Most of the metabolites are found in conjugated forms and are eliminated in bile, while small conjugates are excreted in urine. Circulating metabolites in blood are bound to the proteins, mainly albumin, a fact that affects their rate of clearance and delivery to cells and tissues.

So polyphenols beneficial effects on human health depend both on the intake and bioavailability of the compounds that allow polyphenols to penetrate tissues at a concentration that is active to exert their biological activities (Pandey and Rizvi, 2009); it is also important to address the physiologically relevant concentrations of quercetin that can be achieved through diet.

The influence of the sugar chain in quercetin bioavailability was demonstrated in a human study. The alpha-oligoglucosylation of the sugar moiety of quercetin monoglucoside was prepared by enzymatic modification of isoquercitrin (EMIQ) and the subsequent of alpha-oligoglucosylation of quercetin 3-O-beta-rutinode (rutin). The plasma level of quercetin metabolites was instantly increased by oral intake of EMIQ and its absorption efficiency was significantly higher than that of isquercitrin and rutin. The obtained data indicated that enzymatic alpha-oligoglucosylation to the sugar moiety is effective for enhancing the bioavailability of quercetin glucoside in humans (Murota et al., 2010).

Other recent study conducted to determine whether the variable plasma quercetin response in humans is related to gender, age, body mass index (BMI) and other demographic and lifestyle factors indicated that although plasma levels were highly variable within each group, they were not related to the examined variables (Jin et al., 2010).

HEALTH BENEFITS

The epidemiological evidence for the benefit of consuming a diet rich in foods containing polyphenols is very strong. The biological activity of flavonoids is linked to their ability to interact with membranes, so the relationship between structure and membrane needs to be elucidated. When studying the effects of several flavones and flavonols on liposomal membranes and the relationship between chemical structure and membrane interactivity, the 3-hydroxylation on the C-ring, structural non-modification of the B-ring and 5,7-dihydroxylation of the A ring resulted to provide flavonoids with the greater ability to decrease the fluidity in the deeper hydrophobic regions of lipid bilayers. Due to its chemical structure, quercetin resulted to be one of the most active flavonic compounds in inhibiting the proliferation of tumour cells (with an increased membrane fluidity) and lipid peroxidation. This strong activity disappeared by modifying the C-ring to become rutin (quercetin 3-rutinoside) and isoquercitrin (quercetin 3-glucoside). Moreover, quercetin and its conjugated glucuronide inhibit proliferation and hypertrophy or induce apoptosis in vascular smooth muscle cells in culture (Pérez-Vizcaíno and Duarte, 2010), a mechanism that may account for the antihypertensive and antiatherosclerotic effect of quercetin.

Since the phenolic compounds in dietary sources exhibit potent free radical-scavenging properties, their main role was thought to be as antioxidants involved in protection against lipid peroxidation. However, the most recent studies proved that the mode of action of these compounds is more complex than originally expected (Masella et al., 2005; Haliwell et al., 2005; Romier et al, 2009; D'Archivio et al, 2008). In fact polyphenols might exert several other specific biological effects. They can inhibit cancer cell proliferation and cholesterol uptake (Norato et al., 2009; Leifert et al, 2008), modulate different enzymes including telomerase (Naasani et al., 2003) cycloxygenase (Hussain et al., 2005; O'Leary et al., 2004) and lipoxygenase (Sadik et al., 2003; Schewe et al., 2001; de la Puerta et al., 1999), and interact with several signal transduction pathways (Kong et al., 2000; Spencer et al., 2003; Wiseman et al., 2001; Rosenblat et al, 2009; Masella et al, 2004). Moreover, polyphenols can affect caspasedependent pathways (Monasterio et al., 2004; Way et al., 2005), cell cycle regulation (Fischer and Lane, 2000), and platelet functions (Murphy et al., 2003), and they are also able to prevent endothelial dysfunctions (Carluccio et al., 2010).

High dietary intake of fruits and vegetables is associated with a reduced risk of several common human cancers such as cancers of the lung, breast, prostate, and colon. Flavonoids have been investigated as responsible of this beneficial effect. Pharmacological studies in animal model suggest that flavonoids influence important mechanisms related to carcinogenesis, such as cell cycle control and apoptosis. Cohort and case-control studies that review associations of flavonoids intake with cancer risk reveal consistent evidence that flavonoids, especially quercetin, may reduce the risk of lung cancer (Neuhouser, 2004).

Quercetin also shows protective effects in some models such as the benzo(α)pyrene induced lung carcinogenesis in mice, an effect attributed to its free radical scavenging activity (Pandey and Rizvi, 2009).

Taking in account the therapeutic effect of quercetin on colitis and gastric ulcer, its topical application in the treatment of minor aphthous ulcers was tested. The local administration of a quercetin cream preparation to minor mouth ulcers resulted in a pain relief and complete healing in 35% patients after 2-4 days; this percentage increased until 90% after 4-7 days and reached 100% until 7-10 days. Also the mean ulcer size in the treatment group was statistically significantly minor ($p < 0.004$), thus showing the beneficial effect of quercetin for topic treatment of aphthous ulcers (Hamdy and Ibrahem, 2010).

Oxidative Stress

Free radicals are reactive chemical species with unpaired electron that occur in biological systems. An over-production of these species together with an impaired capability of the bodily antioxidant defense system leads to oxidative stress which is related to several chronic diseases like cancer, neurodegenerative or coronary diseases, between others.

Those compounds capable of delaying or inhibiting the oxidation of several molecules through the inhibition of the initiation or propagation of oxidative chain reactions are known as antioxidants. These molecules are thus capable of counteract the damaging effects of oxidation in animal tissues (Mustafa et al., 2010).

Most of the beneficial effects of polyphenols derive from their antioxidant capacity; the phenolic groups can accept an electron to form relatively stable phenoxyl radicals that disrupt chain oxidation reactions in cellular components. Polyphenol-rich foods and beverages may increase plasma antioxidant capacity by the increase of polyphenols and their metabolites in plasma, by their beneficial effects upon concentration of other reducing agents or by affecting the absorption of pro-oxidative food components, such as iron.

Flavonoids are the main responsible of the antioxidant capability of plants which has already been proved by *in vitro* assays, although the evidence of their action *in vivo* is still limited. Thus, it is possible that the antioxidant effect exerted by these compounds is not the only mechanism to explain their benefit on neuroprotection, endothelial function, atherosclerosis and cardiovascular risk.

The essential requirement for effective radical scavenging activity in the flavonoids structure is the 3',4'-orthodihydroxy configuration in the B-ring and 4-carbonyl group in ring C, which has the good electron donating properties and a radical target (Mustafa et al., 2010). The presence of 3-hydroxyl group or 3 and 5-dihydroxyl groups that give a catechol-like structure increases the stability of the aroxyl radical. The presence of the double bond between C2 and C3 with a 4-keto arrangement is responsible for electron delocalization from ring B and increases the radical scavenging activity (Mustafa et al., 2010).

In addition to its anti-oxidant effect, a large number of enzymes is modulated (mostly inhibited) by quercetin, so it can be predicted its action on several biochemical pathways and therefore, on a huge number of physiological and pathological processes.

The antioxidant effect of quercetin was confirmed by an *in vivo* study on the impact of this flavonol on the indices of peroxidal oxidation of lipids and antioxidant defence system (ADS) of renal allotransplant (RAT) recipients in early postoperative period. It is well known that activation of the free-radical oxidation processes (FROP) in the environment of activity inhibition of ADS plays an important role in pathogenesis of an ischemic-reperfusion damage (IRD) of RAT, causes its dysfunction and shortens long-term survival (Zohrab'ian, 2010).

Together with standard measures, the intraoperative intravenous administration of an antioxidant sample containing lipin and quercetin resulted in an inhibition of the FROP activity, a raise in the ADS potential in the recipient organism and therefore, a promoting of IRD severity reduction and an acceleration of its function restoration.

Cardiovascular Disease

Endothelium and Vascular Smooth Muscle

The endothelium is the inner lining of all blood vessels and functions as a selectively permeable barrier between blood and tissues. Normal endothelial function exerts a fine control of cardiovascular homeostasis as it regulates vasomotor tone, platelet activity, leukocyte adhesion and vascular smooth muscle proliferation via a release of several factors including nitric oxide (NO). Thus endothelial dysfunction is characterized by impaired endothelium-dependent vasodilatation, reduced nitric oxide (NO) activity and a prothrombotic and proinflammatory stated of endothelial cells; this state is an early predictor of cardiovascular disease (Hodgson, 2010; Pérez-Vizcaíno and Duarte, 2010).

Quercetin exerts direct acute vasodilator effects in isolated arteries; in healthy vessels, these effects are endothelium-independent and occur similarly. Quercetin and its methylated metabolites are more potent in coronary arteries and in resistance than in conductance vessels and also in vessels from hypertensive animals (Pérez-Vizcaíno and Duarte, 2010). The effects of quercetin are partially endothelium-dependent and related to the release of endothelium-derived relaxing factors; in this way, quercetin is able to enhance NO status through a very complex mechanism. The glucuronidated and sulfated metabolites of quercetin lack a direct vasodilator effect in the rat aorta (Pérez-Vizcaíno and Duarte, 2010).

Endothelin-1 (ET-1) is a potent vasoconstrictor agent that is released by endothelial cells and which level is elevated when endothelial dysfunction occurs. Moreover, ET-1 itself induces endothelial dysfunction. Quercetin is able to inhibit ET-1 release in human and bovine endothelial cells and therefore reduces ET-1 concentration (Khan et al., 2002; Zhao et al, 1999).

The endothelium-dependent relaxations to insulin which are also impaired in hypertensive rats (SHR) were unaffected after chronic treatment with quercetin (Romero et al., 2010), in contrast to the endothelium-dependent vasodilatation to acetylcholine. The different profile of quercetin against the relaxations induced by these two endothelial NO-releasing agents might be related to the different pathways of acetylcholine and insulin to activate eNOS. Acetylcholine is a classic cholinergic agonist that activates eNOS by a calcium-dependent mechanism. Insulin-stimulated Akt and eNOS phosphorylations were reduced in aortic rings from SHR and WKY rats treated with quercetin, an effect that might be related to a direct inhibitory effect of quercetin on PI3-K (Yoshizumi et al., 2002).

Additionally, apparent changes in endothelial-dependent vasodilatation may occur as a consequence of the opposing effects of the release of endothelium-derived vasoconstrictor prostanoids. Chronic quercetin did not modify the endothelium-dependent vasoconstriction in SHR but markedly inhibited it in NO-deficient (Pérez-Vizcaíno and Duarte, 2010) and in Goldblatt rats (Garcia-Saura et al., 2005).

The sirtuins Sirt2 and its mammalian analog SIRT1 have been implicated in the extended lifespan induced by caloric restriction and more recently in the prevention of vascular senescence (Ota et al., 2010). Activation of SIRT1 has been shown to promote endothelium-dependent vasodilation (Mattagajasingh et al., 2007) and to downregulate angiotensin II receptor expression. Quercetin extends the lifespan of the yeast *Saccharomyces cerevisiae* and the worm *Caenorhabditis elegans* (Belinha et al., 2007; Pietsch et al., 2009).

Many investigations confirm the beneficial effects of quercetin against the development of atherosclerosis via inhibition of cell adhesion molecules such as intercellular adhesion molecule-1 (ICAM-1) and vascular cell adhesion molecule-1 (VCAM-1). However, as explained above, the development of clinically applicable therapeutic interventions must take into account the physiologically relevant conjugates of polyphenols like quercetin (Gómez-Rico, 2006); while quercetin reduced the tumor necrosis factor-alpha (TNF-α) mediated induction of ICAM and VCAM, metabolically prevalent quercetin conjugates were not able to downregulate the pro-inflammatory ICAMs and VCAMs produced by human umbilical artery smooth muscle cells (HUASMCs) exposed to either TNF-α or lipopolysaccharide (LPS). So quercetin has the ability of cells to migrate through endothelia, an important stage of the inflammatory response (Zhang et al, 2009).

Platelets

Although the platelet antiaggregant effect of flavonols was previously described, the *in vivo* antiaggregant effects of quercetin have been questioned as in a human study with onions providing 114mg quercetin per day, no changes were found in platelet aggregation, thromboxane B_2 production, factor VII, or other haemostatic variables (Pérez-Vizcaíno and Duarte, 2010).

Hypertension

In cardiovascular events, hypertension is one of the most powerful risk factor, so treatment of that factor reduces cardiovascular diseases: the larger the reduction in blood pressure is the larger the reduction in cardiovascular risk (Pérez-Vizcaíno and Duarte, 2010). Fruit and vegetable consumption under controlled experimental conditions results in a decrease in blood pressure, although this effect is not so clear under real conditions of use.

Quercetin has demonstrated a reduction on left ventricular hypertrophy in SHR and beneficial effects in several pharmacological models of hypertension (Pérez-Vizcaíno and Duarte, 2010), together with the already mentioned protective effects on endothelial function. These experimental results have been reflected in two recent randomized, double-blind, placebo controlled, crossover clinical trials analyzing the effects of quercetin in blood pressure. The first one was carried on with patients with stage 1 hypertension that had a reduction in systolic, diastolic and mean arterial pressures after quercetin treatment (Edwards et al., 2007); no effect on pre-hypertensives was observed. A more recent study was published with patients with metabolic syndrome that were classified according to their apoE phenotypes (Egert et al., 2010); quercetin decreased systolic blood pressure in the apoE3 group, whereas no effect was observed in patients with the apoE4 phenotype or in healthy volunteers (Conquer et al., 1998).

Atherosclerosis

Atherosclerosis is a multifactorial disease characterized by arterial wall thickening caused by deposition of fatty materials over a long period of time, symptoms being evident in the late stages of the disease. The alteration of the serum profile is one on the first events in the development of atherosclerosis, together with oxidative stress, inflammation and endothelial dysfunction. Consumption of low doses of quercetin reduced the progression of the atherosclerotic lesion development in the apoE deficient mouse (Hayek et al., 1997; Loke et al., 2010), this flavonol being more effective than other representative flavonoids. The underlying mechanism for this protection lies on the prevention of one or several processes involved in this disease such as oxidative stress or inflammation. Although the exact mechanism has not been complete elucidated, quercetin inhibits TNF-α production as well as iNOS expression and NO production in LPS-activated macrophages, an effect associated with the inhibition of the NF-κβ pathway (Pérez-Vizcaíno and Duarte, 2010).

A study carried out on aortic wall samples obtained during autopsy from patients with generalized atherosclerosis proved an increased permeability of endothelial cells with reduced barrier function. Quercetin-3-O—D glucuronide, one of the two main metabolites from quercetin in circulating blood, can permeate through the injured endothelial cells in human atherosclerotic lesions and therefore is localized in the arteries with atherosclerotic lesions (Ishizawa et al., 2011). These findings support the preventive effects of quercetin in cardiovascular diseases.

A protective function in the atherosclerotic process has been found for the HDL-associated enzyme paraoxonase 1 (PON1); therefore it is of interest the study of the impact of dietary factors including flavonoids on the PON1 activity. A recent study was carried on in mice supplemented with daily 0.05 to 2mg quercetin/g diet for 6 weeks and determined the expression of the hepatic PON1 gene and its protein levels. A moderate but significant induction of PON1 mRNA levels aimed the authors to proof the quercetin administration (50, 100 or 150 mg/day for two weeks) effect in healthy human volunteers. Nonetheless, no beneficial effect was obtained in humans, probably due to differences in quercetin metabolism between both mice and humans; in mice, unlike in humans, a large proportion of quercetin is methylated to isorhamnetin which exhibits a potent PON1 inducing activity (Boesch-Saadatmandi et al., 2010).

An at-risk population of 93 overweight-obese volunteers aged 25-65 years, with metabolic syndrome, was the object of a clinical trial to examine the effect of quercetin supplementation of blood pressure, lipid metabolism, markers of oxidative stress, inflammation, and body composition. Quercetin exhibited blood pressure-lowering effect in patients of the apo3/epsilon3 genotype (3.4 mm Hg, $p<0.01$) but not in carriers of the epsilon4 allele. Furthermore, quercetin supplementation resulted in a reduction in HDL cholesterol ($p< 0.01$) and apoA1 ($p< 0.01$) in apo epsilon4 carriers (Egert et el., 2010).

Insulin Resistance

Insulin resistance is defined as an attenuated or inadequate response to insulin and it is associated with a wide variety of conditions including obesity, type-2 diabetes, essential hypertension or cardiovascular disease, between others. Long term effects of diabetes include the development of retinopathy, nephropathy, foot ulcers and several other dysfunctions. Onion polyphenols and specially quercetin, have proved to exert a strong antidiabetic activity and even protect the alterations in diabetic patients during oxidative stress. Quercetin significantly acted in diabetic patients protecting the lipid peroxidation and the inhibition of the antioxidant system (Pandey and Rizvi, 2009).

The effect of quercetin on insulin resistance is not clear; at high doses, quercetin may reduce obesity, although these effects are not demonstrated in human studies (Pérez-Vizcaíno and Duarte, 2010).

Myocardial Ischemia

Atherosclerosis and hypertension are the two main risk factors for myocardial infarction; the reduction of low density lipoprotein (LDL)-cholesterol and atherosclerotic lesions and blood pressure is accompanied by a marked decrease in the risk of coronary disease. Moreover, endothelial dysfunction is another independent factor for myocardial infarction. As explained above, the beneficial effects of quercetin on hypertension, atherosclerosis and endothelial dysfunctions may protect the coronary vessels in the long term.

The pharmacological studies have been followed by epidemiological studies and clinical trials that showed that quercetin intake was inversely related to mortality from coronary heart disease (relative risk 0.42) (Hertog et al., 1993), and to myocardial infarction with a borderline significance. One of the involved mechanisms is the inhibition of metalloproteinase 1 (MMP1) and the disruption of the atherosclerotic plaques (García-Lafuente et al., 2009).

Stroke

The pathophysiological processes in stroke are complex and depend on several factors such as the severity and localization of the ischemic damage in the brain. The main cause of stroke is the interruption of blood flow during vascular obstruction by thromboembolism or thrombosis; therefore hypertension, atherosclerosis, LDL-cholesterol, diabetes and atrial fibrillation are the main risk factors of stroke. As flavonoids, and specially quercetin, act on nearly every one of the above mentioned risk factors, they are supposed to exert a preventive effect on strokes.

Several prospective epidemiological studies reported an inverse association of stroke with flavonol consumption (mainly quercetin), an even a recent meta-analysis found that a high intake of flavonols was inversely related to nonfatal and fatal stroke with a pooled relative risk of 0.80% (Pérez-Vizcaíno and Duarte, 2010). Other studies did not find a relationship between quercetin intake and cerebrovascular disease.

The beneficial effects of quercetin in different parameters related to cardiovascular disease in humans were studied in a multicentre, randomized, double-blind and placebo-controlled study on 248 patients with chronic venous insufficiency (CVI), receiving 720 mg of a standardized extract of red wine leaves (AS195) per day during 12 weeks. At the end of the treatment period, patients significantly decrease lower limb volume when compared to placebo, indicating a clinically relevant effect. Patients reported subjective improvement after treatment with the vegetal extract when compared to placebo, although the rating of efficacy did not correlate well with measured reductions in limb volume. This study concluded that the tested extract was well tolerated and significantly decreased the leg volume in patients with moderate to severe CVI, while secondary efficacy parameters also improved (Rabe et el., 2011).

Anti-Aging Effect

Advanced age leads to detrimental changes in cells and tissues that increase the risk of several diseases and death. One of the most accepted theory to explain the mechanism of aging is the free radical/oxidative stress theory that stands that a certain amount of oxidative damage takes place even under normal conditions; nevertheless, when the efficiency of antioxidative and repair mechanisms decreases, the aging process takes place.

One of the factors occurring in neurodegenerative diseases such as Alzheimer's disease is oxidative stress and damage to brain molecules. Due to the strong antioxidant activity of polyphenols, a protective effect on neurological diseases is shown.

The intake of antioxidant rich diet is capable of reducing the effects of aging. Polyphenols may reduce the adverse events of the aging on nervous system or brain, mainly because of their ability to cross the blood-brain barrier (BBB) that controls the influx of metabolites in the brain.

A recent study was carried out with a standardized extract from *Diospyros kaki* leaves containing more than 77.4% flavonols including 34.6% quercetin, as well as with the isolated compound (Bei et al., 2009). The vegetal extract protects cerebral tissues from ischemia/reperfusion injury, reduces infarct volume and edema, and improves neurological behavior of rats with middle cerebral artery occlusion induced cerebral damage. The standardized extract significantly protects hippocampal CA1 pyramidal neurons from four-vessel occlusion transient global brain ischemia and reperfusion damage in rats. It also protects neurons against the excitotoxic injury induced by glutamate and also ischemic-like damage caused by hypoxia/reoxygen. These results are also found when isolated quercetin was tested and therefore point this flavonoid as responsible, at least in part, of the observed beneficial effects and suggest that it might be potentially used in the prevention and treatment of ischemia/reperfusion injury disorders such as stroke or apoplexy syndrome and other neurodegenerative disease (Bei et al., 2009).

ENERGY

Several diseases such as neurodegenerative disorders, cancer, diabetes, cardiovascular myopathies and the aging process may be due to mitochondrial dysfunction in peripheral tissues and brain (Davis et al., 2009). Quercetin is able to improve endurance time-trial performance on a bicycle ergometer when fed for six weeks in humans, although the biological mechanism for this effect is not known. The study of a short term supplementation with quercetin at a safe dose on mitochondrial biogenesis in brain and soleus muscle and the endurance exercise tolerance revealed that quercetin itself enhance mitochondrial biogenesis in muscle and brain through an increase in mRNa expression of the transcriptional coactivators sirtuin 1(SIRT1) and peroxisome proliferator-activated receptor gamma coactivator (PGC-1 alpha), mtDNA and cytochrome concentration. These changes are associated with an increase in both maximal endurance running capacity and active involvement prolonged exercise activity. The increase in the exercise tolerance is due, at least in part, to an increased oxidative metabolism in both muscular cells and brain, but also to the effect of quercetin as an adenosine A_1 receptor antagonist in brain.

These beneficial effects were tested in healthy but untrained volunteers that randomly received (a) 500 mg of quercetin twice daily dissolved in vitamin-enriched Tang or (b) a nondistinguisable placebo (Tang), in order to determine quercetin effect on maximal aerobic capacity and fatigue during prolonged exercise (Davis et al., 2010). Seven days of quercetin consumption showed a modes increase in peak oxygen uptake (3.9% vs. placebo; $p< 0.05$) along with a substantial (13.2%); $p< 0.05$) increase in ride time to fatigue. These data suggest that quercetin supplementation can increase endurance without exercise training in untrained participants, an effect that may have important implications for athletic and military performance, as well as for health promotion and disease prevention.

Relatively positive effects were also obtained for untrained males receiving 1 g quercetin/day on exercise performance and skeletal muscle mitochondrial biogenesis (Nieman et al., 2010). A randomized crossover design with a supplement of quercetin for 2 weeks was associated with a small but significant improvement in 12-mi treadmill time trial performance and modest but insignificant increases in the relative copy number of mitochondrial DNA and messenger RNA levels of four genes related to mitochondrial biogenesis.

These promising results were not reflected in the study carried out with young persons conducting military physical training, as quercetin supplementation did not influence energy, fatigue or sleep quality after 54 days of supplementation with 1 g/day of quercetin in a soft chew (Bigelman et al., 2011). The same supplementation did not improve peak oxygen uptake or performance on the Army Physical Fitness test, Baumgartner Modified Pill-Up Test, Wingate Anaerobic Test and 36.6 m sprint on healthy volunteers (Bigelman et al., 2010). No beneficial effects were obtained for untrained, sedentary individuals supplemented with 1 g quercetin/day neither for well-trained cyclists on fuel utilization, gross efficiency or perceived effort (Ganio et al., 2010; Dumke et al., 2009).

The effect of quercetin supplementation on fasting resting energy expenditure (REE) and respiratory quotient (RQ) in humans was studied in six healthy, normal-weight women through a randomized, placebo-controlled, double-blinded crossover study (Egert et el., 2011). Patients received capsules of 150 mg quercetin (aglycone) or placebo. The acute response was measured by indirect calorimetry; blood pressure and pulse rate were assessed in 30-min intervals. Baseline (t(0)) REE adjusted for fat-free mass was 4.7 ± 0.26 kJ/min for quercetin and 4.8 ± 0.35 kJ/min for placebo and did not significantly change between baseline and end (t(180)). RQ values decreased slowly and to a similar extent for both treatments. Resting systolic and diastolic blood pressure, pulse pressure as well as resting pulse rate did not change between baseline and end in either treatment group. The obtained results provided no evidence of thermic effect of quercetin in humans.

CONCLUSIONS

People all around the developed countries are becoming more and more concerned about their health based in the consumption of healthy foods, dietary supplements, functional foods and food constituents, so studies on pharmacology of these products is necessary to assess their beneficial effects.

Quercetin (3,3',4',5,7 pentahydroxy flavone) is one of the most studies polyphenolic compounds which has been proved to exert several beneficial effects for human health as antioxidant, anti-inflammatory, antibacterial, anticoagulative and antihypertensive agent; it has also been used in gene expression modulation and in the inhibition of the growth of several cancer cell lines, although its mechanism of action is not completely elucidated for all of these actions. I*n vitro* studies shed light on the mechanisms of action of individual quercetin, but these findings need to be supported by *in vivo* experiments in appropriate animal models of disease and in humans at appropriate doses. Quercetin daily intake comes mainly from diets rich in polyphenolic compounds and its quantity varies depending in feeding habits and countries, but also from several marketed food supplements as an estimated 42% of adults in the United States of America take some form of dietary supplement for their health.

Quercetin is bound to sugars in foods, mainly as –glycosides, and is converted to aglycone in the large intestine by the glycosidase activity of intestinal bacteria. Quercetin aglycone is not detected in human plasma, whereas the two main metabolites quercetin-3-O—D-glucuronide and quercetin-3'-sulfate are accumulated in the range of 10^{-7} to 10^{-6} M after the periodic ingestion of onions with meals for 1 week (Moon et al, 2000). Therefore, the pharmacological function of quercetin should be attributed to its conjugated metabolites (Ishizawa et al., 2011).

Quercetin is a promising compound for the prevention of the most common forms of cardiovascular diseases as it exerts beneficial effects such as the endothelium-independent vasodilator effect, protective effect on NO and endothelial function under oxidative stress conditions, platelet antiaggregant effects, inhibition of LDL oxidation, reduction of adhesive molecules and other inflammatory markers and prevention of neuronal oxidative and inflammatory damage.

Recent *in vivo* and *in vitro* studies suggest that quercetin significantly protects rats from ischemic injury *in vivo* and protects hippocampal neurons from glutamate-induced excitotoxic injury as well as cortical neurons from hypoxia-induced injury *in vitro*, mainly due to its antioxidative activity

These protective actions *in vitro* demonstrate the potential use of quercetin for the prevention and treatment of ischemia/reperfusion injury and other related neurodegenerative diseases, and they should be followed by clinical studies that confirm the protective effects afforded for the prevention of several human diseases in youth and aging adults.

This effect is important not only for the biological effect but also for the fact that the plant source of quercetin is relatively cheap to grow and harvest, and the compound is safe and effective at low dosages (500-1000mg/day) (Davis et al., 2009).

References

Andrikopoulos, N.K.; Dedoussis, G.V.; Falirea, A.; Kalogeropoulos, N.; Hatzinikola, H.S. Deterioration of natural antioxidant species of vegetable edible oils during the domestic deep frying and pan-frying of potatoes. *Int. J. Food Sci. Nutr.* 2002, *53*, 351–363.

Appeldoorn, M.M.; Venema, D.P.; Peters, T.H.F.; Koenen, M.E.; Arts, I.C.W.; Vincken, J.P.; Gruppen, H.; Keijer, J.; Hollman, P.C.H. Some phenolic compounds increase the nitric oxide level in endothelial cells *in vitro*. *J. Agric. Food Chem.* 2009, *57:* 7693–7699.

Aura, A.M.; Martin-Lopez, P.; O'Leary, K.A.; Williamson, G.; Oksman-Caldentey, K.M.; Poutanen, K.; Santos-Buelga, C. *In vitro* metabolism of anthocyanins by human gut microflora. *Eur. J. Nutr.* 2005, *44*, 133–142.

Azuma, K.; Ippoushi, K.; Ito, H.; Higashio, H.; Terao, J. Combination of lipids and emulsifiers enhances the absorption of orally administered quercetin in rats. *J. Agric. Food Chem.* 2002, 50: 1706–1712.

Baiano, A.; Gambacorta, G.; Terracone, C.; Previtali, M.A.; Lamacchia, C.; La Notte, E. Changes in phenolic content and antioxidant activity of Italian extra-virgin olive oils during storage. *J. Food. Sci.* 2009, *74*: C177–183.

Bei, W.; Zang, L.; Guo, J.; Peng, W.; Xu, A.; Good, D.A.; Hu, Y.; Wu, W.; Hu, D.; Zhu, X.; Wei, M.; Li, C. Neuroprotective effects of a standardized flavonoid extract from *Diospyros kaki* leaves. *J. Ethnopharmacol.* 2009, 126: 134-142.

Belinha, I.; Amorim, M.A.; Rodrigues, P.; de Freitas, V.; Moradas-Ferreira, P.; Mateus, N.; Costa, V. Quercetin increases oxidative stress resistance and longevity in Saccharomyces cerevisiae. *J. Agric. Food Chem.* 2007, 55: 2446–2451.

Bieger, J; CCermak, R; Blank, R; de Boer, V.C.; Hollman P.C.; kamphues J.; Wolffram S. Tissue distribution of quercetin in pigs after long-term dietary supplementation. *J. Nutr.* 2008, 138: 1417-1420.

Bigelman, K.A.; Chapman, D.P.; Freese, E.C.; Trilk, J.L.; Cureton, K.J. Effects of 6 weeks of quercetin supplementation on energy, fatigue, and sleep in ROTC cadets. *Mil. Med.* 2011, 176(5):565-72.

Bigelman, K.A.; Fan, E.H.; Chapman, D.P.; Freese, E.C.; Trilk, J.L.; Cureton, K.J. Effects of six weeks of quercetin supplementation on physical performance in ROTC cadets. *Mil. Med.* 2010,175(10):791-8.

Boersma, M.G.; van der Woude, H.; Bogaards, J.; Boeren, S.; Vervoort, J.; Cnubben, N.H.; van Iersel, M.L.; van Bladeren, P.J.; Rietjens, I.M. Regioselectivity of phase II metabolism of luteolin and quercetin by UDP-glucuronosyl transferases. *Chem. Res. Toxicol.* 2002, *15*, 662–670.

Boesch-Saadatmandi, C.; Egert, S.; Schrader, C.; Coumou,l X.; Barouki, R.; Muller, M.J.; Wolffram, S.; Rimbach, G. Effect of quercetin on paraoxonase 1 activity--studies in cultured cells, mice and humans. *J. Physiol. Pharmacol.* 2010, 61(1):99-105.

Bonoli, M.; Bendini, A.; Cerretani, L.; Lercker, G.; Toschi, T.G. Qualitative and semiquantitative analysis of phenolic compounds in extra virgin olive oils as a function of the ripening degree of olive fruits by different analytical techniques. *J. Agric. Food Chem.* 2004, 52: 7026–7032.

Bouaziz, M.; Chamkha, M.; Sayadi, S. Comparative study on phenolic content and antioxidant activity during maturation of the olive cultivar Chemlali from Tunisia. *J. Agric. Food Chem.* 2004, *52*, 5476–5481.

Brenes, M.; Garcia, A.; Dobarganes, M.C.; Velasco, J.; Romero, C. Influence of thermal treatments simulating cooking processes on the polyphenol content in virgin olive oil. *J. Agric. Food Chem.* 2002, *50*: 5962–5967.

Bugianesi, R.; Salucci, M.; Leonardi, C.; Ferracane, R.; Catasta, G.; Azzini, E.; Maiani, G. Effect of domestic cooking on human bioavailability of naringenin, chlorogenic acid, lycopene and betacarotene in cherry tomatoes. *Eur. J. Nutr.* 2004, *43*: 360–366.

Carluccio, M.A.; Siculella, L.; Ancora, M.A.; Massaro, M.; Scoditti, E.; Storelli, C.; Visioli, F.; Distante, A.; De Caterina, R. Olive oil and red wine antioxidant polyphenols inhibit endotelial activation: Antiatherogenic properties of Mediterranean diet phytochemicals. *Arterioscler. Thromb. Vasc. Biol.* 2003, *23*: 622–629.

Carrasco-Pancorbo, A.; Cerretani, L.; Bendini, A.; Segura-Carretero, A.; Lercker, G.; Fernandez-Gutierrez, A. Evaluation of the influence of thermal oxidation on the phenolic composition and on the antioxidant activity of extra-virgin olive oils. *J. Agric. Food Chem.* 2007, *55*: 4771–4780.

Conquer, J.A.; Maiani, G.; Azzini, E.; Raguzzini, A.; Holub, B.J. Supplementation with quercetin markedly increases plasma quercetin concentration without effect on selected risk factors for heart disease in healthy subjects. *J. Nutr.* 1998, 128: 593–597.

Crespy, V.; Morand, C.; Besson, C.; Manach, C.; Demigne, C.; Remesy, C. Comparison of the intestinal absorption of quercetin, phloretin and their glucosides in rats. *J. Nutr.* 2001, *131*: 2109–2114.

Crozier. A.; Jaganath, I.B.; Clifford, M.N. Dietary phenolics: Chemistry, bioavailability and effects on health. *Nat. Prod. Rep.* 2009, *26:* 1001–1043.

Crozier A, Lean MEJ, McDonald MS, Black C. Quantitative analysis of the flavonoid content in commercial tomatoes, onions, lettuce, and celery. *J. Agric. Food Chem.* 1997, 45: 590-595.

D'Archivio, M.; Filesi, C.; Varì, R.; Scazzocchio, B.; Masella, R. Bioavailability of the Polyphenols: Status and Controversies *Int. J. Mol. Sci.* 2010, 11*:* 1321-1342.

D'Archivio, M.; Santangelo, C.; Scazzocchio, B.; Vari, R.; Filesi, C.; Masella, R.; Giovannini, C. Modulatory effects of polyphenols on apoptosis induction: Relevance for cancer prevention. *Int. J. Mol. Sci.* 2008, *9*, 213–228.

Davalos, A.; Castilla, P.; Gomez-Cordoves, C.; Bartolome, B. Quercetin is bioavailable from a single ingestion of grape juice. *Int. J. Food Sci. Nutr.* 2006, 57: 391-398.

Davis, J.M.; Carlstedt, C.J.; Chen, S.; Carmichael, M.D.; Murphy, E.A. The dietary flavonoid quercetin *Int. J. Sport Nutr. Exerc. Metab.* 2010, 20(1): 56-62.

Davis, J.M.; Murphy, E.A.; Carmichael, M.D.; Davis, B. Quercetin increases brain and muscle mitochondrial biogenesis and exercise tolerance. *Am. J. Physiol. Regul. Integr. Comp. Physiol.* 2009, 296: R1071-R1077.

Day, A.J.; Canada, F.J.; Diaz, J.C.; Kroon, P.A.; McLauchlan, R.; Faulds, C.B.; Plumb, G.W.; Morgan, M.R.; Williamson, G. Dietary flavonoid and isoflavone glycosides are hydrolysed by the lactase site of lactase phlorizin hydrolase. *FEBS Lett.* 2000a, *468*: 166–170.

Day, A.J.; Bao, Y.; Morgan, M.R.; Williamson, G. Conjugation position of quercetin glucuronides and effect on biological activity. *Free Radic. Biol. Med.* 2000b, *29*: 1234–1243.

de la Puerta, R.; Ruiz Gutierrez, V.; Hoult, J.R. Inhibition of leukocyte 5-lipoxygenase by phenolics from virgin olive oil. *Biochem. Pharmacol.* 1999, *57*: 445–49.

Del Rio, D.; Costa, L.G.; Lean, M.E.; Crozier, A. Polyphenols and health: What compounds are involved? *Nutr. Metab. Cardiovasc. Dis.* 2010, *20*: 1–6.

Donovan, J.L.; Bell, J.R.; Kasim-Karakas, S.; German, J.B.; Walzem, R.L.; Hansen, R.J.; Waterhouse, A.L. Catechin is present as metabolites in human plasma after consumption of red wine. *J. Nutr.* 1999, *129*: 1662–1668.

Donovan, J.L.; Kasim-Karakas, S.; German, J.B.; Waterhouse, A.L. Urinary excretion of catechin metabolites by human subjects after red wine consumption. *Br. J. Nutr.* 2002, *87*: 31–37.

Dumke, C.L.; Nieman D.C.; Utter, A.C.; Rigby, M.D.; Quindry, J.C.; Triplett, N.T.; McAnulty, S.R.; McAnulty, L.S. Quercetin's effect on cycling efficiency and substrate utilization. *Appl. Physiol. Nutr. Metab.* 2009, 34(6): 993-1000.

DuPont, M.S.; Mondin, Z.; Williamson, G.; Price, K.R. Effect of variety, processing, and storage on the flavonoid glycoside content and composition of lettuce and endive. *J. Agric. Food Chem.* 2000, *48*, 3957–3964.

Edwards, R.L.; Lyon, T.; Litwin, S.E.; Rabovsky, A.; Symons, J.D.; Jalili, T. Quercetin reduces blood pressure in hypertensive subjects. *J. Nutr.* 2007, 137: 2405–2411.

Egert, S.; Rimbach, G.; Müller, M.J. No evidence for a thermic effect of the dietary flavonol quercetin: a pilot study in healthy normal-weight women. *Eur. J. Appl. Physiol.* 2011, 111(5):869-73.

Egert, S.; Boesch-Saadatmandi, C., Wolffram, S., Rimbach, G.; Müller, M.J. Serum lipid and blood pressure responses to quercetin vary in overweight patients by apolipoprotein E genotype. *J. Nutr.* 2010, 140(2): 278-84.

Falany, C.N. Enzymology of human cytosolic sulfotransferases. *Faseb. J.* 1997, *11*: 206–216.

Felgines, C.; Talavera, S.; Texier, O.; Gil-Izquierdo, A.; Lamaison, J.L.; Remesy, C. Blackberry anthocyanins are mainly recovered from urine as methylated and glucuronidated conjugates in humans. *J. Agric. Food Chem.* 2005, *53*: 7721–7727.

Femia, A.P.; Caderni, G.; Ianni, M.; Salvadori, M.; Schijlen, E.; Collins, G.; Bovy, A.; Dolara, P. Effect of diets fortified with tomatoes or onions with variable quercetin-glycoside content on azoxymethane-induced aberrant crypt foci in the colon of rats. *Eur. J. Nutr. 2003,* 42: 346–352.

Ferracane, R.; Pellegrini, N.; Visconti, A.; Graziani, G.; Chiavaro, E.; Miglio, C.; Fogliano, V. Effects of different cooking methods on antioxidant profile, antioxidant capacity, and physical characteristics of artichoke. *J. Agric. Food Chem.* 2008, *56*: 8601–8608.

Ferrazzano, G.F.; Amato, I.; Ingenito, A.; Zarrelli, A., Pinto, G.; Pollio, A. Plant polyphenols and their anti-cariogenic properties: a review. *Molecules* 2011, 16(2): 1486-1507.

Fischer, P.M.; Lane, D.P. Inhibitors of cyclin-dependent kinases as anti-cancer therapeutics. *Curr. Med. Chem. 2000, 7:* 1213–1245.

Forester, S.C.; Waterhouse, A.L. Metabolites are key to understanding health effects of wine polyphenolics. *J. Nutr. 2009,* 139: 1824S–1831S.

Ganio, M.S.; Armstrong, L.E.; Johnson, E.C.; Klau, J.F.; Ballard, K.D., Michniak-Kohn, B., Kaushik, D.; Maresh, C.M. Effect of quercetin supplementation on maximal oxygen uptake in men and women. *J. Sports Sci.* 2010, 28(2):201-8.

Garcia-Lafuente, A.; Guillamon, E.; Villares, A.; Rostagno, M.A.; Martinez, J.A. Flavonoids as anriinflammatory agents: implications in cancer and cardiovascular disease. *Inflamm. Res. 2009,* 58: 537-552.

Garcia-Saura, M.F.; Galisteo, M.; Villar, I.C.; Bermejo, A.; Zarzuelo, A.; Vargas, F.; Duarte, J. Effects of chronic quercetin treatment in experimental renovascular hypertension. *Mol. Cell Biochem.* 2005, 270: 147–155.

Gee, J.M.; DuPont, M.S.; Day, A.J.; Plumb, G.W.; Williamson, G.; Johnson, I.T. Intestinal transport of quercetin glycosides in rats involves both deglycosylation and interaction with the hexose transport pathway. *J. Nutr.* 2000, *130*, 2765–2771.

Gliszczynska-Swiglo, A.; Ciska, E.; Pawlak-Lemanska, K.; Chmielewski, J.; Borkowski, T.; Tyrakowska, B. Changes in the content of health-promoting compounds and antioxidant activity of broccoli after domestic processing. *Food Addit. Contam.* 2006, *23*: 1088–1098.

Gliszczynska-Swiglo, A.; Tyrakowska, B. Quality of commercial apple juices evaluated on the basis of the polyphenol content and the TEAC antioxidant activity. *J. Food Sci.* 2003, *68*: 1844–1849.

Goldberg, D.M.; Yan, J.; Soleas, G.J. Absorption of three wine-related polyphenols in three different matrices by healthy subjects. *Clin. Biochem.* 2003, *36*: 79–87.

Gomez-Alonso, S.; Fregapane, G.; Salvador, M.D.; Gordon, M.H. Changes in phenolic composition and antioxidant activity of virgin olive oil during frying. *J. Agric. Food Chem.* 2003, *51*: 667–672.

Gomez-Rico, A.; Salvador, M.D.; La Greca, M.; Fregapane, G. Phenolic and volatile compounds of extra virgin olive oil (*Olea europaea* L. Cv. Cornicabra) with regard to fruit ripening and irrigation management. *J. Agric. Food Chem.* 2006, *54*: 7130–7136.

Guyot, S.; Marnet, N.; Sanoner, P.; Drilleau, J.F. Variability of the polyphenolic composition of cider apple (*Malus domestica*) fruits and juices. *J. Agric. Food Chem. 2003,* 51: 6240–6247.

Halliwell, B.; Rafter, J.; Jenner, A. Health promotion by flavonoids, tocopherols, tocotrienols, and other phenols: Direct or indirect effects? Antioxidant or not? *Am. J. Clin. Nutr.* 2005, *81:* 268S–276S.

Hayek, T.; Fuhrman, B.; Vaya, J.; Rosenblat, M.; Belinky, P.; Coleman, R.; Elis, A.; Aviram, M. Reduced progression of atherosclerosis in apolipoprotein Edeficient mice following consumption of red wine, or its polyphenols quercetin or catechin, is associated with reduced susceptibility of LDL to oxidation and aggregation. *Arterioscler. Thromb. Vasc. Biol.* 1997, 17: 2744–2752.

Hertog, M.G.; Feskens, E.J.; Hollman, P.C.; Katan, M.B.; Kromhout, D. Dietary antioxidant flavonoids and risk of coronary heart disease: the Zutphen Elderly Study. *Lancet* 1993, 342: 1007–1011.

Hamdy, A.A.; Ibrahem, M.A. Management of aphthous ulceration with topical quercetin: a randomized clinical trial. *J. Contemp. Dent. Pract.* 2010, 11(4):E009-16.

Hodgson, J.M.; Croft, K.D. Tea flavonoids and cardiovascular health. *Mol. Aspects Med.* 2010, 31: 495-502.

Hollman, P.C.; de Vries, J.H.; van Leeuwen, S.D.; Mengelers, M.J.; Katan, M.B. Absorption of dietary quercetin glycosides and quercetin in healthy ileostomy volunteers. *Am. J. Clin. Nutr.* 1995, 62: 1276-1282.

Hussain, T.; Gupta, S.; Adhami, V. M.; Mukhtar, H. Green tea constituent epigallocatechin-3-gallate selectively inhibits COX-2 without affecting COX-1 expression in human prostate carcinoma cells. *Int. J. Cancer* 2005, *113*: 660–669.

Ishizawa, K.; Yoshizumi, M.; Kawai, Y.; Terao, J.; Kihira, Y.; Ikeda, Y. et al. Pharmacology in health foods: Metabolism of quercetin in vivo and its protective effect against arteriosclerosis. *J. Pharmacol. Sci.* 2011, 115: 466–470.

Jemai H, Bouaziz M, Sayadi S. Phenolic composition, sugar contents and antioxidant activity of Tunisian sweet olive cultivar with regard to fruit ripening. *J. Agric. Food Chem.* 2009, 57*:* 2961–2968.

Jin, F.; Nieman, D.C.; Shanely, R.A.; Knab, A.M.; Austin, M.D.; Sha, W. The variable plasma quercetin *Eur. J. Clin. Nutr.* 2010, 64(7):692-7.

Kamaraj, S.; Vinodhkumar, R.; Anandakumar, P.; Jagan, S.; Ramakrishnan, G.; Devaki, T. The effects of quercetin on antioxidant stuatus and tumor markers in the lung and serum of mice treated with benzo(a)pyrene. *Biol. Pharm. Bull.* 2007, 30: 2268-2273.

Khan, N.Q.; Lees, D.M.; Douthwaite, J.A.; Carrier, M.J., Corder, R. Comparison of red wine extract and polyphenol constituents on endothelin-1 synthesis by cultured endothelial cells. *Clin. Sci.* 2002, 103 (Suppl. 48): 72S-75S.

Khatun, M.; Eguchi, S.; Yamaguchi, T.; Takamura, H.; Matoba, T. Effect of the thermal treatment on radical-scavenging activity of some spices. *Food Sci. Technol. Res.* 2006,*12*: 178–185.

Klaiber, R.G.; Baur, S.; Koblo, A.; Carle, R. Influence of washing treatment and storage atmosphere on phenylalanine ammonia-lyase activity and phenolic acid content of minimally processed carrot sticks. *J. Agric. Food Chem.* 2005, *53:* 1065–1072.

Kong, A.N.; Yu, R.; Chen, C.; Mandlekar, S.; Primiano, T. Signal transduction events elicited by natural products: Role of MAPK and caspase pathways in homeostatic response and induction of apoptosis. *Arch. Pharm. Res.* 2000, *23:* 1–16.

Kuhnau, J. The flavonoids. A class of semi-essential food components: Their role in human nutrition. *World Rev. Nutr. Diet* 1976, *24*: 117–191.

Landis-Piwowar, K.R.; Milacic, V.; Dou, Q.P. Relationship between the methylation status of dietary flavonoids and their growth-inhibitory and apoptosis-inducing activities in human cancer cells. *J. Cell Biochem.* 2008, *105:* 514–523.

Leifert, W.R.; Abeywardena, M.Y. Grape seed and red wine polyphenol extracts inhibit cellular cholesterol uptake, cell proliferation, and 5-lipoxygenase activity. *Nutr. Res.* 2008, *28*: 842–850.

Lesser, S.; Cermak, R.; Wolffram, S. Bioavailability of quercetin in pigs is influenced by the dietary fat content. *J. Nutr.* 2004,*134:* 1508–1511.

Loke, W.M.; Proudfoot, J.M.; Hodgson, J.M.; McKinley, A.J.; Hime, N.; Magat, M.; Stocker, R.; Croft, K.D. Specific dietary polyphenols attenuate atherosclerosis in apolipoprotein E-knockout mice by alleviating inflammation and endothelial dysfunction. *Arterioscler. Thromb. Vasc. Biol.* 2010, 30: 749–757.

Macheix, J.J.;Fleuriet, A.; Billot, J. *Fruit Phenolics*; CRC Press: Boca Raton, FL, USA, 1990; pp. 101–126.

Manach, C.; Scalbert, A.; Morand, C.; Remesy, C.; Jimenez, L. Polyphenols: Food sources and bioavailability. *Am. J. Clin. Nutr.* 2004, 79: 727–747.

Masella, R.; Di Benedetto, R.; Vari, R.; Filesi, C.; Giovannini, C. Novel mechanisms of natural antioxidant compounds in biological systems: Involvement of glutathione and glutathione-related enzymes. *J. Nutr. Biochem.* 2005, *16:* 577–586.

Masella, R.; Vari, R.; D'Archivio, M.; Di Benedetto, R.; Matarrese, P.; Malorni, W.; Scazzocchio, B.; Giovannini, C. Extra virgin olive oil biophenols inhibit cell-mediated oxidation of LDL by increasing the mRNA transcription of glutathione-related enzymes. *J. Nutr.* 2004, *134:* 785–791.

Mattagajasingh, I.; Kim, C.S.; Naqvi, A.; Yamamori, T.; Hoffman, T.A.; Jung, S.B.; DeRicco, J.; Kasuno, K.; Irani, K. SIRT1 promotes endothelium-dependent vascular relaxation by activating endothelial nitric oxide synthase. *Proc. Natl. Acad. Sci. USA.* 2007, 104: 14855–14860.

Miglio, C.; Chiavaro, E.; Visconti, A.; Fogliano, V.; Pellegrini, N. Effects of different cooking methods on nutritional and physicochemical characteristics of selected vegetables. *J. Agric. Food Chem.* 2008, *56:* 139–147.

Monasterio, A.; Urdaci, M.C.; Pinchuk, I.V.; Lopez-Moratalla, N.; Martinez-Irujo, J.J. Flavonoids induce apoptosis in human leukemia U937 cells through caspase- and caspase-calpain-dependent pathways. *Nutr. Cancer* 2004, *50:* 90–100.

Moon, J.H.; Nakata, R.; Oshima, S.; Inakuma, T.; Terao, J. Accumulation of quercetin conjugates in blood plasma after the short-term ingestion of onion by women. *Am. J. Physiol. Regul. Integr. Comp. Physiol.* 2000, 279: R461–R467.

Mullen, W.; Edwards, C.A.; Crozier, A. Absorption, excretion and metabolite profiling of methyl-, glucuronyl-, glucosyl- and sulpho-conjugates of quercetin in human plasma and urine after ingestion of onions. *Br. J. Nutr.* 2006, *96:* 107–116.

Mullen, W.; Stewart, A.J.; Lean, M.E.; Gardner, P.; Duthie, G.G.; Crozier, A. Effect of freezing and storage on the phenolics, ellagitannins, flavonoids, and antioxidant capacity of red raspberries. *J. Agric. Food Chem.* 2002, *50*: 5197–5201.

Murota, K.; Matsuda, N.; Kashino, Y.; Fujikura, Y.; Nakamura, T.; Kato, Y.; Shimizu, R.; Okuyama, S.; Tanaka, H.; Koda, T.; Sekido, K.; Terao, J. alpha-Oligoglucosylation of a sugar moiety enhances the bioavailability of quercetin glucosides in humans. *Arch. Biochem. Biophys.* 2010, 501(1):91-7.

Murphy, K.J.; Chronopoulos, A.K.; Singh, I.; Francis, M.A.; Moriarty, H.; Pike, M.J.; Turner, A.H.; Mann, N J.; Sinclair, A.J. Dietary flavanols and procyanidin oligomers from cocoa (Theobroma cacao) inhibit platelet function. *Am. J. Clin. Nutr* 2003, *77:* 1466–1473.

Mustafa, R.A.; Abdul Hamid, A.; Mohamed, S.; Abu Bakar, F. Total Phenolic Compounds, Flavonoids, and Radical Scavenging Activity of 21 Selected Tropical Plants. *J. Food Sci.* 2010, 75(1): C28-C35.

Naasani, I.; Oh-Hashi, F.; Oh-Hara, T.; Feng, W.Y.; Johnston, J.; Chan, K.; Tsuruo, T. Blocking telomerase by dietary polyphenols is a major mechanism for limiting the growth of human cancer cells *in vitro* and *in vivo*. *Cancer Res.* 2003, *63*, 824–830.

Napolitano, A.; Cascone, A.; Graziani, G.; Ferracane, R.; Scalfi, L.; Di Vaio, C.; Ritieni, A.; Fogliano, V. Influence of variety and storage on the polyphenol composition of apple flesh. *J. Agric. Food Chem.* 2004, *52:* 6526–6531.

Nemeth, K.; Piskula, MK. Food content, processing, absorption and metabolism of onion flavonoids. *Crit. Rev. Food Sci. Nutr.* 2007, 47(4): 397-409.

Neuhouser, M.L. Dietary flavonoids and cancer risk: evidence from human population studies. *Nutr. Cancer* 2004, 50(1): 1-7.

Nieman, D.C.; Williams, A.S.; Shanely, R.A.; Jin, F.; McAnulty, S.R.; Triplett, N.T.; Austin, M.D.; Henson, D.A. Quercetin's influence on exercise performance and muscle mitochondrial biogenesis. Med. Sci. Sports Exerc. 2010, 42(2):338-45.

Noratto, G.; Porter, W.; Byrne, D.; Cisneros-Zevallos, L. Identifying peach and plum polyphenols with chemopreventive potential against estrogen-independent breast cancer cells. *J. Agric. Food Chem.* 2009, *57:* 5219–5126.

O'Leary, K.A.; de Pascual-Tereasa, S.; Needs, P.W.; Bao, Y.P.; O'Brien, N.M.; Williamson, G. Effect of flavonoids and vitamin E on cyclooxygenase-2 (COX-2) transcription. *Mutat. Res.* 2004 *551:* 245–254.

Ota, H., Eto, M., Ogawa, S., Iijima, K., Akishita, M., Ouchi, Y. SIRT1/eNOS axis as a potential target against vascular senescence, dysfunction and atherosclerosis. *J. Atheroscler. Thromb.* 2010, 17: 431–435.

Pandey, K.B.; Rizvi, S.I. Plant polyphenols as dietary antioxidants in human health and disease. *Ox. Med. Cell. Longev.* 2009, 2(5): 270-278.

Perez-Jimenez, J.; Serrano, J.; Tabernero, M.; Arranz, S.; Diaz-Rubio, M. E.; Garcia-Diz, L.; Goni, I.; Saura-Calixto, F. Bioavailability of phenolic antioxidants associated with dietary fiber: Plasma antioxidant capacity after acute and long-term intake in humans. *Plant Foods Hum. Nutr.* 2009, *64:* 102–107.

Pérez-Vizcaíno, F.; Duarte, J. Flavonols and cardiovascular disease. *Mol. Aspects Med.* 2010, 31: 478-494.

Pietsch, K.; Saul, N.; Menzel, R.; Sturzenbaum, S.R.; Steinberg, C.E. Quercetin mediated lifespan extension in Caenorhabditis elegans is modulated by age-1, daf-2, sek-1 and unc-43. *Biogerontology* 2009, 10: 565–578.

Piskula, M.K.; Terao, J. Accumulation of (−)-epicatechin metabolites in rat plasma after oral administration and distribution of conjugation enzymes in rat tissues. *J. Nutr.* 1998, *128:* 1172–1178.

Porrini, M.; Riso, P. Factors influencing the bioavailability of antioxidants in foods: A critical appraisal. *Nutr. Metab. Cardiovasc. Dis.* 2008,18: 647–650.

Porrini, M.; Riso, P.; Testolin, G. Absorption of lycopene from single or daily portions of raw and processed tomato. *Br. J. Nutr.* 1998, *80:* 353–361.

Prasain, J.K.; Carlson, S.H.; Wyss, J.M. Flavonoids and age-related disease: Risk, benefits and critical windows. *Maturitas* 2010, 66: 163-171.

Rabe, E.; Stücker, M.; Esperester, A.; Schäfer, E.; Ottillinger, B. Efficacy and tolerability of a red-vine-leaf extract in patients suffering from chronic venous insufficiency--results of a double-blind placebo-controlled study. *Eur. J. Vasc. Endovasc. Surg.* 2011,41(4):540-7.

Rao, S.S.; Lu, C.; Schulze-Delrieu, K. Duodenum as a immediate brake to gastric outflow: A videofluoroscopic and manometric assessment. *Gastroenterology* 1996, *110:* 740–747.

Rizvi, S.I., Mishra, M. Antioxidant effect of quercetin on type 2 diabetes erythrocytes. *J. Food Biochem.* 2009, 33: 404-415.

Rocha-Guzman, N.E.; Gonzlez-Laredo, R.F.; Ibarra-Prez, F.J.; Nava-Bermen, C.A.; Gallegos-Infante, J.A. Effect of pressure cooking on the antioxidant activity of extracts from three common bean (*Phaseolus vulgaris* L.) cultivars. *Food Chem.* 2007, *100:* 31–35.

Rodriguez-Vaquero, M.J.; Alberto, M.R.; Manca-de-Nadra, M.C. Antibacterial effect of phenolic compounds from different wines. *Food Control.* 2007, *18:* 93–101.

Romero, M.; Jimenez, R.; Hurtado, B.; Moreno, J.M.; Rodriguez-Gomez, I.; Lopez-Sepulveda, R.; Zarzuelo, A.; Perez-Vizcaino, F.; Tamargo, J.; Vargas, F.; Duarte, J. Lack of beneficial metabolic effects of quercetin in adult spontaneously hypertensive rats. *Eur. J. Pharmacol.* 2010, 627: 242–250.

Romier, B.; Schneider, Y.J.; Larondelle, Y.; During, A. Dietary polyphenols can modulate the intestinal inflammatory response. *Nutr. Rev.* 2009, *67*: 363–378.

Rosenblat, M.; Aviram, M. Paraoxonases role in the prevention of cardiovascular diseases. *Biofactors* 2009, *35:* 98–104.

Sadik, C.D.; Sies, H.; Schewe, T. Inhibition of 15-lipoxygenases by flavonoids: Structure-activity relations and mode of action. *Biochem. Pharmacol.* 2003, *65:* 773–781.

Sanoner, P.; Guyot, S.; Marnet, N.; Molle, D.; Drilleau, J.P. Polyphenol profiles of French cider apple varieties (*Malus domestica* sp.). *J. Agric. Food Chem.* 1999, 47: 4847–4853.

Scalbert, A.; Williamson, G. Dietary intake and bioavailability of polyphenols. *J. Nutr.* 2000,130: 2073S–85S.

Schewe, T.; Sadik, C.; Klotz, L.O.; Yoshimoto, T.; Kuhn, H.; Sies, H. Polyphenols of cocoa: Inhibition of mammalian 15-lipoxygenase. *Biol. Chem.* 2001, *382:* 1687–96.

Semenza, G. In *Mammalian Ectoenzymes*; Kenny, A.J., Turner, A.J., Eds; Elsevier: Amsterdam, Holand, 1987; pp. 256–287.

Slimestad, R.; Fossen, T.; Vågen, I.M. Onions: a source of unique dietary flavonoids. *J. Agric. Food Chem.* 2007, 55(25): 10067-10080.

Spencer, J.P.; Chowrimootoo, G.; Choudhury, R.; Debnam, E.S.; Srai, S.K.; Rice-Evans, C. The small intestine can both absorb and glucuronidate luminal flavonoids. *FEBS Lett.* 1999, *458*: 224–230.

Spencer, J.P.; Rice-Evans, C.; Williams, R.J. Modulation of pro-survival Akt/protein kinase B and ERK1/2 signaling cascades by quercetin and its *in vivo* metabolites underlie their action on neuronal viability. *J. Biol. Chem.* 2003, *278:* 34783–34793.

Srinivas, K.; King, J.W.; Howard, L.R.; Monrad, J.K. Solubility and solution thermodynamic properties of quercetin and quercetin dihydrate in subcritical water. *J. Food Eng.* 2010, 100: 208-218.

Tamura, M.; Nakagawa, H.; Tsushida, T.; Hirayama, K.; Itoh, K. Effect of pectin enhancement on plasma quercetin and fecal flora in rutin-supplemented mice. *J. Food. Sci.* 2007, *72:* S648–S651.

Tilgmann, C.; Ulmanen, I. Purification methods of mammalian catechol-O-methyltransferases. *J. Chromatogr. B: Biomed. Appl.* 1996, *684*, 147–161.

Tsuchiya, H. Structure-dependent membrane interaction of flavonoids associated with their bioactivity. *Food Chem.* 2010,120: 1089-1096.

Vallejo, F.; Tomas-Barberan, F.; Garcia-Viguera, C. Health-promoting compounds in broccoli as influenced by refrigerated transport and retail sale period. *J. Agric. Food Chem.* 2003, *51:* 3029–3034.

van der Sluis, A.A.; Dekker, M.; de Jager, A.; Jongen, W.M. Activity and concentration of polyphenolic antioxidants in apple: Effect of cultivar, harvest year, and storage conditions. *J. Agric. Food Chem.* 2001, *49:* 3606–3613.

Visioli, F.; Galli, C.; Grande, S.; Colonnelli, K.; Patelli, C.; Galli, G.; Caruso, D. Hydroxytyrosol excretion differs between rats and humans and depends on the vehicle of administration. *J. Nutr.* 2003, *133:* 2612–2615.

Waterhouse, A.L. Wine Phenolics. *Ann. N. Y. Acad. Sci.* 2002, 957: 21–36.

Way, T.D.; Kao, M.C.; Lin, J.K. Degradation of HER2/neu by apigenin induces apoptosis through cytochrome c release and caspase-3 activation in HER2/neu-overexpressing breast cancer cells. *FEBS Lett.* 2005, *579:* 145–52.

Wen, X.; Walle, T. Methylated flavonoids have greatly improved intestinal absorption and metabolic stability. *Drug Metab. Dispos.* 2006a, *34:* 1786–1792.

Wen, X.; Walle, T. Methylation protects dietary flavonoids from rapid hepatic metabolism. *Xenobiotica* 2006b,*36:* 387–397.

Wilkinson, A.P.; Gee, J.M.; Dupont, M.S.; Needs, P.W.; Mellon, F.A.; Williamson, G.; Johnson, I.T. Hydrolysis by lactase phlorizin hydrolase is the first step in the uptake of daidzein glucosides by rat small intestine *in vitro*. *Xenobiotica*, 2003, *33:* 255–264.

Williamson, G.; Manach, C. Bioavailability and bioefficacy of polyphenols in humans. II. Review of 93 intervention studies. *Am. J. Clin Nutr.* 2005, 81: 243S–255S.

Wiseman, S.; Mulder, T.; Rietveld, A. Tea flavonoids: Bioavailability *in vivo* and effects on cell signaling pathways *in vitro*. *Antioxid. Redox Signal.* 2001, *3:* 1009–1021.

Xu, B.; Chang, S.K. Total phenolic, phenolic acid, anthocyanin, flavan-3-ol, and flavonol profiles and antioxidant properties of pinto and Black Beans (*Phaseolus vulgaris L.*) as affected by thermal processing. *J. Agric. Food Chem.* 2009a, *57*: 4754–4764.

Xu, B.; Chang, S.K. Phytochemical profiles and health-promoting effects of cool-season food legumes as influenced by thermal processing. *J. Agric. Food Chem.* 2009b, *57:* 10718–10731.

Xu, X.; Li, W.; Lu, Z.; Beta, T.; Hydamaka, A.W. Phenolic content, composition, antioxidant activity, and their changes during domestic cooking of potatoes. *J. Agric. Food Chem.* 2009, *57:* 10231–10238.

Yoshizumi, M.; Tsuchiya, K.; Suzaki, Y.; Kirima, K.; Kyaw, M.; Moon, J.H.; Terao, J.; Tamaki, T. Quercetin glucuronide prevents VSMC hypertrophy by angiotensin II via the inhibition of JNK and AP-1 signaling pathway. *Biochem. Biophys. Res. Commun.* 2002, 293: 1458–1465.

Zafrilla, P.; Morillas, J.; Mulero, J.; Cayuela, J.M.; Martinez-Cacha, A.; Pardo, F.; Lopez Nicolas, J.M. Changes during storage in conventional and ecological wine: Phenolic content and antioxidant activity. *J. Agric. Food Chem.* 2003, *51:* 4694–4700.

Zhang, Y.; Song, T.T.; Cunnick, J.E.; Murphy, P.A.; Hendrich, S. Daidzein and genistein glucuronides *in vitro* are weakly estrogenic and activate human natural killer cells at nutritionally relevant concentrations. *J. Nutr.* 1999, *129:* 399–405.

Zhao, X.; Gu, Z.; Attele, A.S.; Yuan, C.S. Effects of quercetin on the release of endothelin, prostacyclin and tissue plasminogen activator from human endothelial cells in culture. *J. Ethnopharmacol.* 1999, 67: 279-285.

Zohrab'ian, R.O. Effect of antioxidants lipin and quercetin on indices of lipid peroxidation and antioxidant system in recipients of renal allotransplants. *Klin. Khir.* 2010, 7: 41-4.

In: Quercetin
Editors: Taiki Chikamatsu and Yuudai Hida
ISBN: 978-1 61942- 057-1

Chapter 2

OCCURRENCE IN FOOD, METABOLIC RATE AND HEALTH BENEFITS OF QUERCETIN

María Chávarri, Izaskun Marañón and María Carmen Villarán
Bioprocesses and Preservation Area, Biotechnology and Pharma Unit, TECNALIA R&I; Parque Tecnológico de Álava, Miñano, Alava, Spain

ABSTRACT

Quercetin, the most common member of the flavonoids family, is a group of chemical compounds that can be found in the plant kingdom. Fruits and vegetables - particularly citrus fruits, apples, onions, parsley, tea, and red wine - are the primary dietary sources of quercetin. The flavonol is present in plants in many different glycosidic forms, and the highest concentrations are found in onion where quercetin is bound to 1 or 2 glucose molecules (quercetin-3'-glucoside and quercetin-4'-glucoside). Other important sources of quercetin glycosides are apples (quercetin galactosides) and berries (quercetin arabinoses). In addition to the chemical form of the flavonol, the applied vehicule or the composition of the diet seems to have a substantial effect on quercetin bioavailability. In general, flavonoids have been described as health-promoting, disease-preventing dietary supplements, and have activity as cancer preventive agents. Specifically, quercetin, one of the most prominent dietary antioxidants, is combating the destructive "free radical" molecules that play a part in many diseases. Moreover, quercetin has healthful anti-inflammatory and anti-allergy effects, it can also improve the health of capillaries and it has shown to have anti-cancer effects.

1. INTRODUCTION

Flavonoids are polyphenolic compounds that occur ubiquitously in foods of plant origin. Flavonoids might have evolved to protect plants from oxidative damage from sunlight (ultraviolet rays). More than 6000 different flavonoids have been described widely distributed in plants, although a much smaller number is important from a dietary point of view, and they are categorized as flavonol, flavanol, flavanone, flavone, anthocyanidin and isoflavone. Each flavonoid has distinct properties, and these might help to understand the relationships between their colorful structures and biological activity. There are several studies concerning the production and accumulation of diverse flavonoids in angiosperms, as well as some investigations in cell-free systems in order to examine the major steps leading to various types of flavonoid subgroups by plant enzymes [1-4]. That is a very complex system and, in addition, the initial source of variation in enzyme functions might depend on random mutations that occurred in their genes and the chromosomal rearrangements for enzymes which produce diverse flavonoid pigments as their final functional phytochemicals. The functional variations might occur in different parts of the plant, generating different evolutionary paths [5]. In the 1990s, interest in these compounds truly commenced and has been growing ever since. Flavonoids, and specially quercetin derivatives, have received special attention as dietary constituents in the last years in relation with their possible role in preventing cardiovascular diseases and cancer as it will be explained throughout this chapter. And this health promoting action seems to be related to the antioxidant activity of flavonoids. Quercetin derivatives are a group of chemical compounds that can be found in the plant kingdom and they probably are the most common subgroup of the flavonoids family. Fruit and vegetables are the primary dietary sources of quercetin.

2. Chemistry and Biosynthesis

Flavonoids consist of two benzene rings linked by oxygen containing pyrene ring. Flavonoids containing a hydroxyl group in the 3-position of the pyrene ring are classified as 3-hydroxyflavonoids (flavonols, anthocyanidins, leucoanthocyanidins and catechins), and those lacking it as 3-desoxyflavonoids (flavanones and flavones).

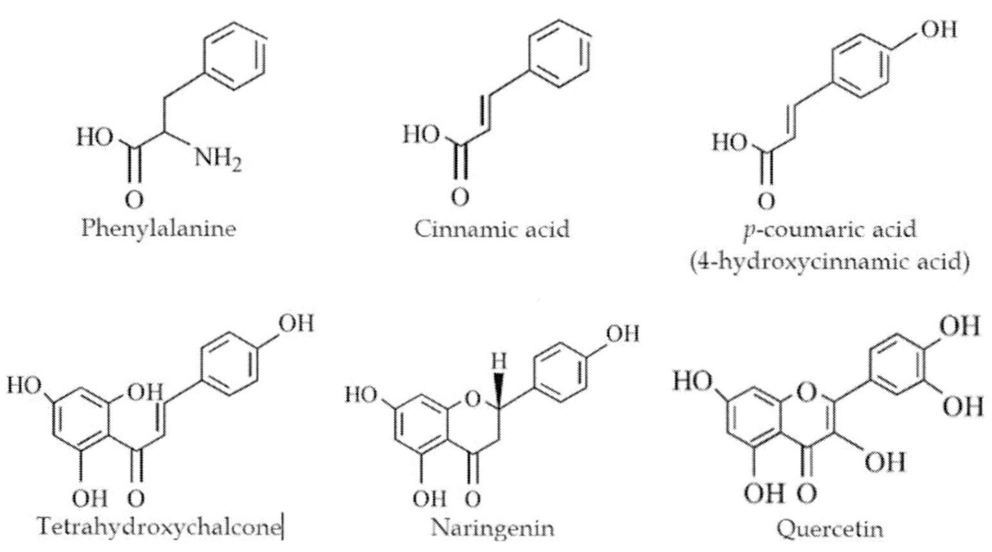

Figure 1. Chemical structure of some of the intermediates in the quercetin biosynthesis from phenylalanine precursor.

In 1975 Wagner and Farkas wrote a concise review on the known methods of flavonoid synthesis [6]. The major steps to the flavonoid skeleton are Fries rearrangement of a suitable substituted phenol acylated with a cinnamic acid, Alkali-catalyzed condesnation of an *ortho*-hydroxyacetophenone with a bezaldehyde derivative leading both to chalcones and flavanones. From an analogous condesnation of an *ortho*-hydroxyacetophenone with a benzoic acid derivative results in dibenzoyl methanes, 2-hydroxyflavanones and flavones. Motohashi and Sakagami wrote in 2009 a more detailed review of several studies related with the many enzymes involved in the secondary metabolism of plants and responsible of the different pathway to flavonoids [7].

The elimination of amino group from the phenylalanine to produce cinnamic acid by the phenylalanine ammonia-lyase (PAL), starts a complex process of enzymatic reactions via *p*-coumaric acid and chalcone (the most common intermediate is a tetrahydrochalcone) to obtain different flavanones, as naringenin, that flavonol synthase (FLS) transforms in flavonols as quercetin (Figure 1). The flavonol glycosides are subsequently synthesized by the flavonoid glucosyl transferase (FGT).

Quercetin or 3,3',4',5,7-pentahydroxylflavone, belongs to the flavonol group and this is the most common flavonol in diet. This compound occurs in plants mainly in leaves and in the outer parts of the plants as glycosides, in which one or more sugar groups is bound to phenolic groups by glycosidic bond, and aglycones (the forms lacking sugar moieties) which occurs less frequently.

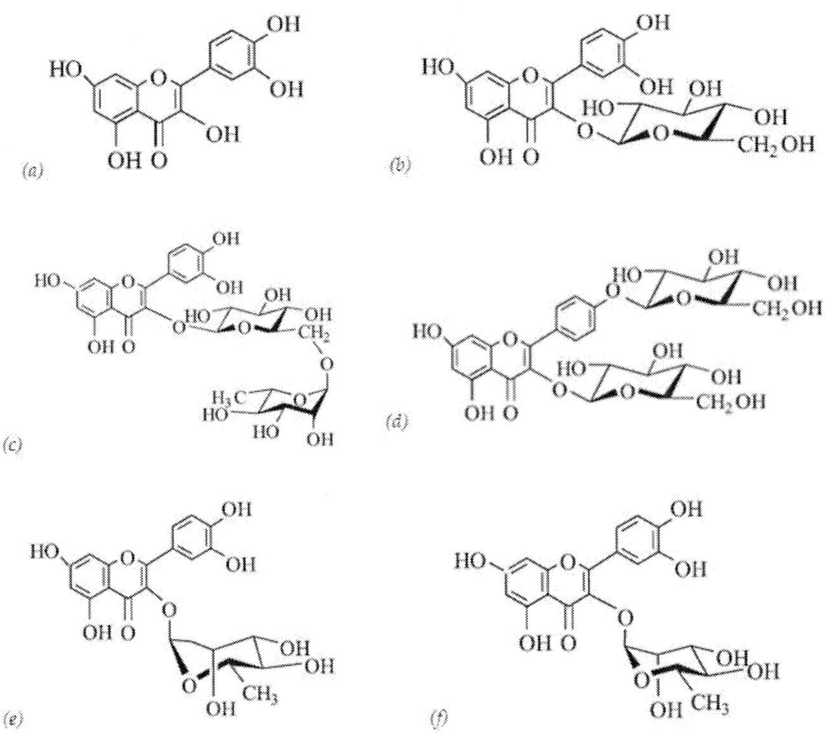

Figure 2. Some representative structures of quercetin subgroup: quercetin (a), quercetin-3-*O*-glucoside (b), rutin (c), quercetin 3,4'-*O*-β-diglucoside (d), quercetin-3-L-rhamnoside (e), and quercetin-3-*O*-rhamnoside (f).

Glucose is the most common sugar bounded to quercetin, but also galactose and rhamnose are frequently found bounded to flavonoids. In general, the preferred position for the sugar group in quercetin glycosides is at the 3-position, but the highest concentrations are found in onion where quercetin is bound to 1 or 2 glucose molecules in 4'-position or 3- and 4'- position.

3. Occurrence in Food

The principal dietary sources of flavonols from plants are apples, beans, blueberries, buckwheat, cranberries, endive, leeks, lettuce, onions, olive, pepper, and tomatoes. Quercetin is preferably founded in onions, apples, citrus fruits, broccoli, parsley, tea and red wine, but it is also present in olive oil, grapes, leek, dark berries and dark cherries.

Almost 180 different glycosides of quercetin have been described in nature, with quercetin-3-rutinoside, also called quercetin-3-rhamnoglucoside or rutin, being one of the most widespread forms (Figure 2). In onion, however, phenolic group at the 4'-position is necessarily bound by a sugar group and thus its major glycosides are quercetin-4'-O-β-glucoside and quercetin-3,4'-O-β-diglucoside (Figure 2). In fact, from the most of 20 detectable flavonols in onion species, these two quercetin conjugates are the main flavonols, which make up to 80–85% of the total flavonoid content [8-10].

Other important source of quercetin glycosides are apples, preferably as quercetin galactosides. Some of the most well studied antioxidant compounds in apples include from the quercetin subgroup quercetin-3-galactoside, quercetin-3-glucoside and rutin, showed in the Figure 2 [11]. The total extractable phenolic content has been investigated and ranges from 110 to 357 mg 100 g^{-1} of fresh apple [12]. It is also known that the concentration of total phenolic compounds is much greater in the peel of apples than in the flesh [13]. Wolfe *et al.* [14] have studied the antioxidant activity of peeled and unpeeled apples, concluding that the activities of unpeeled apples were greater than those of peeled apples. Vitamin C was responsible for less than 0.4% of the antioxidant activity, indicating that other factors, such as phenolics, were the main contributors. [14].

Tea is probably the most important flavanol source in many countries. It combines a high level of consumption with a relatively high flavanol content. Furthermore, it is the only plant food for human consumption found so far which contains (–)-epigallocatechin gallate (EGCG). However, quercetin level in black tea, for example, is around 15 mg kg-1 fresh weight [15-16] and also low for the green tea [17].

The *citrus fruit* peel and seeds are very rich in phenolic compounds, such as phenolic acids and flavonoids. The peels are richer in flavonoids than are the seeds, but these products are not used so it is necessary to study these byproducts as natural antioxidants ingredients to be used in foods formulations. The 7-*O*-glycosylflavanones are the most abundant flavonoids in all citrus fruits (hesperetin or naringenin, for example), more than flavonols as quercetin [18]. Naringin, hesperidin, and neohesperidin are also the main flavonoid markers of citrus juice, as well as quercetin [19].

Table 1. Total phenolics, flavonoids and anthocyanins content of berries

Berries/genus and species	Phenolics mg g^{-1} fresh weight	Flavonoids mg g^{-1} fresh weight	Anthocyanins mg g^{-1} fresh weight
Bilberry (*Vaccinium myrtillus*)	525	44	300
Blackberry (*Rubus fructicosus*)	486	276	83-326
Blueberry (*Vaccinium corymbosum*)	261-585	50	25-495
Cranberry (*Vaccinium macrocarpon*)	315	157	67–140
Lingonberry (*Vaccinium vitis-idea*)	652	74	77
Raspberry (*Rubus ideaous*)	121	6.0	99
Redcurrant (*Ribes rugrum*)	1400	9.0	22
Strawberry (*Fragaria x. ananassa*)	313	-	54

The phenolic compounds in *wine* are responsible of the taste, color and mouthfeel of wine. Red wine is richer in phenols abundant in the skin and seeds, such as anthocyanin, proanthocyanidins and flavonols, whereas the phenols in white wine will essentially originate from the pulp, and these will be the phenolic acids together with lower amounts of catechins and stilbenes.

Red wines will also have the phenols found in white wines. Quercetin is a yellow pigment in wines and, like other flavonoids, his concentration in grape berries increases as they are exposed to sunlight. However, quercetin is a flavonol present in a very low concentration in wine and, in the most of cases in a not detectable level using the usual analytical tools as Liquid Chromatography [20]. According to the studies from the Università degli Studi di Parma, the quercetin remaining in the winemaking byproducts is significant enough even to study his exploitation as a potential source of this health-promoting phenolic compound [21].

The predominant flavonoid in broccoli is kaempferol followed by quercetin. Taking as reference the work published by Koh *et al.* in 2009 [22], the level of quercetin in commercial broccoli samples ranged from 0.03 to 13.70 mg 100 g^{-1} of fresh weight, and the total phenolic activity ranged from 48.15 to 157.77 mg 100 g^{-1} fresh weight. Similarly to other vegetal products, these variations in the levels of flavonoids can be attributed to numerous factors including: genotype, agronomic environment, developmental stage at harvest and post-harvest handling conditions [22].

Phenolic compounds are the major group of phytochemicals in *berry fruits* including flavonoids (anthocyanins, flavonols, flavones, flavanols, flavanones, and isoflavonoids), stilbenes, tannins, and phenolic acids. Many phenolic compounds of berries are responsable for the color (i.e. anthocyanins) and flavor (i.e. tannins), but several factors as species, variety, geographic region, storage conditions, ripeness, climate and others play an important role in the concentration of berries specific phenolic compounds. Redcurrant, blackberry, and bilberry show remarkable high contents of phenolics, flavonoids, and anthocyanins, as it is showed in the Table 1 [23].

4. QUERCETIN CONSUMPTION

So the daily intake is closely related with an equilibrate diet including fruit and vegetables but only some specific products are relevant in order to achieve a considerable dose level. Quercetin levels in vegetables were generally below 10 mg kg^{-1}, except for onions (280-490 mg kg^{-1}), broccoli (30 mg kg^{-1}) and beans (45-60 mg kg^{-1}), so the differences between countries, and even regions, usually are too big to establish a accurate value. Moreover, it exist differences between the different varieties of a same product. And there is other important factor of influence: the concentration of flavonoids and their specific profile depends of the environmental conditions. The biosynthesis of flavonoids increase considerably due to a wide range of environmental stresses, mainly because of the UV radiation. In fact, seasonal variations impact greatly in the flavonol content, having the most significative differences in the leafy vegetables as lettuce (2-30 mg kg^{-1} quercetin), and the flavonol content could be three to five times higher in summer than other seasons [15].

Finally, the quercetin content in the dietary product will be different according to the conservation conditions after harvest and the cooking process selected for the food elaboration.

Although flavonoids have been reported to be generally stable under refrigerated conditions after harvest, as in the broccoli samples investigated by Vallejo *et al.* [26], Koh *et al.* demonstrated that the total flavonoid content decreased up to 59% during transportation as compared to broccoli at harvest [22].

The study or Rodrigues *et al.* about the cooking process of onion bulbs shows that moderate microwave cooking did not affect to the flavonol content, but intense microwave treatment cause flavonol losses of 16% and 18% for quercetin 3,4'-diglucoside and quercetin 4'-glucoside, respectively. Boiling onions for 30 min leaded losses of quercetin glycosides, which leached to the boiling water without being degraded at 37% and 29% for quercetin 3,4'-diglucoside and quercetin 4'-glucoside, respectively [27].

Table 2. Main dietary quercetins and their possible sources in the diet

Flavonol	Source	Content (mg kg^{-1})	Reference
Quercetin-3,4V-glucoside	Onion	284-486	[24]
Quercetin-3-glucoside			
Quercetin-3-rhamnoside (Rutin)	Black tea	10-25	[16]
Quercetin-3-galactoside	Apple	21-72	[24]
Quercetin-3-rhamnoside			
Quercetin-3-arabinoside			
Quercetin-3-glucoside			
Quercetin-3-rhamnoglucoside	Black currant	44	[25]
Quercetin-3-rhamnoside			
Quercetin-3-galactoside			

5. Metabolic Fate of Quercetin

Important sites of flavonoid metabolism are the gastrointestinal lumen, cells of the intestinal wall, and the liver. The metabolism of flavonoids is a matter of interest because metabolism often affects the biological activity of a compound and its ability to enter cells.

5.1. Intestinal Absorption and Metabolism

In order to understand the physiological effects of quercetin, it is important to take into account their intestinal absorption and metabolism. Quercetin absorption from the intestine occurs by several different pathways. In general, flavonoid aglycones can be easily absorbed into the intestinal cells as their lipophilicity facilitates the passage across the mucosal phospholipid bilayer of cells. Lactase phlorizin hydrolase (LPH), which is expressed on the brush border membrane of the small intestinal epithelium, has a crucial role in the absorption of flavonoids bearing β-glycoside linkages. Day *et al.* [28] demonstrated that LPH was capable of hydrolyzing various flavonoid glycosides, such as quercetin-4′-glucoside, quercetin-3-glucoside, genistein-7-glucoside and daidzein-7-glucoside, to form aglycones.

On the other hand, flavonoid monoglucosides can be transported by sodium glucose transporter-1 (SGLT-1) [29] on the brush border membrane of the intestinal cells. Wolffram *et al.* [30] demonstrated that SGLT-1 was involved in the uptake of quercetin-3-glucoside in rat small intestinal cells. Most flavonoid glycosides entering the enterocytes are deglycosylated by β-glucosidases, namely, the broad-specificity cytosolic β-glucosidase [31]. The flavonoids appear to be subjected to glucuronidation, sulfation and methylation in the intestinal epithelial cells before entering circulation [32–34]. In either case, quercetin aglycone is immediately metabolized into its conjugated forms by the action of phase II enzymes including uridine-5′-diphosphate glucuronosyltransferase (UGT) and/or phenol sulfotransferase (PST). Methylation of the hydroxyl groups at the 3′- or 4′-positions in the conjugated form can also be achieved by catechol-*O*-methyl transferase (COMT) [35].

The flavonoid conjugates then access into hepatocytes where they are further methylated, glucuronidated or sulfated [36, 37]. These flavonoid conjugates are excreted into the urine and also into bile fluid, thereby returning to the intestinal lumen [38]. Once there, they may again be reabsorbed by the intestinal cells, mainly in the large intestine. The lymphatic system also contributes to the transport of quercetin metabolites around the body [39]. Irrespective of the pathway, no quercetin aglycone is present in the blood circulation. Day *et al.* [40] identified the major metabolites present in human plasma as follows; quercetin 3'-*O*-β-D-glucuronide (Q3'GA), quercetin 4'-*O*-β-D-glucuronide (Q4'GA), quercetin 3-*O*-β-D-glucuronide (Q3GA), 3'-*O*-methyl quercetin 4'-*O*-β-D-glucuronide, 3'-*O*-methyl quercetin 3-*O*-β-D-glucuronide and quercetin 3'-*O*-sulfate. The maximum concentration of quercetin metabolites in human plasma was approximately 1.5 μM, reached within 2 h after the intake of onion (50 mg quercetin equivalent) and then decreasing gradually to an undetectable level [41]. Repeated ingestion of onion, however, resulted in the accumulation of quercetin metabolites, reaching a plasma concentration of 0.6 μM after a 1 week trial [42]. It is therefore likely that continuous intake is necessary to maintain the plasma concentration of quercetin metabolites at pharmacologically relevant levels.

Meanwhile, significant amounts of dietary flavonoids reach the large intestine, because the absorption rate of the flavonoids in the small intestine is typically low. The intestinal microbes have high levels of β-glucosidase and β-glucuronidase activity [43–45], and the glycosylated and/or conjugated flavonoids are quickly hydrolyzed to aglycones or methylated forms by the enzymatic activity in the large intestine. Matsukawa *et al.* [46] showed that only quercetin and monomethylated quercetin (isorhamnetin and tamarixetin) were detected in the cecal contents and feces of rats fed quercetin-3-glucoside.

In general, the metabolic conversion of quercetin reduces its free radical-scavenging activity and other physiological functions, compared with the activity of its aglycone. Some metabolites, however, still possess considerable activity, such as Q3GA (free radical-scavenging activity, suppression of cyclooxygenase-2 expression in lymphocytes), and Q3'GA and Q4'GA (inhibition of oxidative enzymes such as xanthine oxidase (XOD) and lipoxygenase (LOX)) [41]. Consequently, specific forms of the flavonoids are present in the small and large intestines and plasma, and each of them can produce distinct biological effects on the intestinal epithelial cells.

5.2. Bioavailability

The bioavailability and metabolism of flavonoids, especially quercetin and (+)-catechin, were investigated by several groups in the 1960s and 1970s [47, 48]. In most of these studies, rather high doses of flavonoids were given to laboratory animals and the main focus was on the bioavailability of flavonoid degradation products produced by the gastrointestinal microflora. Today, sensitive methods allowing serum and urine analyses are available for many flavonoids. These methods allow estimations of flavonoid bioavailability in human beings at appropriate dietary intake levels.

It is evident that the bioavailability of flavonoids varies greatly between different subgroups and compounds. This is hardly surprising, considering the differences in their chemical properties (i.e., polarity).

Specifically in quercetin, following single or repeat oral administration of 75–1000 mg quercetin (~300–4000 mg kg^{-1} body weight), total plasma quercetin concentrations (i.e., free and conjugated quercetin and its metabolites) between 12.2 and up to 100 nmol mL^{-1} were detected in Wistar and Lister rats [49, 50, 51, 52]. Although free quercetin was not detected in the plasma with single dosing (1 g kg^{-1} body weight), unconjugated quercetin was present at levels of 0.56 nmol mL^{-1} (0.17 μg mL^{-1}) in male Wistar rats following repeat-dose administration (10 days at 1 g kg^{-1} body weight) [51]. In another study, free quercetin was found in the plasma, albeit only at a concentration of 0.9 μmol L^{-1} (0.27 μg mL^{-1}), following single intragastric treatment of male Sprague–Dawley rats with 50 mg quercetin kg^{-1} body weight [53]. Conversely, in weanling rats administered quercetin in the diet at 0.45% for a period of 6 weeks (equivalent to doses of up to 58.5 mg day^{-1} during the last week of treatment), plasma samples did not contain any detectable levels of the aglycone [54].

Hollman *et al.* [55] compared the bioavailability of quercetin from major dietary sources in human subjects. Plasma levels of quercetin were measured after a single large dose of onions, which contain glucose conjugates of quercetin, apples, which contain both glucose- and non-glucose- quercetin glycosides, or pure quercetin-3-rutinoside, the major quercetin glycoside in tea. The areas under the plasma concentration ± time curves were measured and the relative bioavailability of quercetin could then be calculated. The relative bioavailability of quercetin from apples and of pure quercetin rutinoside was both 30% relative to onions. Although the dose of quercetin given with the onions was lower (225 μmol vs 325 μmol), peak plasma levels were higher (0.74 μM) for onions than for apples and for pure rutinoside (both 0.30 μM). Peak levels were achieved less than 0.7 hr after ingestion of onions, 2.5 hr after apples and 9 hr after the rutinoside. Half-lives of elimination were similar (24 hr) for onions and apples. These data show that quercetin glucosides from onions are absorbed rapidly; the rutinoside is absorbed slowly, whereas the overall absorption rate of various glycosides from apples is intermediate. Thus, the sugar moiety of quercetin glycosides is an important determinant of their absorption and bioavailability.

The effect of sugar moiety on the absorption of quercetin was confirmed when pure quercetin glucoside (300 μmoles) or pure quercetin rutinoside (300 μmoles) was administered to healthy human volunteers [56]. The peak concentration of quercetin (C_{max}) in plasma (3 μM) was 20 times higher and reached (T_{max}) more than ten times faster after intake of the glucoside than after the rutinoside. The bioavailability of the rutinoside was only 20% of that of the glucoside. These pharmacokinetic data suggest that quercetin glucoside was absorbed from the small intestine, whereas quercetin rutinoside was absorbed from the colon after deglycosylation.

Conjugation with glucose enhances absorption from the small gut. Because of the long half-lives of elimination, repeated consumption of quercetin-containing foods will cause accumulation of quercetin in blood and increase the antioxidant capacity of blood plasma [57].

In earlier human trials the unconjugated quercetin aglycone was not identified in plasma samples following oral administration of the flavonol [58, 59, 60, 61], more recent trials utilizing improved detection methods have demonstrated trace quantities of the aglycone in the plasma of one subject ingesting fried onions [62] and mean plasma levels of up to 8 ng mL^{-1} in another study in which participants were provided 500 mg quercetin three times daily for a period of 5 days (120–350 ng mL^{-1} of total quercetin) [63]. Following single-dose administration of 10 mg quercetin per 70 kg of body weight dissolved in different beverages (i.e., vegetable juice, white wine, or grape juice), mean plasma aglycone levels of up to 25 ng mL^{-1} were identified, with the highest plasma levels observed when quercetin was provided in wine [64]. Also, the food matrix in which quercetin is administered appears to play a significant role in the bioavailability of the free aglycone following ingestion [64].

While both animal and human studies have demonstrated that following oral consumption of quercetin as much as 60% of the dose is absorbed (as total quercetin), extensive metabolism as a result of the first-pass effect ensures that the free unconjugated quercetin aglycone circulates in plasma at extremely low concentrations.

However, it is necessary to take into account that there are many factors that influence the extent and rate of absorption of phenols: (*i*) their uptake and interactions in the small intestine including conjugation, (*ii*) the potential for metabolism by the bacterial microflora of the colon and subsequent absorption of the resulting metabolites, and (*iii*) biliary excretion after hepatic biotransformation and/or conjugation [65]. Absorption of phenols, via the small intestine, is influenced by physiochemical factors such as molecular size, lipophilicity, solubility, pK_a, and biological factors including gastric and intestinal transit time, lumen pH, membrane permeability and biliary excretion after first pass metabolism [66, 67]. In the case of quercetin, there are a limited number of studies concerning the effect of food components on its intestinal absorption despite the importance for judging the bioavailability. Piskula and Terao [68] found that quercetin´s solubility in vehicles for administration to rats greatly affected the efficiency of quercetin absorption. Thus, the solubility of quercetin in bulk foods may be a key factor for the bioavailability, because quercetin aglycone is not freely soluble in water. Azuma *et al.* [69] indicated that a combination of lipids (phosphatidylcholine and soybean oil) and emulsifiers (sucrose fatty ester) can elevate the absorption of quercetin aglycone in rat plasma. De Vries *et al.* [70] recently demonstrated that wine is not superior to onion or black tea as a dietary source of quercetin. Addition of milk does not affect the quercetin absorption from black tea in human [71]. All dietary factors affecting the quercetin absorption should be clarified because modulation of quercetin bioavailability is likely to be critical for evaluating its physiological function.

On the other hand, to circumvent the bacterial degradation in the colon, the absorption of quercetin from regular foods was studied in ileostomy subjects, who lack a colon with the bacterial flora [72]. Absorption of the quercetin glucosides from onions (52%) was far better than that of the pure aglycone (24%) while absorption of pure rutin (quercetin-3-β-*O*-rhamnosylglucoside), a major glycoside in tea, was 17%. Thus, some glycosides can be absorbed in man without prior hydrolysis by microorganisms.

5.3. Distribution

Several authors reported on the distribution of quercetin following oral administration to determine possible target organs of the antioxidant activity of quercetin. Although acute treatment of Wistar rats with quercetin resulted in equal distribution of systemically-absorbed quercetin across all major tissues [73], in rats fed quercetin in the diet for a period of 11 weeks, quercetin was observed to concentrate in several organs (i.e., lung, testes, kidney, thymus, heart, liver), with the highest concentrations of quercetin and its methylated derivatives, particularly isorhamnetin, detected in the pulmonary tissue [74]. Quercetin was primarily identified in its conjugated form in the tissue samples; however, free quercetin was extracted from some organs (i.e., lungs, liver, kidney, and testes) at concentrations up to 40% of total extracted quercetin.

5.4. Excretion

Systemically-absorbed quercetin may be eliminated in the urine [75, 76, 77, 78, 79, 51, 80, 81] or alternatively, may be secreted into the bile and excreted in the feces [77]. Also quercetin can undergo microbial degradation in the colon to phenolic acids and CO_2, which is exhaled in the breath [77, 82, 73]. Unabsorbed quercetin and the phenolic acid microfloral degradation products are eliminated in the feces [75, 77, 51].

The urinary excretion of quercetin has been investigated in several studies. Aziz *et al.* [83] studied human plasma and urinary contents of the flavonols quercetin and isorhamnetin after ingestion of onions by five subjects. Peak plasma concentrations for quercetin and quercetin and isorhamnetin glucosides occurred at 1.5–2 hr after ingestion. Over 24 hr, urinary excretion of isorhamnetin glucoside (a minor onion flavonol) was 17%, but the urinary excretion of quercetin and quercetin glucoside, the major onion flavonols, was < 1% of ingested dose. Thus, for these flavonols, the glucoside form seems to be absorbed intact, but quercetin is absorbed to a very limited extent. In rats fed a diet containing 0.25% quercetin, the concentrations of quercetin and methylated metabolites were approximately 3-fold in bile compared with urine. The high molecular weight of quercetin glucuronides and sulfates and their extensive binding to protein [84-86] could favor their biliary excretion [87].

6. Health Benefits

In 1936 Szent-Györgyi observed that a mixture of two flavonoles decreased capillary permeability and fragility in humans and proposed the name vitamin P [88]. However, the term vitamin P was abandoned because these flavonoids ultimately did not meet the definition of a vitamin. A multitude of in vitro studies has shown that flavonoids can inhibit, and sometimes induce, a large variety of mammalian enzyme systems. The effects of mainly flavones and flavonoids on 24 different enzymes or enzyme systems were described previously [89]. Some of these enzymes are involved in important pathways that regulate cell division and proliferation, platelet aggregation, detoxification, and inflammatory and immune response. Thus it is not surprising that effects of flavonoids have been found in cell systems and animals, on different stages in the cancer process, on the immune system, and on hemostasis [89].

Worries about the mutagenicity of flavonoids in bacterial systems [90] triggered much research on flavonol quercetin. However, mutagenicity of flavoinoids in vivo in mammals was never found [91, 92]. Animal studies of the carcinogenicity of quercetin were also negative except in one case [89]. However, the anticarcinogenic and antiproliferative effects of quercetin and other flavonoids are becoming increasingly evident [93].

The protective effects of flavonoids in biological systems are ascribed to their capacity to transfer electrons free radicals, chelate metal catalysts [94], activate antioxidant enzymes [95], reduce α-tocopherol radicals [96], and inhibit oxidases [97]. Although this multidimensional effect is likely responsible for the consistent overall effectiveness of these compounds in diverse experimental systems, it poses difficulties in delineating structure-activity relationships. A number of structure-activity studies employ oxidases and/or transition metals as reactive oxygen species (ROS) generators, both of which confound the identification of relationships between chemical structure and free radical scavenging. Over the past fifteen years, a considerable number of *in vitro* studies have sought to arrive at a common hierarchy of flavonoids in terms of substitutions and antioxidant activity. These data enable a better understanding of the antioxidant and prooxidant effects of flavonoids, and offer reasonable predictions of the influence of structural modifications that ensue during metabolism.

6.1. Antioxidant

Antioxidants are compounds that protect cells against the damaging effects of reactive oxygen species, such as singlet oxygen, superoxide, peroxyl radicals, hydroxyl radicals and peroxynitrite. An imbalance between antioxidants and reactive oxygen species results in oxidative stress, leading to cellular damage. Oxidative stress has been linked to cancer, aging, atherosclerosis, ischemic injury, inflammation and neurodegenerative diseases (Parkinson's and Alzheimer's). Flavonoids may help provide protection against these diseases by contributing to the total antioxidant defence system of the human body.

The most well-known property of polyphenols is their antioxidant capacity [98-100]. Within the flavonoid family, quercetin is the most potent scavenger of ROS, including superoxide (O_2^-) [101, 102], and reactive nitrogen species (RNS) like nitric oxide (NO) [103, 104] and peroxynitrite ($ONOO^-$) [105, 106]. These antioxidative capacities of quercetin are attributed to the presence of two antioxidant pharmacophores within the molecule that have the optimal configuration for free radical scavenging, i.e. the catechol group in the B ring and the OH group at position 3 of the AC ring [107]. Moreover, because polyphenols are redox-sensitive compounds [108], depending on cell type, dose, and/or time of treatment, they can also act as pro-oxidants, enhancing reactive oxygen species production, especially H_2O_2, and, therefore, reducing cell growth [99].

6.2. Anti-Inflamatory Properties

Quercetin is known to possess strong anti-inflammatory capacities [109, 110]. Quercetin is showed anti-inflammatory action by its direct antioxidant action and inhibition of inflammatory mediators and enzymes, such as lipoxygenase (LPS). Specifically, quercetin inhibits LPS-induced TNFα production in macrophages [111] and LPS-induced IL8 production in lung cells (A549) [112]. Moreover, in glial cells it was even shown that quercetin can inhibit LPS-induced mRNA levels of two cytokines, i.e. TNFα and IL-1α [113].

A possible explanation for these anti-inflammatory effects of quercetin may be found in the interplay between oxidative stress and inflammation. Indeed, it has already been shown that quercetin can inhibit the production as well as the gene expression of TNFα via modulation of NF-κB in human peripheral blood mononuclear cells [114].

6.3. Anti-Cancer Properties

Quercetin and related flavonoids have attracted much attention as potential anti-carcinogens. Their cancer-preventive effects have been attributed to various mechanisms including their anti-oxidative activity, the inhibition of enzymes that activate carcinogens, the modification of signal transduction pathways, and interactions with receptors and other proteins [115–117].

The cancer-preventive activity of flavonoids has been attributed to, amongst others, the induction of important phase II enzymes [118], which play a central role in the defense system of cells, by detoxifying reactive genotoxic substances and by contributing significantly to the cellular protection against redox cycling and oxidative stress [119, 120].

The transcription of genes encoding detoxifying enzymes such as glutathione *S*-transferases and NAD(P)H:quinine oxidoreductase 1 (NQO1) [121] is shown to be regulated by the electrophile-responsive element (EpRE), an upstream enhancer element of certain phase II genes [122]. Quercetin is reported to be a strong inducer of EpRE-mediated gene transcription [123, 124, 118].

Several proteins have been identified as specific targets of quercetin. Signalling pathways targeted by quercetin include the MAPK pathways and the oncogenic AKT [125, 126, 127]. Specifically, MEK1 is an important downstream component of oncogenic RAS signalling and thus is potentially a good target for disrupting MAPK signalling. The development of pharmacological inhibitors of MEK1, such as PD184352, has shown that MEK1 possesses a unique binding pocket adjacent to its ATP-binding site [128], and computer modelling has indicated that quercetin [125] could dock with this allosteric pocket. In fact, quercetin showed a much stronger inhibitory effect against MEK1 kinase activity than the well-known MEK1 inhibitor, PD098059 [125]. Lee et al. [125], Raf and MEK may be direct molecular targets for the chemopreventive effects of quercetin, too.

Another signalling pathways target by quercetin is AKT pathway. Tumour-specific changes in metabolism were discovered by Warburg in the 1920s. These metabolic changes consist of increased glucose consumption, decreased oxidative phosphorylation and lactate production [129]. AKT and mTOR are key players in reprogramming metabolic pathways in cancer cells. AKT is also thought to be involved in pathways that control the availability of nutrients acting through AMPactivated protein kinase (AMPK), which controls glucose and lipid metabolism by sensing changes in nutrient and extracellular energy levels. This suggests that the AKT-mediated oncogenic pathway could be regulated by nutrients. PI3K is an upstream regulator of AKT–mTOR signalling and also interacts with quercetin [127]. Based on X-ray crystallography, quercetin [130] has been shown to directly bind and suppress PI3K activity.

Various cellular receptors have been reported to be involved in the cancer-preventive activities of quercetin. An aryl hydrocarbon receptor (AhR) is a candidate target receptor for the chemopreventive effects of flavonols and flavones. The AhR is a DNA-binding transcription factor which can be activated and/or inhibited by flavonoids. The AhR is a ligand-dependent transcription factor that can be activated by synthetic and naturally occurring chemicals. One of the authors and his colleagues demonstrated that flavonols, such as quercetin and kaempferol, antagonised TCDD-induced AhR transformation in a cell-free system, using rat liver cytosol [131]. Quercetin was also found to suppress AhR transformation in primary cultured rat hepatocytes, and the suppressive effect of quercetin was stronger than that of a-naphthoflavone, a known antagonist of the AhR. The results of Fukuda *et al.* [132] indicate that quercetin is a potent antagonist for the AhR and might therefore exert preventive effects on the AhR-dependent carcinogenicity evoked by exposure to Polycyclic aromatic hydrocarbons.

Numerous *in vivo* studies on the chemopreventive and anti-genotoxic effects of quercetin have been published. For instance, one study published in "Carcinogenesis" in 1991 found that quercetin reduced the incidence of colonic neoplasia in rodent models of mutagen-induced colon cancer [133]. There is also abundant evidence the colon could be one of the target sites for quercetin [134-145]. This may be due to the fact that quercetin is virtually unabsorbed in the form of aglycone, but is subjected to conjugation reactions such as glucuronidation and sulfation, [146] though some of the metabolites may retain anti-oxidant activity [147].

6.4. Cardiovascular Health

Large numbers of studies have been conducted so far, showing the contributive role of quercetin to prevent cardiovascular diseases [148-152]. Epidemiological data have clearly shown a negative relationship between consumption of plant-based foods, such as fruits, vegetables and legumes and cardiovascular diseases risk [153-156]. It has been hypothesized that bioactive components with antioxidant capacities present in these foods may contributed to lower incidence of cardiovascular disease.

The effects of quercetin and related flavonoids modulating endothelial function and dysfunction have been widely studied [157]. Quercetin relaxes vascular smooth muscle [158] and its chronic daily treatment reduced blood pressure and endothelial dysfunction in experimental models of hypertension, characterized by an activation of the renin–angiotensin system, such as in spontaneously hypertensive rats (SHRs) [159-161], in rats made hypertensive by chronic inhibition of nitric oxide (NO) synthase [162] or in renovascular hypertensive rats [163]. Interestingly, quercetin and its methylated metabolites are more potent in coronary arteries [164] and in resistance than in conductance vessels [165] and also in vessels from hypertensive animals [166]. Furthermore, it has been recently found that quercetin prevents endothelial dysfunction, O_2^- production, and overexpression of cytosolic $p47^{phox}$ induced by angiotensin II in rat aorta [167]. Moreover, chronic quercetin also reduces blood pressure and improves endothelial function in deoxicorticosterone acetate-salt rats, a low renin model of hypertension in which Endothelin-1 (ET-1) plays a predominant role. The effects of quercetin were associated with a reduction in systemic and vascular oxidative stress and restoration of aortic Cu/Zn Superoxide dismutase expression [168, 169]. Since the sustained O_2^- production by angiotensin II could be an effect derived from the increased ET-1 synthesis [170] it is possible that inhibition in angiotensin II-mediated O_2^- production induced by both quercetin and isorhamnetin [167] are a result of decreased ET-synthesis and/or interference with ET-1 signaling pathways. In fact, quercetin decreased ET-1 synthesis in cultured bovine aortic endothelial cells [171] and vascular smooth muscle cells [172]. To summarize, there is solid evidence that, in vitro, quercetin and related flavonols exert: (1) endothelium-independent vasodilator effects, (2) protective effect on nitric oxide and endothelial function under conditions of oxidative stress, (3) platelet antiaggregant effects, (4) inhibition of LDL oxidation, (5) reduction of adhesion molecules and other inflammatory markers and (6) prevention of neuronal oxidative and inflammatory damage.

REFERENCES

[1] Martens, S., A. Preuß, and U. Matern, Multifunctional flavonoid dioxygenases: Flavonol and anthocyanin biosynthesis in Arabidopsis thaliana L. *Phytochemistry,* 2010. 71(10): p. 1040-1049.

[2] Yang, B., et al., Flavonol glycosides in wild and cultivated berries of three major subspecies of Hippophaë rhamnoides and changes during harvesting period. *Food Chemistry,* 2009. 115(2): p. 657-664.

[3] Figueiredo-González, M., et al., Pattern recognition of three Vitis vinifera L. red grapes varieties based on anthocyanin and flavonol profiles, with correlations between their biosynthesis pathways. *Food Chemistry,* 2012. 130(1): p. 9-19.

[4] Graham, T.L., Flavonoid and flavonol glycoside metabolism in Arabidopsis. Plant Physiology and Biochemistry. 36(1-2): p. 135-144.

[5] Rice-Evans, C.A. and L. Packer, *Flavonoids in Health and Disease. Antioxidants in Health and Disease,* ed. L. Packer and J. Fuchs. Vol. 7. 1998, New York: Marcel Dekker, Inc. 542.

[6] Wagner, H. and L. Farkas, *Synthesis of flavonoids, in The Flavonoids.* Part I, J.B. Harbone, T.J. Mabry, and H. Mabry, Editors. 1975, Academic Press: New York. p. 127-213.

[7] Motohashi, N. and H. Sakagami, Bioactive Heterocycles VII. Flavonoids and Anthocyanins in Plants, and Latest Bioactive Heterocycles II, in *Topics in Heterocyclic Chemistry, N. Motohashi,* Editor. 2009, Springer: Verlag Berlin Heidelberg. p. 19-23.

[8] Price, K.R., J.R. Bacon, and M.J.C. Rhodes, Effect of Storage and Domestic Processing on the Content and Composition of Flavonol Glucosides in Onion (Allium cepa). *Journal of Agricultural and Food Chemistry,* 1997. 45(3): p. 938-942.

[9] Beesk, N., et al., Distribution of quercetin-3,4'-O-diglucoside, quercetin-4'-O-monoglucoside, and quercetin in different parts of the onion bulb (Allium cepa L.) influenced by genotype. *Food Chemistry,* 2010. 122(3): p. 566-571.

[10] Bonaccorsi, P., et al., Flavonol Glucoside Profile of Southern Italian Red Onion (Allium cepa L.). *Journal of Agricultural and Food Chemistry,* 2005. 53(7): p. 2733-2740.

[11] Boyer, J. and R. Liu, Apple phytochemicals and their health benefits. *Nutrition Journal,* 2004. 3(1): p. 1-15.

[12] Podsędek, A., et al., Compositional characterisation of some apple varieties. *European Food Research and Technology,* 2000. 210(4): p. 268-272.

[13] Burda, S., W. Oleszek, and C.Y. Lee, Phenolic compounds and their changes in apples during maturation and cold storage. *Journal of Agricultural and Food Chemistry*, 1990. 38(4): p. 945-948.

[14] Wolfe, K., X. Wu, and R.H. Liu, Antioxidant Activity of Apple Peels. *Journal of Agricultural and Food Chemistry,* 2003. 51(3): p. 609-614.

[15] Hollman, P.C.H. and I.C.W. Arts, Flavonols, flavones and flavanols – nature, occurrence and dietary burden. *Journal of the Science of Food and Agriculture,* 2000. 80(7): p. 1081-1093.

[16] Hertog, M.G.L., P.C.H. Hollman, and B. van de Putte, Content of potentially anticarcinogenic flavonoids of tea infusions, wines, and fruit juices. *Journal of Agricultural and Food Chemistry,* 1993. 41(8): p. 1242-1246.

[17] Perva-Uzunalic, A., et al., Extraction of active ingredients from green tea (Camellia sinensis): Extraction efficiency of major catechins and caffeine. *Food Chemistry,* 2006. 96(4): p. 597-605.

[18] Yusof, S., H.M. Ghazali, and G.S. King, Naringin content in local citrus fruits. *Food Chemistry,* 1990. 37(2): p. 113-121.

[19] Belajová, E. and M. Suhaj, Determination of phenolic constituents in citrus juices: Method of high performance liquid chromatography. *Food Chemistry,* 2004. 86(3): p. 339-343.

[20] López, M., et al., Analysis of phenolic constituents of biological interest in red wines by high-performance liquid chromatography. *Journal of Chromatography A*, 2001. 922(1-2): p. 359-363.

[21] Careri, M., et al., Direct HPLC Analysis of Quercetin and trans-Resveratrol in Red Wine, Grape, and Winemaking Byproducts. *Journal of Agricultural and Food Chemistry,* 2003. 51(18): p. 5226-5231.

[22] Koh, E., et al., Content of ascorbic acid, quercetin, kaempferol and total phenolics in commercial broccoli. *Journal of Food Composition and Analysis.* 22(7-8): p. 637-643.

[23] Paredes-López, O., et al., Berries: Improving Human Health and Healthy Aging, and Promoting Quality Life—A Review. *Plant Foods for Human Nutrition (Formerly Qualitas Plantarum),* 2010. 65(3): p. 299-308.

[24] Hertog, M.G.L., P.C.H. Hollman, and M.B. Katan, Content of potentially anticarcinogenic flavonoids of 28 vegetables and 9 fruits commonly consumed in the Netherlands. *Journal of Agricultural and Food Chemistry,* 1992. 40(12): p. 2379-2383.

[25] Vuorinen, H., K. Määtta, and R. Törrönen, Content of the flavonols myricetin, quercetin, and kaempferol in finnish berry wines. *Journal of Agricultural and Food Chemistry,* 2000. 48(7): p. 2675-2680.

[26] Vallejo, F., F. Tomás-Barberán, and C. García-Viguera, Health-Promoting Compounds in Broccoli as Influenced by Refrigerated Transport and Retail Sale Period. *Journal of Agricultural and Food Chemistry,* 2003. 51(10): p. 3029-3034.

[27] Rodrigues, A.S., et al., Effect of curing and cooking on flavonols and anthocyanins in traditional varieties of onion bulbs. *Food Research International,* 2009. 42(9): p. 1331-1336.

[28] Day A.J., Canada F.J., Diaz J.C., Kroon P.A., McLauchlan R., Faulds C.B., et al. Dietary flavonoid and isoflavone glycosides are hydrolysed by the lactase site of lactase phlorizin hydrolase. *FEBS Lett.,* 2000. 468: p. 166–70.

[29] Walgren R.A., Lin J.T., Kinne R.K. and Walle T. Cellular uptake of dietary flavonoid quercetin 4′-beta-glucoside by sodium-dependent glucose transporter SGLT1. *J. Pharmacol. Exp. Ther.,* 2000. 294: p. 837–43.

[30] Wolffram S., Block M. and Ader P. Quercetin-3-glucoside is transported by the glucose carrier SGLT1 across the brush border membrane of rat small intestine. *J. Nutr.,* 2002. 132: p. 630–5.

[31] Nemeth K., Plumb G.W., Berrin J.G., Juge N., Jacob R., Naim H.Y., et al. Deglycosylation by small intestinal epithelial cell beta-glucosidases is a critical step in the absorption and metabolism of dietary flavonoid glycosides in humans. *Eur. J. Nutr.,* 2003. 42: p. 29–42.

[32] Crespy V., Morand C., Manach C., Besson C., Demigne C. and Remesy C.. Part of quercetin absorbed in the small intestine is conjugated and further secreted in the intestinal lumen. *Am. J. Physiol.,* 1999. 277: p. G120–6.

[33] Piskula M.K. and Terao J. Accumulation of (−)-epicatechin metabolites in rat plasma after oral administration and distribution of conjugation enzymes in rat tissues. *J. Nutr.,* 1998. 128: p. 72–8.

[34] Radominska-Pandya A., Little J.M., Pandya J.T., Tephly T.R., King C.D., Barone G.W., et al. UDP-Glucuronosyltransferases in human intestinal mucosa. *Biochim. Biophys. Acta.*, 1998. 1394: p. 199–208.

[35] Murakami A., Ashida H. and Terao J. Multitargeted cancer prevention by quercetin. *Cancer Lett.,* 2008. 269(2): p. 315-25.

[36] Donovan J.L., Crespy V., Manach C., Morand C., Besson C., Scalbert A, et al. Catechin is metabolized by both the small intestine and liver of rats. *J. Nutr.,* 2001. 131: p. 1753–7.

[37] O'Leary K.A., Day A.J., Needs P.W., Mellon F.A., O'Brien N.M. and Williamson G. Metabolism of quercetin-7- and quercetin-3-glucuronides by an in vitro hepatic model: the role of human beta-glucuronidase, sulfotransferase, catechol-O-methyltransferase and multi-resistant protein 2 (MRP2) in flavonoid metabolism. *Biochem. Pharmacol.,* 2003. 65: p. 479–91.

[38] Matsukawa N., Matsumoto M. and Hara H. High biliary excretion levels of quercetin metabolites after administration of a quercetin glycoside in conscious bile duct cannulated rats. *Biosci. Biotechnol. Biochem.,* 2009. 73: p. 1863–5.

[39] Murota K. and Terao J. Quercetin appears in the lymph of unsaturated rats at its phase II metabolites after administered into the stomach. *FEBS Lett.,* 2005. 579 : p. 5343–5346.

[40] Day A.J., Mellon F.A., Barron D., Sarrazin G., Morgan M.R.A. and Williamson G. Human metabolism of dietary flavonoids; identification of plasma metabolites of quercetin. *Free Radic. Res.,* 2001. 212: p. 941–952.

[41] Williamson G., Baron D., Shimoi K. and Terao J. In vitro biological properties of flavonoid conjugates found in vivo. *Free Radic. Res.,* 2005. 39: p. 457–469.

[42] Moon J-H., Nakata R., Oshima S., Inakuma T. and Terao J. Accumulation of quercetin conjugates in blood plasma after the short-term ingestion of onion by women. *Am. J. Physiol. Regul. Integr. Comp. Physiol.,* 2000. 279: p. R461–R467.

[43] Bokkenheuser V.D. and Winter J. Hydrolysis of flavonoids by human intestinal bacteria. *Prog. Clin. Biol. Res.,* 1988. 280: p. 143–5.

[44] Kim D.H., Jung E.A., Sohng I.S., Han J.A., Kim T.H. and Han M.J. Intestinal bacterial metabolism of flavonoids and its relation to some biological activities. *Arch. Pharm. Res.,* 1998. 21: p. 17–23.

[45] Aura A.M., O'Leary K.A., Williamson G., Ojala M., Bailey M., Puupponen-Pimia R., et al. Quercetin derivatives are deconjugated and converted to hydroxyphenylacetic acids but not methylated by human fecal flora in vitro. *J. Agric. Food Chem.,* 2002. 50: p. 1725–30.

[46] Matsukawa N., Matsumoto M., Shinoki A., Hagio M., Inoue R. and Hara H. Nondigestible saccharides suppress the bacterial degradation of quercetin aglycone in the large intestine and enhance the bioavailability of quercetin glucoside in rats. *J. Agric. Food Chem.,* 2009. 57(20): p. 9462-8.

[47] Scheline R. CRC *handbook of mammalian metabolism of plant compounds.* Boca Raton (FL) 7 CRC Press; 1991.

[48] Griffiths L.A. and Barrow A. Metabolism of flavonoid compounds in germ-free rats. *Biochem. J.,* 1972. 130: p. 1161-2.

[49] Manach, C., Morand, C., Demigne, C., Texier, O., Regerat, F. and Remesy, C. Bioavailability of rutin and quercetin in rats. *FEBS Lett.,* 1997. 409: p. 12–16.

[50] Manach, C., Texier, O., Morand, C., Crespy, V., Régérat, F., Demigné, C. and Rémésy, C. Comparison of the bioavailability of quercetin and catechin in rats. *Free Radic. Biol.,* 1999. 27: p. 1259–1266.

[51] Nakamura, Y., Ishimitsu, S. and Tonogai, Y. Effects of quercetin and rutin on serum and hepatic lipid concentrations, fecal steroid excretion and serum antioxidant properties. *J. Health Sci.* (Tokyo), 2000. 46: p. 229–240.

[52] Carbonaro, M., Grant, G. Absorption of quercetin and rutin in rat small intestine. *Ann. Nutr. Metab.,* 2005. 49: p. 178–182.

[53] Justino, G.C., Santos, M.R., Cana´rio, S., Borges, C., Florencio, M.H. and Mira, L. Plasma quercetin metabolites: Structure-antioxidant activity relationships. *Arch. Biochem. Biophys.,* 2004. 432: p. 109–121.

[54] Graf, B.A., Ameho, C., Dolnikowski, G.G., Milbury, P.E., Chen, C.Y. and Blumberg, J.B. Rat gastrointestinal tissues metabolize quercetin. *J. Nutr.,* 2006. 136: p. 39–44.

[55] Hollman, P.C., Van Trijp, J.M., Mengelers, M.J., De Vries, J.H. and Katan, M.B. Bioavailability of the dietary antioxidant flavonol quercetin in man. *Cancer Lett.,* 1997. 114: p. 139–140.

[56] Hollman, P.C. and Katan, M.B. Health effects and bioavailability of dietary flavonols. *Free Radic. Res.,* 1999. 31 (Suppl.): p. S75–S80.

[57] Hollman, P.C. and Katan, M.B. Dietary Flavonoids: Intake, Health Effects and Bioavailability. *Food and Chemical Toxicology,* 1999. 37: p. 937-942.

[58] Manach, C., Morand, C., Crespy, V., Demigne, C., Texier, O., Regerat, F. and Remesy, C. Quercetin is recovered in human plasma as conjugated derivatives which retain antioxidant properties. *FEBS Lett.,* 1998. 426: p. 331–336.

[59] Erlund, I., Kosonen, T., Alfthan, G., Maenpaa, J., Perttunen, K., Kenraali, J., Parantainen, J. and Aro, A. Pharmacokinetics of quercetin from quercetin aglycone and rutin in healthy volunteers. *Eur. J. Clin. Pharmacol.,* 2000. 56: p. 545–553.

[60] Walle, T., Otake, Y., Walle, U.K. and Wilson, F.A. Quercetin glucosides are completely hydrolyzed in ileostomy patients before absorption. *J. Nutr.,* 2000. 130: p. 2658–2661.

[61] Graefe, E.U., Wittig, J., Mueller, S., Riethling, A.K., Uehleke, B., Drewelow, B., Pforteh, Jacobasch, G., Derendorf, H. and Veit, M. Pharmacokinetics and bioavailability of quercetin glycosides in humans. *J. Clin. Pharmacol.,* 2001. 41: p. 492–499.

[62] Mullen, W., Boitier, A., Stewart, A.J. and Crozier, A. Flavonoid metabolites in human plasma and urine after the consumption of red onions: Analysis by liquid chromatography with photodiode array and full scan tandem mass spectrometric detection. *J. Chromatogr.* A, 2004. 1058: p. 163–168.

[63] Wang, L. and Morris, M.E. Liquid chromatography-tandem mass spectroscopy assay for quercetin and conjugated quercetin metabolites in human plasma and urine. *J. Chromatogr.* B, 2005. 821: p. 194–201.

[64] Goldberg, D.M., Yan, J. and Soleas, G.J. Absorption of three winerelated polyphenols in three different matrices by healthy subjects. *Clin. Biochem.,* 2003. 36: p. 79–87.

[65] Lin, J.H., Chiba, M. and Baillie, T.A. Is the role of the small intestine in first-pass metabolism overemphasized? *Pharmacol. Rev.,* 1999.51 (2): p. 135–158.

[66] Higuchi, W.I., Ho, N.F., Park, J.Y. and Komiya, I. 1981. *Rate-limiting steps and factors in drug absorption.* In: Prescott, L.F., Nimno, W.S. (Eds.), Drug Absorption. ADIS Press, New York, pp. 35–60.

[67] Ho, N.F., Park, J.Y., Ni, P.F. and Higuchi, W.I. 1983. Advancing quantitative and mechanistic approaches in interfacing gastrointestinal drug absorption studies in animals and humans. In: *Animal Models for Oral Drug Delivery.* In Situ and in Vivo Approaches. 1983:27-106 Am. Pharmaceut. Assoc. Washington, D.C.

[68] Piskula, M. K. and Terao, J. Quercetin's solubility affects its accumulation in rat plasma after oral administration. *J. Agric. Food Chem.,* 1998. 46: p. 4313–4317.

[69] Azuma, K., Ippoushi, K., Ito, H., Higashio, H. and Terao, J. Combination of lipids and emulsifiers enhances the absorption of orally administered quercetin in rats. *J. Agric. Food Chem.,* 2002. 50: p. 1706–1712.

[70] de Vries J.H., Hollman P.C., van Amersfoort I., Olthof M.R., Katan M.B. Red wine is a poor source of bioavailable flavonols in men. *J. Nutr.,* 2001. 131: p. 745-8.

[71] Hollman P.C., Van Het Hof, K.H., Tijburg L.B. and Katan MB. Addition of milk does not affect the absorption of flavonols from tea in man. *Free Radic. Res.,* 2001. 34: p. 297-300.

[72] Hollman, P.C., de Vries, J.H., Leeuwen, S.D., Mengelers, M.J. and Katan, M.B. Absorption of dietary quercetin glycosides and quercetin in healthy ileostomy volunteers. *Am. J. Clin. Nutr.,* 1995. 62 (6): p. 1276–1282.

[73] Abrahamse, S.L., Kloots, W.J. and van Amelsvoort, J.M.M. Absorption, distribution, and secretion of epicatechin and quercetin in the rat. *Nutr. Res.,* 2005. 25: p. 305–317.

[74] de Boer, V.C., Dihal, A.A., van der Woude, H., Arts, I.C., Wolffram, S., Alink, G.M., Rietjens, I.M., Keijer, J. and Hollman, P.C. Tissue distribution of quercetin in rats and pigs. *J. Nutr.,* 2005. 135: p. 1718–1725.

[75] Gugler, R., Leschik, M., Dengler, H.J. Disposition of quercetin in man after single oral and intravenous doses. *Eur. J. Clin. Pharmacol.,* 1975. 9: p. 229–234.

[76] Onishi, M., Hatcher, J.F., Nunoya, T., Pamukcu, A.M. and Bryan, G.T. In vitro metabolism of quercetin by rat liver and kidney preparations. *Proc. Am. Assoc. Cancer Res. Annu. Meet.,* 1982. 23: p. 90 (Abstract no. 353).

[77] Ueno, I., Nakano, N. and Hirono, I. Metabolic fate of [14C] quercetina in the ACI rat. *Jpn. J. Exp. Med.,* 1983. 53: p. 41–50.

[78] de Vries, J.H., Hollman, P.C., Meyboom, S., Buysman, M.N., Zock, P.L., Van Staveren, W.A. and Katan, M.B. Plasma concentrations and urinary excretion of the antioxidant flavonols quercetin and kaempferol as biomarkers for dietary intake. *Am. J. Clin. Nutr.,* 1998. 68: p. 60–65.

[79] Young, J.F., Nielsen, S.E., Haraldsdottir, J., Daneshvar, B., Lauridsen, S.T., Knuthsen, P., Crozier, A., Sandstrom, B. and Dragsted, L.O. Effect of fruit juice intake on urinary quercetin excretion and biomarkers of antioxidative status. *Am. J. Clin. Nutr.,* 1999. 69: p. 87–94.

[80] Wang, F.M., Yao, T.W. and Zeng, S. Determination of quercetin and kaempferol in human urine after orally administrated tablet of Ginkgo biloba extract by HPLC. *J. Pharm. Biomed. Anal.,* 2003. 33: p. 317–321.

[81] Wang, F.M., Yao, T.W. and Zeng, S. Disposition of quercetin and kaempferol in human following an oral administration of Ginkgo biloba extract tablets. *Eur. J. Drug Metab. Pharmacokinet.,* 2003. 28: p. 173–177.

[82] Walle, T., Walle, U.K. and Halushka, P.V. Carbon dioxide is the major metabolite of quercetin in humans. *J. Nutr.,* 2001. 131: p. 2648–2652.

[83] Aziz, A. A., Edwards, C. A., Lean, M. E. J., and Crozier, A. Absorption and excretion of conjugated flavonols, including quercetin-40-O-ß-glucoside and isorhamnetin-40-O-ß-glucoside by human volunteers after the consumption of onions. *Free Radic. Res.,* 2000. 29: p. 257– 269.

[84] Spencer, C.M., Cai, Y., Martin, R., Gaffney, S.H., Goulding, P.N., Magnolato, P.N., et al. Polyphenol complexation—some thoughts and observations. *Phytochemistry,* 1988. 27: p. 2397- 409.

[85] Manach, C., Morand, C., Texier, O., Favier, M.L., Agullo, G., Demigne, C., et al. Quercetin metabolites in plasma of rats fed diets containing rutin or quercetin. *J. Nutr.,* 1995. 125: p. 1911- 22.

[86] Boulton, D.W., Walle, U.K. and Walle, T. Extensive binding of the bioflavonoid quercetin to human plasma proteins. *J. Pharm. Pharmacol,* 1998. 50: p. 243-9.

[87] Fleck, C. and Braunlich H. Factors determining the relationship between renal and hepatic excretion of xenobiotics. *Arzneimittelforschung,* 1990. 40: p. 942-6.

[88] Rusznyàk, S. and Szent-Györgyi A. Vitamin P: flavonols as vitamins. *Nature,* 1936. 138: p. 27.

[89] Middleton E. and Kandaswami, C. The impact of plant flavonoids on mammalian biology: implications for immunity, inflammation and cancer. In: Harborne JB, ed. *The Flavonoids: Advances in Research since 1986.* London: Chapman and Hall. 619-652.

[90] Sugimura, T., Nagao M., Matsushima T., et al. Mutagenicity of flavone derivatives. *Proc. Jpn. Acad.,* 1977. 53: p. 194-197.

[91] Aeschbacher H.U. and Meier H, Ruch E. Nonmutagenicity in vivo of the food flavonol quercetin. *Nutr. Cancer,* 1982. 4: p. 90-98.

[92] MacGregor J.T., Wehr C.M., Manners G.D., Jurd I., Minkler, J.L. and Carrano, A.V. In vivo exposure to plant flavonols. Influence of frequencies of micronuclei in mouse erythrocytes and sister-chromatid exchange in rabbit lymphocytes. *Mutat. Res.,* 1983. 124 (3-4): p. 255-270.

[93] Huang M.T. and Ferraro T. 1992. Phenolic compounds in food and cancer prevention. In: Huang MT, Ho C, Lee CY, eds. Phenolic compounds in Food and their Effects on Health II. *Antioxidants and Cancer Prevention.* Washington DC: American Chemical Society, 8-34.

[94] Ferrali, M., Signorini, C., Caciotti, B., Sugherini, L., Ciccoli, L., Giachetti, D. and Comporti, M. Protection against oxidative damage of erythrocyte membranes by the flavonoid quercetin and its relation to iron chelating activity. *FEBS Lett.,* 1997. 416: p. 123–129.

[95] Elliott, A.J., Scheiber, S.A., Thomas, C. and R.S. Pardini, Inhibition of glutathione reductase by flavonoids. *Biochem. Pharmacol.,* 1992. 44: p. 1603–1608.

[96] Hirano, R., Sasamoto, W., Matsumoto, A., Itakura, H., Igarashi, O., and Kondo, K. Antioxidant ability of various flavonoids against DPPH radicals and LDL oxidation. *J. Nutr. Sci. Vitaminol.* (Tokyo), 2001. 47: p. 357–362.

[97] Cos, P., Ying, L., Calomme, M., Hu, J.P., Cimanga, K., Van Poel, B., Pieters, L., Vlietnck, A.J. and D. Vanden Berghe. Structure-activity relationship and classification of flavonoids as inhibitors of xanthine oxidase and superoxide scavengers. *J. Nat. Prod.,* 1998. 61: p. 71–76.

[98] Nijveldt, R.J., van Nood, E., van Hoorn, D.E., Boelens, P.G., van Norren, K. and van Leeuwen, P.A. Flavonoids: a review of probable mechanisms of action and potential applications. *Am. J. Clin. Nutr.,* 2001. 74: p. 418-25.

[99] Ramos, S. Cancer chemoprevention and chemotherapy: dietary polyphenols and signaling pathways. *Mol. Nutr. Food Res.,* 2008. 52: p. 507-26.

[100] Scalbert, A. and Williamson, G. Dietary intake and bioavailability of polyphenols. *J. Nutr.,* 2000. 130: p. 2073S-85S.

[101] Hanasaki, Y., Ogawa, S., Fukui, S. The correlation between active oxygens scavenging and antioxidative effects of flavonoids. *Free Radic. Biol. Med.,* 1994. 16: p. 845–850.

[102] Cushnie, T.P. and Lamb, A.J. Antimicrobial activity of flavonoids. *Int. J. Antimicrob. Agents,* 2005. 26: p. 343–356.

[103] van Acker, S.A., Tromp, M.N., Haenen, G.R.M.M., van der Vijgh, W.J., Bast, A. Flavonoids as scavengers of nitric oxide radical. *Biochem. Biophys. Res. Commun.,* 1995. 214: p. 755–759.

[104] Haenen, G.R.M.M. and Bast, A. Nitric oxide radical scavenging of flavonoids. *Methods Enzymol.,* 1999. 301: p. 490–503.

[105] Haenen, G.R.M.M., Paquay, J.B., Korthouwer, R.E., Bast, A. Peroxynitrite scavenging by flavonoids. *Biochem. Biophys. Res. Commun.,* 1997. 236: p. 591–593.

[106] Heijnen, C.G., Haenen, G.R.M.M., van Acker, F.A., van der Vijgh, W.J. and Bast, A. Flavonoids as peroxynitrite scavengers: the role of the hydroxyl groups. *Toxicol.* In Vitro, 2001. 15: p. 3–6.

[107] Heijnen, C.G., Haenen, G.R.M.M., Oostveen, R.M., Stalpers, E.M. and Bast, A. Protection of flavonoids against lipid peroxidation: the structure activity relationship revisited. *Free Radic. Res.,* 2002. 36: p. 575–581.

[108] Ju, J., Lu, G., Lambert, J.D. and Yang, C.S. Inhibition of carcinogenesis by tea constituents. *Semin. Cancer Biol.,* 2007. 17: p. 395-402.

[109] Read, M.A. Flavonoids: naturally occurring anti-inflammatory agents. *Am. J. Pathol.,* 1995. 147: p. 235–237.

[110] Orsolic, N., Knezevic, A.H., Sver, L., Terzic, S., Basic, I. Immunomodulatory and antimetastatic action of propolis and related polyphenolic compounds. *J. Ethnopharmacol.,* 2004. 94: p. 307–315.

[111] Manjeet, K.R. and Ghosh, B. Quercetin inhibits LPS-induced nitric oxide and tumor necrosis factor-alpha production in murine macrophages. *Int. J. Immunopharmacol.,* 1999. 21: p. 435–443.

[112] Geraets, L., Moonen, H.J.J., Brauers, K., Wouters, E.F.M., Bast, A., Hageman, G.J. Dietary flavones and flavonoles are inhibitors of poly(ADP-ribose)polymerase-1 in pulmonary epithelial cells. *J. Nutr.,* 2007. 137: p. 2190–2195.

[113] Bureau, G., Longpré, F., Martinoli, M.G. Resveratrol and quercetin, two natural polyphenols, reduce apoptotic neuronal cell death induced by neuroinflammation. *J. Neurosci. Res.,* 2008. 86: p. 403–410.

[114] Nair, M.P., Mahajan, S., Reynolds, J.L., Aalinkeel, R., Nair, H., Schwartz, S.A. and Kandaswami, C. The flavonoid quercetin inhibits proinflammatory cytokine (tumor necrosis factor alpha) gene expression in normal peripheral blood mononuclear cells via modulation of the NF-kappabeta system. *Clin. Vaccine Immunol.,* 2006. 13: p. 319–328.

[115] Canivenc-Lavier, M.C., Vernevaut, M.F., Totis, M., Siess, M.H., Magdalou, J., and M. Suschetet. Comparative effects of flavonoids and model inducers on drug-metabolizing enzymes in rat liver. *Toxicology,* 1996. 114: p. 19–27.

[116] Shih, H., Pickwell, G.V. and Quattrochi, L.C. Differential effects of flavonoid compounds on tumor promoter-induced activation of the human CYP1A2 enhancer. *Arch. Biochem. Biophys.,* 2000. 373: p. 287–294.

[117] Moon, Y.J., Wang, X., Morris, M.E., Dietary flavonoids: effects on xenobiotic and carcinogen metabolism, *Toxicol.* In Vitro, 2006. 20: p. 187–210.

[118] Lee-Hilz, Y.Y., Boerboom, A.M.J.F., Westphal, A.H., van Berkel, W.J.H., Aarts, J.M.M.J.G. and Rietjens, I.M.C.M. Pro-oxidant activity of flavonoids induces EpRE-mediated gene expression. *Chem. Res. Toxicol.,* 2006. 19: p. 1499–1505.

[119] Chen, C. and Kong, A.N.T. Dietary chemopreventive compounds and ARE/EpRE signaling. *Free Radical Biol. Med.,* 2004. 36: p. 1505–1516.

[120] Itoh, K., Tong, K.I. and Yamamoto, M. Molecular mechanism activating Nrf2-Keap1 pathway in regulation of adaptive response to electrophiles. *Free Radical Biol. Med.,* 2004. 36: p. 1208–1213.

[121] Dinkova-Kostova, A.T., Holtzclaw, W.D. and Kensler, T.W. The role of Keap1 in cellular protective responses. *Chem. Res. Toxicol.,* 2005. 18: p. 1779–1791.

[122] Jaiswal, A.K., Nrf2 signaling in coordinated activation of antioxidant gene expression. *Free Radical Bio Med.,* 2004. 36: p. 199- 207.

[123] Valerio, L.G., Kepa, J.K., Pickwell, G.V. and Quattrochi, L.C. Induction of human NAD(P)H: quinone oxidoreductase (NQO1) gene expression by the flavonol quercetin. *Toxicol. Lett.,* 2001. 119: p. 49–57.

[124] Boerboom, A.M.J.F., Vermeulen, M., van der Woude, H., Bremer, B.I., Lee-Hilz, Y.Y., Kampman, E., van Bladeren, P.J., Rietjens, I.M.C.M. and Aarts, J.M.M.J.G. Newly constructed stable reporter cell lines for mechanistic studies on electrophile-responsive element-mediated gene expression reveal a role for flavonoid planarity. *Biochem. Pharmacol.,* 2006. 72: p. 217–226.

[125] Lee, K. W., N.J. Kang, Y.S. Heo, E.A. Rogozin, A. Pugliese, M.K. Hwang, G.T. Bowden, A.M. Bode, H.J. Lee and Z. Dong. Raf and MEK protein kinases are direct molecular targets for the chemopreventive effect of quercetin, a major flavonol in red wine. *Cancer Res.,* 2008. 68: p. 946–955.

[126] Hwang, M. K., Song, N. R., Kang, N. J., Lee, K. W. and Lee, H. J. Activation of phosphatidylinositol 3-kinase is required for tumor necrosis factor-alpha-induced upregulation of matrix metalloproteinase-9: its direct inhibition by quercetin. *Int. J. Biochem. Cell Biol.,* 2009. 41: p. 1592–1600.

[127] Lee, K. M., Hwang, M. K., Lee, D. E., Lee, K. W. and Lee, H. J. Protective effect of quercetin against arseniteinduced COX-2 expression by targeting PI3K in rat liver epithelial cells. *J. Agric. Food Chem.,* 2010. 58: p. 5815–5820.

[128] Ohren, J. F. et al. Structures of human MAP kinase kinase 1 (MEK1) and MEK2 describe novel noncompetitive kinase inhibition. *Nature Struct. Mol. Biol.,* 2004. 11: p. 1192–1197.

[129] Engelman, J. A. and Cantley, L. C. Chemoprevention meets glucose control. *Cancer Prev. Res. (Phila),* 2010. 3: p. 1049–1052.

[130] Walker, E. H. et al. Structural determinants of phosphoinositide 3-kinase inhibition by wortmannin, LY294002, quercetin, myricetin, and staurosporine. *Mol. Cell,* 2000. 6: p. 909–919.

[131] Ashida, H., Fukuda, I., Yamashita, T. and Kanazawa, K. Flavones and flavonols at dietary levels inhibit a transformation of aryl hydrocarbon receptor induced by dioxin. *FEBS Lett.,* 2000. 476: p. 213–217.

[132] Fukuda, I., Mukai, R., Kawase, M., Yoshida, K. and Ashida, H. Interaction between the aryl hydrocarbon receptor and its antagonists, flavonoids. *Biochem. Biophys. Res. Commun.,* 2007. 359: p. 822–827.

[133] Deschner, E.E., Ruperto, J., Wong, G. and Newmark, H.L. Quercetin and rutin as inhibitors of azoxymethanol-induced colonic neoplasia. *Carcinogenesis,* 1991. 12: p. 1193–6.

[134] Khanduja, K.L., Gandhi, R.K., Pathania, V. and Syal, N. Prevention of N-nitrosodiethylamine-induced lung tumorigenesis by ellagic acid and quercetin in mice. *Food Chem. Toxicol.,* 1999. 37: p. 313–318.

[135] Gee, J.M., Hara, H. and Johnson, I.T. Suppression of intestinal crypt cell proliferation and aberrant crypt foci by dietary quercetin in rats. *Nutr. Cancer,* 2002. 43: p. 193–201.

[136] Matsukawa, Y., Nishino, H., Okuyama, Y., Matsui, T., Matsumoto, T., Matsumura, S., Shimizu, Y., Sowa, Y. and Sakai, T. Effects of quercetin and/or restraint stress on formation of aberrant crypt foci induced by azoxymethane in rat colons. *Oncology,* 1997. 54: p. 118–121.

[137] M.A. Pereira, C.J. Grubbs, L.H. Barnes, H. Li, G.R. Olson, I. Eto, M. Juliana, L.M. Whitaker, G.J. Kelloff, V.E. Steele and R.A. Lubet. Effects of the phytochemicals, curcumin and quercetin, upon azoxymethane-induced colon cancer and 7,12-dimethylbenz[a]anthracene-induced mammary cancer in rats. *Carcinogenesis,* 1996. 17: p. 1305–1311.

[138] Deschner, E.E., Ruperto, J.F., Wong, G.Y. and H.L. Newmark. The effect of dietary quercetin and rutin on AOM-induced acute colonic epithelial abnormalities in mice fed a high-fat diet. *Nutr. Cancer,* 1993. 20: p. 199–204.

[139] Mahmoud, N.N., Carothers, A.M., Grunberger, D., Bilinski, R.T., Churchill, M.R., Martucci, C., Newmark, H.L. and M.M. Bertagnolli. Plant phenolics decrease intestinal tumors in an animal model of familial adenomatous polyposis. *Carcinogenesis,* 2000. 21: p. 921–927.

[140] Makita, H., Tanaka, T., Fujitsuka, H., Tatematsu, N., Satoh, K., Hara, A. and H. Mori. Chemoprevention of 4-nitroquinoline 1-oxide-induced rat oral carcinogenesis by the dietary flavonoids chalcone, 2-hydroxychalcone, and quercetin. *Cancer Res.,* 1996. 56: p. 904–909.

[141] Verma, A.K., Johnson, J.A., Gould, M.N. and M.A. Tanner. Inhibition of 7,12-dimethylbenz(a)anthracene- and N-nitrosomethylurea-induced rat mammary cancer by dietary flavonol quercetin. *Cancer Res.,* 1998. 48: p. 5754–5758.

[142] Kato, R., Nakadate, T., Yamamoto, S. and T. Sugimura. Inhibition of 12-O-tetradecanoylphorbol-13-acetate-induced tumor promotion and ornithine decarboxylase activity by quercetin: possible involvement of lipoxygenase inhibition. *Carcinogenesis,* 1983. 4: p. 1301–1305.

[143] Dihal, A.A., de Boer, V.C., van der Woude, H., Tilburgs, C., Bruijntjes, J.P., Alink, G.M., Rietjens, I.M., Woutersen, R.A. and R.H. Stierum. Quercetin, but not its

glycosylated conjugate rutin, inhibits azoxymethane-induced colorectal carcinogenesis in F344 rats. *J. Nutr.,* 2006. 136: p. 2862–2867.

[144] Volate, S.R., Davenport, D.M., Muga, S.J. and M.J. Wargovich. Modulation of aberrant crypt foci and apoptosis by dietary herbal supplements (quercetin, curcumin, silymarin, ginseng and rutin). *Carcinogenesis,* 2005. 26: p. 1450–1456.

[145] Femia, A.P., Caderni, G., Ianni, M., Salvadori, M., Schijlen, E., Collins, G., Bovy, A. and P. Dolara. Effect of diets fortified with tomatoes or onions with variable quercetin-glycoside content on azoxymethane-induced aberrant crypt foci in the colon of rats. *Eur. J. Nutr.,* 2003. 42: p. 346–352.

[146] Murota, K. and J. Terao. Quercetin appears in the lymph of unsaturated rats at its phase II metabolites after administered into the stomach. *FEBS Lett.,* 2005. 579: p. 5343–5346.

[147] Shirai, M., Kawai, Y., Yamanishi, R., Kinoshita, T., Chuman, H. and J. Terao. Effect of a conjugated quercetin metabolite, quercetin 3-glucuronide, on lipid hydroperoxide-dependent formation of reactive oxygen species in differentiated PC-12 cells. *Free Radic. Res.,* 2006. 40: p. 1047–1053.

[148] Stoclet, J.C., Chataigneau, T., Ndiaye, M., et al. Vascular protection by dietary polyphenols. *Eur. J. Pharmacol.* 2004. 500(1-3): p. 299-313.

[149] Manach, C., Mazur, A., Scalbert, A. Polyphenols and prevention of cardiovascular diseases. *Curr. Opin Lipidol.,* 2005. 16(1): p. 77-84.

[150] Arts, I.C., Hollman, P.C. Polyphenols and disease risk in epidemiologic studies. Am J Clin Nutr., 2005. 81(1 Suppl): p. 317S-325S.

[151] Hubbard, G.P., Wolffram, S., Lovegrove, J.A., et al. The role of polyphenolic compounds in the diet as inhibitors of platelet function. *Proc. Nutr. Soc.,* 2003. 62(2): p. 469-78.

[152] Scalbert, A., Manach, C., Morand, C., et al. Dietary polyphenols and the prevention of diseases. *Crit. Rev. Food Sci. Nutr.,* 2005. 45(4): p. 287-306.

[153] Dauchet, L., Amouyet, P., and Dallongeville, J. Fruit and vegetable consumption and risk of stroke. A meta-analysis of cohort studies. *Neurology,* 2005. 65: p. 1193−1197.

[154] Hu, F. B. Plant-based foods and prevention of cardiovascular disease: an overview. *The American Journal of Clinical Nutrition,* 2003. 78(3): p. 544S−551S.

[155] Ness, A. R. and Powles, J. W. Fruit and vegetables, and cardiovascular disease: A review. *International Journal of Epidemiology,* 1997. 26(1): p. 1−13.

[156] Nothlings, U., Schulze, M. B., Weikert, C., Boeing, H., van der Schouw, Y. T., Bamia, C., et al. Intake of vegetables, legumes, and fruit, and risk for all-cause, cardiovascular, and cancer mortality in a European diabetic population. *The Journal of Nutrition,* 2008. 138: p. 775−781.

[157] Perez-Vizcaino, F., Duarte, J. and Andriantsitohaina, R. Endothelial function and cardiovascular disease: effects of quercetin and wine polyphenols. *Free Radic. Res.,* 2006. 40: p. 1054–1065.

[158] Duarte J, Pérez Vizcaino F, Utrilla P, Jiménez J, Tamargo J and Zarzuelo A. Vasodilatory effects of flavonoids in rat aortic smooth muscle. Structure-activity relationships. *Gen. Pharmacol.,* 1993. 24: p. 857–62.

[159] Duarte J, Pérez-Palencia R, Vargas F, et al. Antihypertensive effects of the flavonoid quercetin in spontaneously hypertensive rats. *Br. J. Pharmacol.,* 2001. 133: p. 117–24.

[160] Machha, A. and Mustafa, M.R. Chronic treatment with flavonoids prevents endothelial dysfunction in spontaneously hypertensive rat aorta. *J. Cardiovasc. Pharmacol.,* 2005. 46: p. 36–40.

[161] Sánchez, M., Galisteo, M., Vera, R., et al. Quercetin downregulatesNADPH oxidase, increases eNOS activity and prevents endothelial dysfunction in spontaneously hypertensive rats. *J. Hypertens.,* 2006. 24: p. 75–84.

[162] Duarte, J., Jimenez, R., O'Valle, F., et al. Protective effects of the flavonoid quercetin in chronic nitric oxide deficient rats. *J. Hypertens.,* 2002. 20: p. 1843–54.

[163] Garcia-Saura, M.F., Galisteo, M., Villar, I.C., et al. Effects of chronic quercetin treatment in experimental renovascular hypertension. *Mol. Cell Biochem.,* 2005. 270: p. 147–55.

[164] Ibarra, M., Perez-Vizcaino, F., Cogolludo, A., Duarte, J., Zaragoza-Arnaez, F., Lopez-Lopez, J.G. and Tamargo, J. Cardiovascular effects of isorhamnetin and quercetin in isolated rat and porcine vascular smooth muscle and isolated rat atria. *Planta Med.,* 2002. 68: p. 307–310.

[165] Perez-Vizcaino, F., Ibarra, M., Cogolludo, A.L., Duarte, J., Zaragoza-Arnaez, F., Moreno, L., Lopez-Lopez, G. and Tamargo, J. Endothelium-independent vasodilator effects of the flavonoid quercetin and its methylated metabolites in rat conductance and resistance arteries. *J. Pharmacol. Exp. Ther.,* 2002. 302: p. 66–72.

[166] Ibarra, M., Moreno, L., Vera, R., Cogolludo, A., Duarte, J., Tamargo, J. and Perez-Vizcaino, F. Effects of the flavonoid quercetin and its methylated metabolite isorhamnetin in isolated arteries from spontaneously hypertensive rats. *Planta Med.,* 2003. 69: p. 995–1000.

[167] Sánchez, M., Lodi, F., Vera, R., et al. Quercetin and isorhamnetin prevent endothelial dysfunction, superoxide production, and overexpression of p47phox induced by angiotensin II in rat aorta. *J. Nutr.,*2007. 137: p. 910–5.

[168] Galisteo, M., Garcia-Saura, M.F., Jiménez, R., et al. Effects of chronic quercetin treatment on antioxidant defence system and oxidative status of deoxycorticosterone acetate-salt-hypertensive rats. *Mol. Cell Biochem.,* 2004. 259: p. 91–9.

[169] Galisteo, M., Garcia-Saura, M.F., Jiménez, R., et al. Effects of quercetin treatment on vascular function in deoxycorticosterone acetate-salt hypertensive rats. Comparative study with verapamil. *Planta. Med.,* 2004. 70: p. 334–41.

[170] Laplante, M.A., Wu, R., Moreau, P. and de Champlain, J. Endothelin mediates superoxide production in angiotensin II-induced hypertension in rats. *Free Radic. Biol. Med.,* 2005. 38: p. 589–96.

[171] Khan, N.Q., Lees, D.M., Douthwaite, J.A., Carrier, M.J. and Corder R. Comparison of red wine extract and polyphenol constituents on endothelin-1 synthesis by cultured endothelial cells. *Clin. Sci.* (Lond), 2002. 103: p. 72S–5S.

[172] Ruef, J., Moser, M., Kübler, W. and Bode, C. Induction of endothelin-1 expression by oxidative stress in vascular smooth muscle cells. *Cardiovasc. Pathol.,* 2001. 10: p. 311–5.

In: Quercetin
Editors: Taiki Chikamatsu and Yuudai Hida

ISBN: 978-1 61942- 057-1

Chapter 3

QUERCETIN: SOURCES, BIOAVAILABILITY AND EFFECTS ON CANCER CELLS

***Eduardo Cremonese Filippi-Chiela*[1], *Guido Lenz*[1,2,*] *and Lauren L. Zamin*[3]**
[1]Department of Biophysics and [2]Center of Biotechnology, Universidade Federal do Rio Grande do Sul, Porto Alegre, RS, Brazil
[3]Universidade Federal da Fronteira Sul, Cerro Largo, RS, Brazil

ABSTRACT

Quercetin (3,3',4',5,7-pentahydroxyflavone, Quer) is the most abundant of the flavonoids found in nature and has a long history of consumption by humans. The main source of Quer is green tea (*Camellia sinensis*), red onion, grapes, apples, berries, cherries, broccoli, citrus fruits, caper, lovage among others. In plants, Quer exhibits strong antioxidant properties, possibly protecting against harmful ultraviolet rays. Research concerning the health benefits of Quer has shown that this compound is cardioprotective and neuroprotective, mainly by acting as antioxidant, antiinflamatory, vasodilating, antihypertensive and antithrombotic. In addition, Quer is considered a potential anti-cancer agent, although some recent data suggest that it can also increase cancer growth. The mechanism by which Quer can exert its effects is not completely elucidated. Some *in vitro* and *in vivo* works showed that Quer can interact with proteins involved in cell signaling, cell cycle and apoptosis. Owing to the large number of potential health beneficial effects of Quer, its consumption has increased, and the addition of this compound to various traditional food products has grown. However, prior to the use of Quer as food supplementation or medicine a better understanding of the real health benefits, the pharmacokinetics (i.e. bioavailability, metabolism and toxicity), pharmacodynamics and the safety of this compound is fundamental. This chapter will focus in the sources, bioavailability and potential antitumoral effect of Quer, discussing data from different cell systems, animal models, and human studies.

---

* Corresponding author: Dr. G. Lenz Departamento de Biofísica and Center of Biotechnology–UFRGS Av. Bento Gonçalves, 9500. Prédio 43431–Lab. 107 CEP 91501-970, Porto Alegre, RS, BRASIL TEL: +55 51 3308 7620; FAX +55 51 3308 7309 e-mail: lenz@ufrgs.br.

1. Introduction

The first observation regarding the flavonoids biological activities was published in 1936 by Rusznyak and Szent-Gyorgyi. Initially, flavonoids were considered vitamins (vitamin P) because of their effect on capillary permeability, but this was later dismissed. The interest in these compounds decayed after they were shown not to be required as micronutrients for human health in the 1940s [Joint-Committee-Nomenclature-ASBC-AIN, 1950]. However, after the publication of epidemiological studies associating a reduced incidence of cancer and cardiovascular disease with a high intake of food rich in flavonoids, a large expansion of the field took place, in the 1990s [Hertog et al., 1993; Keli et al., 1996]. Among all of the flavonoids, Quercetin (Quer) has attracted much attention because it is ubiquitously present in plant-derived foods and has a great potential as anticancer, antioxidant, antiinflamatory and cardioprotective compound [Murakami et al., 2008; Russo et al., 2011].

This review will focus on Quer, the most abundant flavonoid found in vegetal kingdom, whose properties have been associated with the prevention of several diseases, including cancer. We selected and analyzed key aspects of Quer sources, bioavailability, and health effects, mainly its antitumoral activity in cancer from Nervous System. We apologize in advance for the many citations omitted and hope that the present chapter may help to predict future developments in these fields.

2. Chemistry and Source of Quer

In the last twenty years the interest in secondary plant metabolism compounds has grown in part due to the epidemiological data that indicated an inverse correlation between fruit and vegetable consumption and the incidence of chronic diseases [Hertog et al., 1993; Hertog et al., 1995; Huxley and Neil, 2003]. One of the most important and widely distributed phytochemical family in plants is flavonoids. Flavonoids are poliphenolic compounds that have a basic chemical structure of diphenylpropanes (C6–C3–C6) consisting of two aromatic rings linked through three carbons [Bravo, 1998; Croft, 1998]. They can be further subdivided into six major subclasses, based upon variations in the heterocyclic C-ring including flavones, flavonols, flavanones, catechins, anthocyanidins, and isoflavones [Bravo, 1998; Croft, 1998]. Among them, flavonols and flavones are of particular importance in the human diet as antioxidants and due to their association with health benefits [Haghi and Hatami, 2010].

Quer (3,3',4',5,7-pentahydroxyflavone) (Figure 1) belongs to the class of flavonols and is one of the predominant flavonoids present in food (Table 1 and reviewed in USDA Database for the Flavonoid Content of Selected Foods). It mainly occurs in plants as glycoside, i.e. linked through one of the hydroxyl groups of the flavonol to a sugar group such as glucose (isoquercitrin), galactose (hyperoside), rhamnose (quercetrin), rutinose (rutin) or xylose [Havsteen, 1983; Middleton and Kandaswami, 1993; Scalbert and Williamson, 2000; Spanos and Wrolstad, 1992]. In plants, these compounds are involved in energy production [Theoharides et al., 2001] and exhibit strong anti-oxidant properties, possibly protecting plants against harmful ultraviolet rays [Wiczkowski et al., 2003].

The physical properties of Quer and other flavonols are attributable to their hydrophobic, co-planar structure. Their water-solubility increases with increasing number of sugar groups.

The chemical activities of Quer can be ascribed to its electron-donating property (reducing activity) which is due to the presence of a phenolic hydroxyl group. This property is essential for exerting anti-oxidant activity by scavenging free radicals [Murakami et al., 2008]

Table 1. Sources of Quer

Product	Concentration	Reference
Apple (*Malus pumila* Mill)	36 mg/kg	Hertog et al., 1992
Apricot (*Prunus armeniaca* L.)	25 mg/kg	Hertog et al., 1992
Broccoli (*Brassica oleracea* L. cv. Italica L.)	30 mg/kg	Hertog et al., 1992
Calendula officinalis flower	1.1 mg/g	Haghi and Hatami, 2010
Camellia sinensis leaf (green)	2.8 mg/g	Haghi and Hatami, 2010
Capers (*Capparis* sp.)	Not determinate	Sharaf et al., 2000 and 1997
French beans (*Phaseolus vulgaris* L.)	32-45 mg/kg	Hertog et al., 1992
Ginkgo biloba leaf	1.36 mg/g	Haghi and Hatami, 2010
Grape, red (*Vitis vinifera* L.)	15 mg/kg	Hertog et al., 1992
Grape, white (*Vitis vinifera* L.)	12 mg/kg	Hertog et al., 1992
Guava mature leaves (*Psidium guajava*)	2883 mg/kg	Vargas et al., 2006
Kale (*Brassica oleracea* L. cv. Acephala DC).	110 mg/kg	Hertog et al., 1992
Lettuce leaf (*Lactuca sativa*)	0.8 mg/g	Haghi and Hatami, 2010
Olive leaf (*Olea europaea*)	0.5 mg/g	Haghi and Hatami, 2010
Onion (*Allium cepa* L.)	284-486 mg/kg	Hertog et al., 1992
Pear (*Pyrus communis* L.)	6.4 mg/kg	Hertog et al., 1992
Red currant (*Ribes rubrum-hybriden*)	13 mg/kg	Hertog et al., 1992
Red wine	0.45-57.6 µg/mL	Careri et al., 2003
Slicing beans (*Phaseolus vulgaris* L.)	28-30 mg/kg	Hertog et al., 1992
Strawberry (*Fragaria ananassa* Duch.)	8.6 mg/kg	Hertog et al., 1992
Sweet cherry (*Prunus Cerasus* L.)	15 mg/kg	Hertog et al., 1992
Turnip tops (*Brassica campretis* L.)	7.3 mg/kg	Hertog et al., 1992

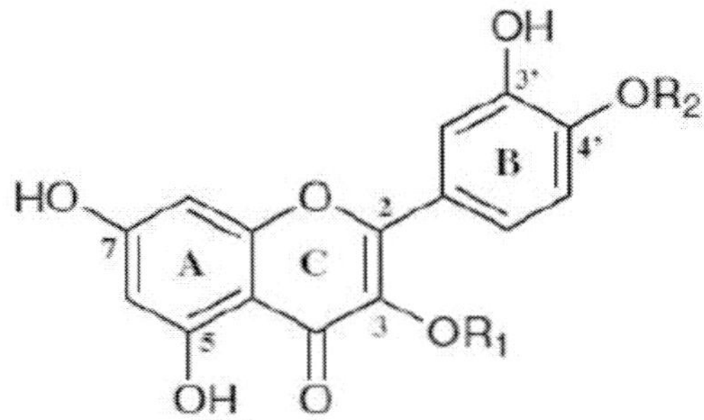

R_1=H, R_2=H; Quercetin.
R_1=β-D-glucose, R_2=H; Isoquercitrin.
R_1=β-D-galactose, R_2=H; Hyperoside.
R_1=β-D-rutinose, R_2=H; Rutin.
R_1=H, R_2=β-D-glucose; G4'G.
R_1=R_2=β-D-glucose; Q3.4'-diG.

Figure 1. Quer and related molecules structure.

3. Metabolism of Quer

3.1. Absorption

Potential health effects of bioactive plant compounds depend on their bioavailability following oral administration. At present, the pharmacokinetics of Quer has not been fully characterized, although a number of studies have been carried out both in animals and humans [Ishizawa et al., 2011; de Boer et al., 2005; Egert et al., 2008]. As already mentioned, in plant used as food, Quer is mainly present as various glycosides. However, because of the hydrophilic character of its glycosides, only Quer without a sugar group, i.e. the aglycon, was initially suggested (and now confirmed) to be taken up in the gastro-intestinal tract by passive diffusion [Kuhnau, 1976; Griffiths, 1982]. Upon ingestion, Quer monoglycoside, in which only one glucose molecule is bound to Quer, such as isoquercitrin, is absorbed in the small intestine as Quer aglycone following hydrolysis with lactose phorizin hydrolase at the brush border membranes [Murota et al, 2000]. In the case of other glycosides which contain one sugar other than glucose (such as hyperoside) or disaccharides/oligosaccharides (such as rutin), absorption occurs in the large intestine as Quer aglycone through deconjugation caused by the activity of enterobacteria. In either case, Quer aglycone is immediately metabolized into its conjugated forms by the action of phase II enzymes [van der Woude et al., 2004]. Although Quer metabolites are mostly returned to the digestive tract via multidrug resistance-associated protein 2, some are transported through the portal vein into the liver, where they undergo secondary metabolism. The lymphatic system also contributes to the transport of Quer metabolites around the body [Murota and Terao, 2005]. Day et al. (2001) identified the major Quer metabolites present in human plasma as follows: quercetin 3′-O- β -D-glucuronide, quercetin 4′-O- β -D-glucuronide, quercetin 3-O- β -D-glucuronide, 3′-O-methyl quercetin 4′-O- β -D-glucuronide, 3′-O-methyl quercetin 3-O- β -D-glucuronide and quercetin 3′-O-sulfate.

3.2. Distribution

Regarding the tissue distribution, a study in rats fed with Quer in the diet (50 or 500 mg/kg body weight) for 11 weeks observed that Quer concentrated in lungs, testes, kidneys, thymus, heart and liver, with the highest concentrations in the pulmonary tissue and the lowest in the brain, white fat, and spleen [de Boer et al. 2005]. In a short-term study in pigs wich received 500 mg/kg (body weight) for 3 consecutive days, liver and kidney contained high concentrations of Quer and its metabolites, whereas brain, heart, and spleen had low concentrations [de Boer et al. 2005] (see also Table 2).

In both rats and humans, Quer and its derivatives were shown to possess strong affinity for serum albumin [Manach et al., 1995; McAnlis et al., 1999; Sengupta and Sengupta, 2003].

3.3. Excretion

Systemically-absorbed Quer may be eliminated in the urine [Gugler et al., 1975; Ueno et al., 1984; de Vries et al., 1998; Wang et al., 2003]. A substantial portion of the metabolites may be secreted into the bile [Murota and Terao, 2003] and excreted in the feces [Ueno et al., 1984]. Quer can undergo microbial degradation in the colon to phenolic acids and CO_2, which is exhaled in the breath [Ueno et al., 1984; Walle et al., 2001; Abrahamse et al., 2005]. Unabsorbed Quer and the phenolic acid microfloral degradation products are eliminated in the feces [Gugler et al., 1975; Ueno et al., 1984; Nakamura et al., 2000].

3.4. Bioavailability

National dietary record-based cohort assessments (e.g., from Australia, the Netherlands, Finland, Italy, Croatia, Japan, and the United States) of the intake of Quer from the habitual diet indicated mean consumption levels in the range of less than 5 mg to ~40 mg Quer/day [Hertog et al., 1995; Rimm et al., 1996; Knekt et al., 1997; Kimira et al., 1998; Johannot and Somerset, 2006; Lin et al., 2006]. However, daily levels of Quer as high as 200–500 mg may be attained by high-end consumers of fruits and vegetables, especially in cases where the individuals consume the peel portion of Quer-rich fruits and vegetables, such as tomatoes, apples, and onions (illustrated in Table 1) [Jones and Hughes, 1982; USDA, 2000]. In some countries, Quer is available as a dietary supplement with manufacturers' recommendations daily doses of 200–1200 mg Quer. Recent reviews of the data related to the potential toxicity of Quer support its safety as a dietary supplement and for the addition to foods [Harwood et al., 2007; Okamoto, 2005].

Data on bioavailability of Quer aglycone or Quer glycosides vary substantially between studies, according to the methods applied for Quer measurement, and in different species (reviewed in Table 2). Quer intervention trials in humans have so far shown inconclusive and even conflicting results [Williamson and Manach, 2005].

Table 2. Overview of literature on the Quer concentration, bioavailability and effects in different model systems

Specie	Dosage/ Administration route	Concentration Obtained	Effects/Reference
Caenorhabditis elegans n=20	Quer 200 μM incorporated into the culture medium	[Quer] in the worm: 19.85 μg /mg protein. Quer metabolites found in the worm: Quercetin 3-O-glucoside; Quercetin glycoside; Quercetin sulfate glycoside; Quercetin; Isorhamnetin	↑ reproductive capacity of *C. elegans* (9%), ↑ the thermoresistance (17%), ↑ the oxidative stress resistance, marked ↓ the oxidation of proteins and ↑ lifespam(11%). *Surco-Laos et al., 2011.*
Mice n=36	5% of Quer diet for 8 weeks (calculated as 5.3 g/(kg body wt · day) Quer intake)	The peak plasma [Quer] was 152 μM at 6 weeks.	MiaPaCa-2 cells (human pancreatic cancer cell line) were injected subcutaneously into the flank of nude mice. Eight weeks of 5% Quer intake did not reduce tumor growth. *Zhang et al., 2010.*
Human study: n=36 (18 women, 18 men) between 19 and 40 years	50, 100, or 150 mg/day for 2 weeks/ Oral	[Plasma] (median change): 50 mg/day: 92.2 nmol/L 100 mg/day: 171.8 nmol/L 150 mg/day: 316.2 nmol/L Elimination rates 50 mg/day: 0.09 nmol/minL 100 mg/day: 0.15 nmol/minL 150 mg/day: 0.29 nmol/minL	No adverse effects were found. There were no significant gender-specific differences in Quer concentrations at baseline and after Quer supplementation. Irrespective of the dose applied, Quer supplementation did not significantly affect fasting serum concentrations of triacylglycerols or total, LDL, or HDL cholesterol. *Egert et al., 2008*
Pigs: *Expt 1* - short-term feeding – 1 day; n=3 *Expt 2* - long-term feeding – 4 weeks, n=7	*Expt. 1*: 25 mg Quer/kg *Expt. 2:* 50 mg Quer/kg Oral	*Expt.1:* [Quer] (nmol/g wet tissue): Liver 6.20; Kidney 2.84; Jejunum 2.36; Lung 0.39; Muscle (longissimus dorsi) 0.11; Plasma 1.48 μmol/L *Expt. 2:* [Quer] (nmol/g wet tissue): Colon 13.92; Kidney 6.31; Jejunum 5.51; Liver 2.83; Lymph node 2.23; Mesentery 0.57; Lung 0.28; White adipose tissue 0.17; Muscle (longissimus dorsi) 0.09; Brain 0.02 Plasma 0.67 μmol/L	*Bieger et al., 2008*
Human study: n=41 prehypertensive and stage 1 hypertensive	365 mg Quer aglycone taken twice per day for 4 weeks	Plasma [Quer] was 695 ± 103 nmol/L after placebo treatment and increased to 1419 ± 189 nmol/L after Quer treatment	No adverse effects were found. Quer supplementation ↓ systolic, diastolic, and mean arterial pressure in stage 1 hypertensive subjects, but not in prehypertensive subjects. Concentrations of

Specie	Dosage/ Administration route	Concentration Obtained	Effects/Reference
42-52 years			plasma triglycerides and total, LDL, VLDL, and HDL cholesterol, and fasting blood glucose concentrations did not change after Quer supplementation. Antioxidant capacity and oxidative stress were not altered by Quer supplementation. *Edwards et al., 2007*
Rats and Pigs *Expt 1* - Six rats/group *Expt 2* – Three Pigs	*Expt 1* - The diet was supplemented with 0.1 or 1% Quer for 11 week *Expt 2* - 500 mg/kg (body wt day) on diet for 3 days	*Expt 1* – Quer (0.1%): Plasma 7.7 µmol/L; Lung 1.04 nmol/g tissue; also found (>1 nmol/g tissue) on Testes, Kidney, Heart, Liver, Brown fat, Thymus, Muscle and Bone. Quer (1%): Plasma 40.4 µmol/L; found in the organs cited above in higher concentration and in the Brain. *Expt 2* – Plasma Quer: 1.1 µmol/L also found on Liver, Kidney, Brain, Heart and Spleen	*de Boer et al., 2005*
Human Study n=10	*Expt 1:* 100 mg ^{14}C-Quer Oral. *Expt 2:* 0.3 mg ^{14}C-Quer iv	*Expt 1:* An early peak [plasma] of 890 nmol/L was reached 30 min after the dose. After 8 h there was a second peak of 1160 nmol/L. The [plasma] then declined exponentially over the entire study period of 72 h. *Expt 2:* [Plasma] started with 100 nmol/L and quickly fall of total radioactivity over the first 4 h. The overall recoveries in urine and feces were 3.5–8.3% after the oral and 21.3–30.2% after the iv dose. The $^{14}CO_2$ formation/exhalation accounted for 23.0–81.1% of the administered ^{14}C-labeled Quer doses, both oral and iv.	*Walle et al., 2001*

Abbreviations: iv–intravenous; Expt-experiment; wt-weight.

Table 3. Effect of Quer on tumor *in vitro* and *in vivo* models

Tumor type	Mechanism of actions	References
	In vitro	
Breast Cancer Cell lines: MDA-MB-231, MCF-7, HCC1937	Quer suppressed COX-2 expression and PGE2 production; inhibited angiogenesis, cell migration and invasion; induced cell cycle arrest, apoptosis	Chien et al., 2009; Choi et al., 2008; Chou et al., 2010; Gulati et al., 2006; Huang et al., 2011; Lin et al., 2008; Seo et al., 2011; Xiao et al., 2011
Colorectal cancer Cell lines: HT-29, Caco-2, SW480, HCT-116, IEC-6, FHC, VACO-235, COLO 201, LS-174T, T84, DLD-1, LT97, rat and mouse colonocytes	Quer inhibited cell growth; decreased cell migration; induced cell cycle arrest, cytotoxicity, apoptosis, differentiation, and autophagy	Dihal et al., 2006; Gee et al., 2002; Goncalves et al., 2010; Johnson, 2002; Kaindl et al., 2008; Kim et al., 2005; Kuntz et al., 1999; Kuo, 1996; Mertens-Talcott and Percival, 2005; Psahoulia et al., 2007; Ramos, 2008; Shan et al., 2009; Soobrattee et al., 2006; van der Woude et al., 2003; van Erk et al., 2005; Yang et al., 2000
Hepatoma Cell lines: HepG2, HA22T/VGH	Quer induced cell cycle arrest and apoptosis	Chang et al., 2009; Granado-Serrano et al., 2006; Mu et al., 2007; Tanigawa et al., 2008
Leukemia Cell lines: MOLT-4, HL-60	Quer reduced total cell number and viability, induced cell cycle arrest and apoptosis	Avci et al., 2011; Lee et al., 2011b; Mertens-Talcott and Percival, 2005; Niu et al., 2011
Lung cancer Cell line: A549, H460, H2009 and H1299, NCI-H209	Quer induced growth cell inhibition, cell cycle arrest and apoptosis	Chen et al., 2007; Hung, 2007; Nguyen et al., 2004; Yang et al., 2006; Yeh et al., 2011
Melanoma Cell lines: B16, DB-1, Mel-Juso, M14, and G361	Quer inhibited cell growth and induced apoptosis	Ferrer et al., 2005; Rosner et al., 2006; Thangasamy et al., 2010; Zhang et al., 2005
Prostatic cancer Cell lines: LNCaP, PC-3	Quer induced cell death, apoptosis	Lee et al., 2008; Senthilkumar et al., 2010; Senthilkumar et al., 2011
Pancreatic cancer Cell lines: EPP85-181P, EPP85-181RDB, BxPc-3, MIA-PaCa2	Quer inhibited cell growth and induced apoptosis	Borska et al., 2010; Lee et al., 2002

Tumor type	Mechanism of actions	References
Sarcoma Osteosarcoma cell lines: MG-63, U2-OS/MTX300 Liposarcoma cell line: SW872	Quer decreased cell number, induced apoptosis and cell cycle arrest	Huang et al., 2006; Liang et al., 2011; Suh et al., 2010; Xie et al., 2011
	In vivo	
Breast Cancer MDA-MB-231 implanted in a nude mouse model; 4T1 cell implanted in Balb/c mice	Quer decreased breast cancer cell proliferation and prolonged survival	Du et al., 2010; Schlachterman et al., 2008
Melanoma B16 implanted in mice	Quer inhibited metastasis	Ferrer et al., 2005
Pancreatic cancer MIA-PaCa2 cells implanted in a nude mouse model	Quer inhibited growth of cancer stem cell-enriched xenografts associated with reduced proliferation, angiogenesis, cancer stem cell-marker expression and induction of apoptosis	Zhou et al., 2010
Sarcoma Sarcoma-180 ascitic tumors	Quer increased longevity	Indap et al.., 2006

Table 4. Effect of Quer on Nervous System tumor with possible mechanism of action

Model/Tumor Type	Dose/Administration	Mechanism of action/Reference
Human U87MG glioblastoma cell line	10-50 μM added to the culture medium	Quer ↓ the expression and enzymatic activity of PLD 1, subsequently inhibiting proliferation and invasion of glioma cells. Quer ↓ NFkB-induced PLD1 expression via ↓ of NFkB transactivation. Quer ↓ activation and expression of MMP-2, a key modulator of glioma cell invasion, induced by PA, a product of PLD activity. *Park and Min, 2011*.
Rat C6 astroglioma cell line	1, 2, 5, 10, 20 and 50 μM added to the culture medium	The lowest concentration causing a significant loss of cells was 20 μM. However, Quer at 5–10 μM was not cytotoxic, even protecting C6 cells from H_2O_2-induced (500 μM) damage. *Seibert et al., 2011*.
Human brain astrocytoma cells MOGGCCM	5, 15, 30, 45 μM alone or in combination with Tmz 5, 10, 25, 50, 100 μM. Drugs were added to the culture medium	Tmz induced autophagy, while Quer ↑ necrosis in a dose-dependent manner. The combinations of both drugs were much more effective in programmed cell death induction. At a low (5μM) concentration, Quer potentiated the pro-autophagic effect of Tmz, while after treatment with a higher drug concentration (30 μM), autophagy switched to apoptosis. Tmz attenuated the toxic effect of quercetin. Apoptosis was mediated by the mitochondrial pathway and activation of caspase 3 and cytochrome C release, but no changes in caspase 8 expression was observed. It was accompanied by ↓ mitochondrial membrane potential and inhibition of Hsp27 and Hsp72 expression. Autophagy was correlated with ↑ level of LC3II. Tmz and Quer also inhibited migratory phenotype of MOGGCCM cells and changed the nuclei morphology from a circular to an irregular shape. *Jakubowicz-Gil et al., 2010*.
Human U87 glioblastoma cell line	50 μM added to the culture medium	Quer effectively blocked TPA-induced migration/invasion while simultaneously inhibiting COX-2/PGE2 production, MMP-9 enzyme activity, and peroxide production in U87 cells. *Chiu et al., 2010*.
Human U87 and U138 glioblastoma cell line; mouse GL261 glioma cell line and Rat C6 glioma cell line	25 and 100 μM alone or in combination with Rsv. Both drugs were added to the culture medium	Quer ↓ cell number in a dose dependent manner in all cell lines tested. In combination with Rsv, induced apoptosis and ↓ the Akt phosphorylation after 72h of treatment in C6 cells. Quer and Rsv chronically administered (12 days) presented a strong synergism in inducing senescence-like growth arrest. *Zamin et al., 2009*.
Human DAOY medulloblastoma cell line	1, 2.5, 5, 10, 20 μmol/L added to the culture medium	Quer and others flavonoids inhibited DAOY cell migration by affecting both Met and Akt (but not ERK-1/2) as well as the cell actin cytoskeleton, and these effects may prevent invasion and metastasis by these cells. *Labbé et al., 2009*.
Human glioblastoma cell lines U87-MG, A172, and	50, 100, 200 μM added to the culture medium	Quer did not cause cytotoxicity 24 h after treatment. Combining Quer with TRAIL strongly ↑ TRAIL-mediated apoptosis in U87-MG, U251, A172, and LN229 glioma cells; U373 cells

Model/Tumor Type	Dose/Administration	Mechanism of action/Reference
LN229, U251 and U373		could not be sensitized by Quer to TRAIL-mediated apoptosis. TRAIL-induced apoptosis was enhanced by Quer-induced reduction of survivin protein levels. Upon treatment with Quer, the protein level of survivin was strongly ↓ in U87-MG, U251, and A172 but not in U373 glioma cells. Quer suppressed survivin via increasing proteasomal degradation and via repressing phosphorylated Akt, known to coregulate survivin protein levels. *Siegelin et al., 2009.*
Human glioblastoma A172 cell line	10, 20, 30, 50 and 100 μM added to the culture medium	Quer resulted in loss of cell viability in a dose- and time-dependent manner. Quer did not ↑ ROS generation and the Quer-induced cell death was also not affected by antioxidants, suggesting that ROS generation is not involved in loss of cell viability. Quer ↓ phosphorylation of ERK and Akt. Transient transfection with constitutively active forms of MEK and Akt protected against the Quer-induced loss of cell viability. Querinduced depolarization of mitochondrial membrane potential and ↑ caspase activity. Quer ↓ survivin expression. *Kim et al., 2008.*
Human neuroblastoma SK-N-AS cell line and neuronal cell culture prepared from cortices of 18-day-old Wistar rat	3, 15, 30, 45 μM added to the culture medium	Quer induced apoptosis and necrosis in both the neuroblastoma cell line and neurons. Neurons were much more sensitive to cell death (both apoptotic and necrotic) upon Quer treatment than the cancer cell line. Quer ↓ Hsp27 expression in neurons and neuroblastoma cells and Hsp72 expression in cancer cells. *Jakubowicz-Gil et al., 2008.*
Human glioblastoma U138MG cell line	10, 30, and 100 μM added to the culture medium	Quer inhibited the ecto-5-NT/CD73 activity and modulated its expression, resulting in a decreased extracellular adenosine production with a consequent tumor progression reduction. *Braganhol et al., 2007.*
Human glioblastoma U138MG cell line	3, 10, 30 or 100 μM added to the culture medium	↓cell proliferation and viability in a dose- and time-dependent manner, induced necrosis and apoptosis, caused cell cycle arrest at G2 checkpoint and ↓ the mitotic index. By the other side, Quer protected hypocampal organotypic slices cultures from cell death induced by OGD. *Braganhol et al., 2006.*

Abreviattions: 12-O-tetradecanoylphorbol-13-acetate (TPA), Cyclooxygenase (COX), Ecto-5-nucleotidase/CD73 (ecto-5-NT/CD73), Extracellular signal-regulated Kinase (ERK), Metalloproteinase (MMP), Oxygen and Glucose Deprivation (OGD), Prostaglandin E2 (PGE2), Phosphatidic Acid (PA), Phospholipase D (PLD), Reactive Oxygen Species (ROS), Resveratrol (Rsv), Temozolomide (Tmz), Tumor Necrosis Factor–related Apoptosis-inducing Ligand (TRAIL).

4. Biological Effects of Quer

Effects of Quer in human health are described in several systems. Looking for "Quercetin" in PubMed (http://www.ncbi.nlm.nih.gov/pubmed/), we found 8301 references (at 09/10/2011). There are many biological effects attributed to Quer such as antioxidant [Boots et al., 2008], antihypertensive [Mackraj et al., 2008; Edwards et al., 2007; Perez-Vizcaino et al., 2009], antitumoral [Murakami et al., 2008; Zamin et al., 2009], anti-inflammatory [Lee et al., 2010; Chuang et al., 2010], neuroprotective [Braganhol et al., 2006; Ossola et al., 2009], cardioprotective [Annapurna et al., 2009] and ameliorates hyperglycemia-related diseases [Rivera et al., 2008; Fang et al., 2008; Ahn et al., 2008; Yang et al., 2011], as shown *in vitro*, in animal models and, to some extent, in humans. These and others biological effects are summarized in Figure 2. In the next section we will focus on the recent studies concerning the antitumoral effect of Quer in tumors from the Nervous System.

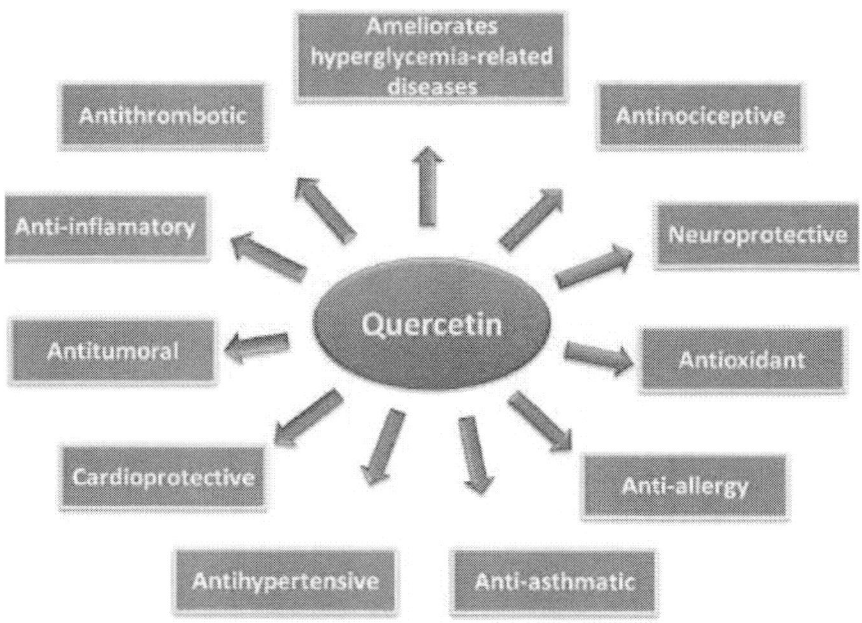

Figure 2. Examples of biological actions and possible clinical applications of Quer.

4.1. Antitumoral Effect of Quer

The idea that human death rate for cancer was associated to nutritional factors ingestion was proposed in 1981 [Doll and Peto, 1981]. This hypothesis was based on epidemiological studies that show an inverse relationship between fruits and vegetables consumption and risk of cancer. This may be explained by the presence, in the diet, of phytochemicals with potential chemotherapeutic and chemopreventive properties [Reddy et al., 2003]. The phytochemicals are a class of heterogeneous molecules, including vitamins (carotenoids) and food polyphenols, such as flavonoids, phytoalexins, phenolic acids, indoles and sulfur-rich compounds [Russo, 2007; Surh, 2003]. As already mentioned, Quer is the most abundant flavonoid in the Vegetable Kingdom and is considered the prototype of a naturally-occurring chemopreventive agent because its described biological activities (antioxidant, anti-inflammatory, anti-proliferative, pro-apoptotic and anti-angiogenic). Quer was suggested to act on all stages of carcinogenesis from initiation to invasion and metastasis and act on different genetic, biochemical and immunological aspects that underpin the development and maintenance of tumors [Lee et al., 2011a].

An abundant literature suggests that Quer can be efficient in treating several types of cancer (more than 1200 papers on Pubmed) by inducing cell death or cell cycle arrest preferentially in cancer cells *versus* their normal counterparts. The mechanism of action is through a process involving the down-regulation of selective oncogenes (such as Mcl-1, Ras, MEK, PI3K) and/or the up-regulation of tumor suppressor genes (p53, p21), which, in turn, enhance selective pathways leading to the elimination of cancer cells and preservation of normal non-tumoral tissue [Russo et al., 2011]. Table 3 summariz the effects of Quer against various tumor cell types *in vitro* and *in vivo*.

However, some *in vivo* studies did not find an antitumoral effect of Quer. Singh et al., (2010) examined the effects of Quer on estrogen-induced breast cancer *in vivo*. The ACI rat model of estrogen-induced breast cancer was used. Female ACI rats were given Quer via the diet (2.5 g/kg food) for a period of 240 days. At the end of the experiments, Quer did not prevent oxidative changes in the breast and did not confer protection against breast cancer [Singh et al., 2010]. In another study Quer did not show significant inhibitory effect on the growth of established mammary tumor inoculated in C3H/J mice [Indap et al., 2006].

There are, however, studies that show an increased risk of tumors development with Quer administration, despite not being mutagenic or teratogenic [Verschoyle et al., 2007]. In a study conducted by Pamukcu et al., (1980), albino Norwegian rats were fed a diet supplemented with 0.1 % Quer for 406 days. By the conclusion of the experiment, 80 % of treated rats had developed intestinal tumors and 20 % had bladder tumors. No tumors of either type were seen in control animals. Mean survival time was similar in treated and untreated animals [Pamukcu et al., 1980].

4.1.1. Antitumoral Effect of Quer on Nervous System

Gliomas are the most common primary brain tumors and have an incidence of 5–8/100, 000 individuals. Gliomas are classified by World Health Organization, according to their morphological characteristics, into astrocytic, oligodendroglial, mixed tumor (oligoastrocytic) and ependymal tumor [Sarkar et al., 2009]. The most malignant and most aggressive glioma is Glioblastoma, whose median survival of patients is only 12 months after diagnosis, even using surgery, chemo and radiotherapy [Avgeropoulos and Batchelor, 1999]. Gliomas are characterized by diffuse infiltrations of the surrounding Central Nervous System (CNS) tissue [Russell et al., 1989] and this characteristic is one of the main reasons for the lack of successful treatment [Tonn and Goldbrunner, 2003]. Nevertheless, the therapeutic strategy for gliomas has remained essentially unchanged for decades due to a limited understanding of the biology of the disease. There is an urgent need to develop mechanism-based approaches for the management of glioma, i.e. to develop strategies which can eliminate only the damaged (pre-malignant) or malignant cells without harming normal CNS tissue [Mukhtar and Ahmad, 1999].

Neuroblastoma (NB) is the most common pediatric extracraneal tumor and its origin has been clearly associated to the development of the sympathetic Nervous System [De Preter et al., 2006]. NB accounts for approximately 15% of pediatric cancer deaths with an estimated incidence of 1 per 7000 births in the USA [Hiyama et al., 2008]. Histologically, NB is mainly composed by neuroblasts at different stages of differentiation, and a variable amount of Schwannian-like stroma [Shimada et al., 2001]. This embryonal cancer of postganglionic sympathetic Nervous System arises from adrenal gland and less frequently metastasizes in other places such as chest, neck, lymph nodes, pelvis, liver, and bone. The prognosis is variable and depends on several factors. NB is characterized by its intriguing clinical behaviors that include spontaneous differentiation and regression, maturation into benign ganglioneuroma, and deadly metastatic tumor. Despite aggressive conventional treatments and diagnosis techniques in neurosurgery, the survival rate for patients with NB remains poor. The majority of children older than 1 year of age with tumor in advanced stage die from progressive disease, while only 40% of children over 4 years old with NB survive for 5 years, emphasizing the urgent need for the development of innovative therapeutic strategies for treatment of malignant NB [Ogawa et al., 2011; Roy Choudhury et al., 2012].

One of the first studies showing the antiproliferative effect of Quer in Nervous System tumors was published in 1983, using a mouse NB and glioma hybrid cell model. In this study Quer inhibited both cell proliferation and K^+ current with effective doses inducing half-maximum effects of 10 μM and 70 μM respectively [Rouzaire-Dubois et al., 1993]. Since them, several reports have been published, reinforcing the potential of Quer as a drug against these tumor types. Some of these works are listed in the Table 4, together with the main mechanisms of action. It is important to note that these data are all obtained *in vitro*, and until now, *in vivo* studies concerning Nervous System tumor and Quer was not reported.

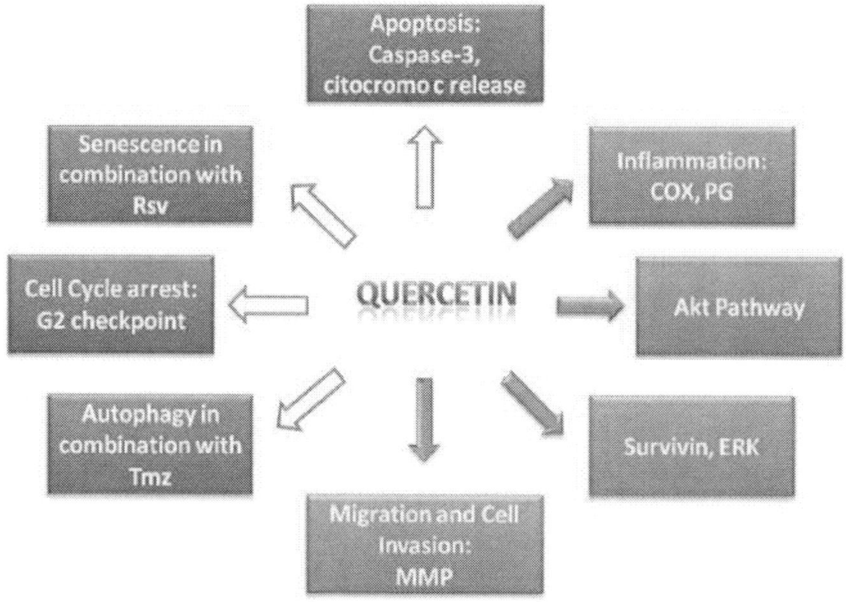

Figure 3. Selection of some antitumoral effects of Quer on Nervous System studies. Filled arrows indicate the events that are inhibited by Quer and empty arrows indicate the events that are activated by Quer. For more details see the text and the table 3.

Two decades of molecular studies have identified important genetic events in human Glioblastomas, including inactivation of the p53 and retinoblastoma tumour suppressor pathways, dysregulation of growth factor signalling via amplification and mutational activation of receptor tyrosine kinase (RTK) genes and the activation of the phosphatidylinositol-3-OH kinase (PI(3)K) pathway [Furnari et al., 2007; Cancer Genome Atlas Network, 2008]. Quer was initially identified as a PI3K inhibitor, being used further to design the synthetic compound LY294002, a widely used PI3K inhibitor [Vlahos et al., 1994]. Several reports have described the effect of Quer in decreasing AKT phosphorylation, a downstream target of these receptors (Table 4), in Nervous System tumors. Although not yet demonstrated in gliomas, the ability of Quer in increased p53 expression and/or phosphorylation has been demonstrated in other tumors [Xavier et al., 2011; Seo et al., 2011; Vidya et al., 2010].

CONCLUSION

In this review we discussed several aspects regarding the beneficial health effects of Quer. This molecule has emerged as an attractive compound to treat or prevent several diseases, including cancer. However, as discussed here, the most part of the results indicating the beneficial effect of Quer were obtained *in vitro*. In this view, further investigations concerning Quer metabolism, bioavailability, mechanism of action and *in vivo* effects should be done to better understand the effects and the risk of the intake of this flavonoid. We hope that the studies that are in progress elucidate those aspects to, perhaps, culminate with the regular use of Quer (or related compound) in human disease.

REFERENCES

Abrahamse, S. L., Kloots, W. J., Van Amelsvoort, J. M. M. (2005). Absorption, distribution, and secretion of epicatechin and quercetin in the rat. *Nutri. Res.*, 25 (3), 305–317.

Ahn, J., Lee, H., Kim, S., Park, J., Ha, T. (2008). The anti-obesity effect of quercetin is mediated by the AMPK and MAPK signaling pathways. *Biochem. Biophys. Res. Commun.*, 373(4), 545-549.

Annapurna, A., Reddy, C. S., Akondi, R. B., Rao, S. R. (2009). Cardioprotective actions of two bioflavonoids *J. Pharm. Pharmacol.*, 61(10*)*, 1365-1374.

Avgeropoulos, N. G., Batchelor, T. T. (1999). New treatment strategies for malignant gliomas. *Oncologist*, 4, 209–224.

Avci, C. B., Yilmaz, S., Dogan, Z. O., Saydam, G., Dodurga, Y., Ekiz, H. A., Kartal, M., Sahin, F., Baran, Y., Gunduz, C. (2011). Quercetin-induced apoptosis involves increased hTERT enzyme activity of leukemic cells. *Hematology,* 16(5), 303-307.

Boots, A. W., Haenen, G. R., Bast, A. (2008). Health effects of quercetin: from antioxidant to nutraceutical. *Eur J. Pharmacol,* 585, 325–337.

Borska, S., Drag-Zalesinska, M., Wysocka, T., Sopel, M., Dumanska, M., Zabel, M., Dziegiel, P. (2010). Antiproliferative and pro-apoptotic effects of quercetin on human pancreatic carcinoma cell lines EPP85-181P and EPP85-181RDB. *Folia Histochem. Cytobiol.,* 48(2*)*, 222-229.

Braganhol, E., Tamajusuku, A. S., Bernardi, A., Wink, M. R., Battastini, A. M. (2007). Ecto-5'-nucleotidase/CD73 inhibition *Biochim. Biophys. Acta,* 770(9), 1352-1359.

Braganhol, E., Zamin, L. L., Canedo, A. D., Horn, F., Tamajusuku, A. S., Wink, M. R., Salbego, C., Battastini, A. M. (2006). Antiproliferative effect of quercetin in the human U138MG glioma cell line. *Anticancer Drugs,* 17(6), 663-671.

Bieger, J., Cermak, R., Blank, R., de Boer, V. C., Hollman, P. C., Kamphues, J., Wolffram, S. (2008). Tissue distribution of quercetin in pigs after long-term dietary supplementation. *J. Nutr.,* 138(8*)*, 1417-1420.

Bravo, L. B. (1998). Polyphenols: chemistry, dietary sources, metabolism, and nutritional significance. *Nutr. Rev.,* 56, 317–333.

Cancer Genome Atlas Research Network. (2008). Comprehensive genomic characterization defines human glioblastoma genes and core pathways. *Nature,* 455(7216*)*, 1061-1068.

Careri, M., Corradini, C., Elviri, L., Nicoletti, I., Zagnoni, I. (2003). Direct HPLC Analysis of Quercetin and trans-Resveratrol in Red Wine, Grape, and Winemaking Byproducts. *J. Agric. Food Chem.,* 51, 5226- 5231.

Chang, Y. F., Hsu, Y. C., Hung, H. F., Lee, H. J., Lui, W. Y., Chi, C. W., Wang, J. J. (2009). Quercetin induces oxidative stress and potentiates the apoptotic action of 2-methoxyestradiol in human hepatoma cells. *Nutr. Cancer,* 61(5), 735-745.

Chen, W., Wang, X., Zhuang, J., Zhang, L., Lin, Y. (2007). Induction of death receptor 5 and suppression of survivin contribute to sensitization of TRAIL-induced cytotoxicity by quercetin in non-small cell lung cancer cells. *Carcinogenesis,* 28(10), 2114-2121.

Chiu, W. T., Shen, S. C., Chow, J. M., Lin, C. W., Shia, L. T., Chen, Y. C. (2010). Contribution of reactive oxygen species to migration/invasion of human glioblastoma cells U87 via ERK-dependent COX-2/PGE(2) activation. *Neurobiol. Dis.,* 37(1), 118-129.

Chien, S. Y., Wu, Y. C., Chung, J. G., Yang, J. S., Lu, H. F., Tsou, M. F., Wood, W. G., Kuo, S. J., Chen, D. R. (2009). Quercetin-induced apoptosis acts through mitochondrial- and caspase-3-dependent pathways in human breast cancer MDA-MB-231 cells. *Hum. Exp. Toxicol.* 28(8), 493-503.

Choi, E. J., Bae, S. M., Ahn, W. S. (2008). Antiproliferative effects of quercetin through cell cycle arrest and apoptosis in human breast cancer MDA-MB-453 cells. *Arch. Pharm. Res.,* 31(10), 1281-1285.

Chou, C. C., Yang, J. S., Lu, H. F., Ip, S. W., Lo, C., Wu, C. C., Lin, J. P., Tang, N. Y., Chung, J. G., Chou, M. J., Teng, Y. H., Chen, D. R. (2010). Quercetin-mediated cell cycle arrest and apoptosis involving activation of a caspase cascade through the mitochondrial pathway in human breast cancer MCF-7 cells. *Arch. Pharm. Res.,* 33(8), 1181-1191.

Chuang, C. C., Martinez, K., Xie, G., Kennedy, A., Bumrungpert, A., Overman, A., Jia, W., McIntosh, M. K. (2010). Quercetin is equally or more effective than resveratrol in attenuating tumor necrosis factor-alpha-mediated inflammation and insulin resistance in primary human adipocytes. *Am. J. Clin. Nutr.,* 92, 1511-1521.

Croft, K. D. (1998). The chemistry and biological effects of flavonoids and phenolic acids. *Ann. NY Acad. Sci.,* 854, 435–442.

Day, A. J., Mellon, F. A., Barron, D., Sarrazin, G., Morgan, M. R. A., Williamson, G. (2001). Human metabolism of dietary flavonoids; identification of plasma metabolites of quercetin. *Free Radic Res.*, 212 941–952.

De Boer, V. C., Dihal, A. A., Van der Woude, H., Arts, I. C., Wolffram, S., Alink, G. M., Rietjens, I. M., Keijer, J., Hollman, P. C. (2005). Tissue distribution of quercetin in rats and pigs. *J. Nutr.*, 135 (7), 1718–1725.

De Preter, K., Vandesompele, J., Heimann, P., Yigit, N., Beckman, S., Schramm, A., Eggert, A., Stallings, R. L., Benoit, Y., Renard, M., De Paepe, A., Laureys, G., Påhlman, S. Speleman, F. (2006). Human fetal neuroblast and neuroblastoma transcriptome analysis confirms neuroblast origin and highlights neuroblastoma candidate genes. *Genome Biol.,* 7, R84.

De Vries, J. H., Hollman, P. C., Meyboom, S., Buysman, M. N., Zock, P. L., Van Staveren, W. A., Katan, M. B. (1998). Plasma concentrations and urinary excretion of the antioxidant flavonols quercetin and kaempferol as biomarkers for dietary intake. *Am. J. Clin. Nutr.,* 68, 60–65.

Dihal, A. A., Woutersen, R. A., Van Ommen, B., Rietjens, I. M., Stierum, R. H. (2006). Modulatory effects of quercetin on proliferation and differentiation of the human colorectal cell line Caco-2. *Cancer Lett,,* 238, 248-259.

Doll, R., Peto, R. (1981). The causes of cancer: quantitative estimates of avoidable risks of cancer in the United States today. *J. Natl. Cancer Inst.,* 66, 1191–1308.

Du, G., Lin, H., Wang, M., Zhang, S., Wu, X., Lu, L., Ji, L., Yu, L. (2010). Quercetin greatly improved therapeutic index of doxorubicin against 4T1 breast cancer by its opposing effects on HIF-1α in tumor and normal cells. *Cancer Chemother. Pharmacol.,* 65(2*),* 277-287.

Edwards, R. L., Lyon, T., Litwin, S. E., Rabovsky, A., Symons, J. D., Jalili, T. (2007). Quercetin reduces blood pressure in hypertensive subjects. *J. Nutr.,* 137(11), 2405-2411.

Egert, S., Wolffram, S., Bosy-Westphal, A., Boesch-Saadatmandi, C., Wagner, A. E., Frank, J., Rimbach, G., Mueller, M. J. (2008). Daily quercetin *J. Nutr.,* 138(9*),* 1615-21.

Fang, X. K., Gao, J., Zhu, D. N. (2008). Kaempferol and quercetin isolated from Euonymus alatus improve glucose uptake of 3T3-L1 cells without adipogenesis activity. *Life Sci.,* 82, 615–622.

Ferrer, P., Asensi, M., Segarra, R., Ortega, A., Benlloch, M., Obrador, E., Varea, M. T., Asensio, G., Jordá, L., Estrela, J. M. (2005). Association between pterostilbene and quercetin inhibits metastatic activity of B16 melanoma. *Neoplasia,* 7(1), 37-47.

Furnari, F. B., Fenton, T., Bachoo, R. M., Mukasa, A., Stommel, J. M., Stegh, A., Hahn, W. C., Ligon, K. L., Louis, D. N., Brennan, C., Chin, L., DePinho, R. A., Cavenee, W. K. (2007). Malignant astrocytic glioma: genetics, biology, and paths to treatment. *Genes Dev.,* 21, 2683–2710.

Gee, J. M., Hara, H., Johnson, I. T. (2002). Suppression of intestinal crypt cell proliferation and aberrant crypt foci by dietary quercetin in rats. *Nutr. Cancer,* 43, 193-201.

Goncalves, P., Araujo, J. R., Martel, F. (2010). Butyrate uptake and effect on proliferation, differentiation, viability and apoptosis of Caco-2 cells: influence of polyphenols. *FASEB J.,* 24, 965-910.

Granado-Serrano, A. B., Martín, M. A., Bravo, L., Goya, L., Ramos, S. (2006). Quercetin induces apoptosis via caspase activation, regulation of Bcl-2, and inhibition of PI-3-

kinase/Akt and ERK pathways in a human hepatoma cell line (HepG2). *J. Nutr.,* 136(11*)*, 2715-2721.

Griffiths, L. A. (1982). Mammalian metabolism of flavonoids. In: Harborne, J. B., Mabry, T. (Eds.), The Flavonoids: Advances in Research. Chapman and Hall, London, pp. 681–718.

Gugler, R., Leschik, M., Dengler, H. J. (1975). Disposition of quercetin in man after single oral and intravenous doses. *Eur. J. Clin. Pharmacol.,* 9, 229–234.

Gulati, N., Laudet, B., Zohrabian, V. M., Murali, R., Jhanwar-Uniyal, M. (2006). The antiproliferative effect of Quercetin in cancer cells is mediated via inhibition of the PI3K-Akt/PKB pathway. *Anticancer Res.,* 26(2A), 1177-1181.

Haghi, G., Hatami, A. (2010). Simultaneous Quantification of Flavonoids and Phenolic Acids in Plant Materials by a Newly Developed Isocratic High-Performance Liquid Chromatography Approach. *J. Agric. Food Chem.,* 58, 10812–10816.

Harwood, M., Danielewska-Nikiel, B., Borzelleca, J. F., Flamm, G. W., Williams, G. M., Lines, T. C. (2007). A critical review of the data related to the safety of quercetin and lack of evidence of *in vivo* toxicity, including lack of genotoxic/carcinogenic properties. *Food Chem. Toxicol.,* 45, 2179–2205.

Havsteen, B. (1983). Flavonoids, a class of natural products of high pharmacological potency. *Biochem. Pharmacol.,* 32, 1141–1148.

Hertog, M. G., Hollman, P. C. H., Kahn, M. B. (1992). Content of Potentially Anticarcinogenic Flavonoids of 28 Vegetables and Fruits Commonly Consumed in The Netherlands. *J. A. Food Chem.*, 40, 2379-2383.

Hertog, M. G., Feskens, E. J., Hollman, P. C., Katan, M. B., Kromhout, D. (1993). Dietary antioxidant flavonoids and risk of coronary heart disease: The Zutphen elderly study. *Lancet,* 342, 1007–1011.

Hertog, M. G., Kromhout, D., Aravanis, C., Blackburn, H., Buzina, R., Fidanza, F., Giampaoli, S., Jansen, A., Menotti, A., Nedeljkovic, S., Pekkarinen, M., Simic, B. S., Toshima, H., Feskens, E. J.M., Hollman, P. C. H., Katan, M. B. (1995). Flavonoid intake and long-term risk of coronary heart disease and cancer in the seven countries study. *Arch. Intern. Med.,* 155, 381–386.

Hiyama, E., Iehara, T., Sugimoto, T., Fukuzawa, M., Hayashi, Y., Sasaki, F., Sugiyama, M., Kondo, S., Yoneda, A., Yamaoka, H., Tajiri, T., Akazawa, K., Ohtaki, M. (2008). Effectiveness of screening for neuroblastoma at 6 months of age: a retrospective population-based cohort study. *Lancet,* 371(9619*)*, 1173–1180.

Huang, H. C., Lin, C. L., Lin, J. K. (2011). 1,2,3,4,6-penta-O-galloyl-β-D-glucose, quercetin, curcumin and lycopene induce cell-cycle arrest in MDA-MB-231 and BT474 cells through downregulation of Skp2 protein. *J. Agric. Food Chem.,* 59(12*)*, 6765-6775.

Huang, S. L., Hsu, C. L., Yen, G. C. (2006). Growth inhibitory effect of quercetin on SW 872 human liposarcoma cells. *Life Sci.,* 79(2*)*, 203-209.

Hung, H. (2007). Dietary quercetin inhibits proliferation of lung carcinoma cells. *Forum Nutr.,* 60, 146-157.

Huxley, R. R., Neil, H. A. (2003). The relation between dietary flavonol intake and coronary heart disease mortality: a meta-analysis of prospective cohort studies. *Eur. J. Clin. Nutr.,* 57, 904–908.

Indap, M. A., Bhosle, S. C., Shinde, A. D., Barkume, M. S., Ingle, A. D. (2006). Tumour response to quercetin, a bioflavonoid with some promises in therapies. *Indian J. Pharm. Sci.,* 68, 570-574.

Ishizawa, K., Yoshizumi, M., Kawai, Y., Terao, J., Kihira, Y., Ikeda, Y., Tomita, S., Minakuchi, K., Tsuchiya, K., Tamaki, T. (2011). Pharmacology in health *J. Pharmacol. Sci., 115(4),* 466-470.

Jakubowicz-Gil, J., Langner, E., Wertel, I., Piersiak, T., Rzeski, W. (2010). Temozolomide, quercetin and cell death in the MOGGCCM astrocytoma cell line. *Chem. Biol. Interact., 188(1),* 190-203.

Jakubowicz-Gil, J., Rzeski, W., Zdzisińska, B., Piersiak, T., Weiksza, K., Glowniak, K., Gawron, A. (2008). Different sensitivity *Acta Neurobiol. Exp.,* 68(4), 463-476.

Johannot, L., Somerset, S. M. (2006). Age-related variations in flavonoid intake and sources in the Australian population. *Public Health Nutr..* 9, 1045–1054.

Johnson, I. T. (2002). Anticarcinogenic effects of diet-related apoptosis in the colorectal mucosa. *Food Chem. Toxicol.,* 40, 1171-1178.

Joint-Committee-Nomenclature-ASBC-AIN, 1950. Term ''vitamin P'' recommended to be discontinued. *Science,* 112, 268.

Jones, E., Hughes, R. E. (1982). Quercetin, flavonoids and the life-span of mice. *Exp. Geronto.l,* 17, 213–217.

Kaindl, U., Eyberg, I., Rohr-Udilova, N., Heinzle, C., Marian, B. (2008). The dietary antioxidants resveratrol and quercetin protect cells from exogenous pro-oxidative damage. *Food Chem. Toxicol.,* 46, 1320-1326.

Keli, S. O., Hertog, M. G., Feskens, E. J., Kromhout, D. (1996). Dietary flavonoids, antioxidant vitamins, and incidence of stroke: the Zutphen study. *Arch. Intern. Med.,* 156, 637–642.

Kim, E. J., Choi, C. H., Park, J. Y., Kang, S. K., Kim, Y. K. (2008). Underlying mechanism of quercetin *Neurochem. Res.*, 33(6), 971-979.

Kim, W. K., Bang, M. H., Kim, E. S., Kang, N. E., Jung, K. C., Cho, H. J., Park, J. H. (2005). Quercetin decreases the expression of ErbB2 and ErbB3 proteins in HT-29 human colon cancer cells. *J. Nutr. Biochem.,* 16, 155-162.

Kimira, M., Arai, Y., Shimoi, K., Watanabe, S. (1998). Japanese intake of flavonoids and isoflavonoids from foods. *J. Epidemiol.,* 8, 168–175.

Knekt, P., Jarvinen, R., Seppanen, R., Heliovaara, M., Teppo, L., Pukkala, E., Aromaa, A. (1997). Dietary intake of flavonoids and the risk of lung cancer and other malignant neoplasms. *Am. J. Epidemiol.,* 146, 223–230.

Kuhnau, J. (1976). The flavonoids. A class of semi-essential food components: their role in human nutrition. *World Rev. Nutr. Diet,* 24, 117–191.

Kuntz, S., Wenzel, U., Daniel, H. (1999). Comparative analysis of the effects of flavonoids on proliferation, cytotoxicity, and apoptosis in human colon cancer cell lines. *Eur. J. Nutr.,* 38, 133-142.

Kuo, S. M. (1996). Antiproliferative potency of structurally distinct dietary flavonoids on human colon cancer cells. *Cancer Lett.,* 110, 41-48.

Labbé, D., Provençal, M., Lamy, S., Boivin, D., Gingras, D., Béliveau, R. (2009). The flavonols quercetin, kaempferol, and myricetin inhibit hepatocyte growth factor-induced medulloblastoma cell migration. *J. Nutr.,* 139(4), 646-652.

Lee, D. H., Szczepanski, M., Lee, Y. J. (2008). Role of Bax in quercetin *Biochem. Pharmacol.,* 75(12), 2345-2355.

Lee, K. M., Hwang, M. K., Lee, D. E., Lee, K. W., Lee, H. J. (2010). Protective effect of quercetin against arsenite-induced COX-2 expression by targeting PI3K in rat liver epithelial cells. *J. Agric. Food Chem.,* 58, 5815-5820.

Lee, K. W., Bode, A. M., Dong, Z. (2011)a. Molecular targets of phytochemicals for cancer prevention. *Nat. Rev. Cancer,* 11, 211–218.

Lee, L. T., Huang, Y. T., Hwang, J. J., Lee, P. P., Ke, F. C., Nair, M. P., Kanadaswam, C., Lee, M. T. (2002). Blockade of the epidermal growth factor receptor tyrosine kinase activity by quercetin and luteolin leads to growth inhibition and apoptosis of pancreatic tumor cells. *Anticancer Res.*, 22(3*),* 1615-1627.

Lee, W. J., Chen, Y. R., Tseng, T. H. (2011)b. Quercetin induces FasL-related apoptosis, in part, through promotion of histone H3 acetylation in human leukemia HL-60 cells. *Oncol. Rep.* 25(2), 583-591.

Liang, W., Li, X., Li, C., Liao, L., Gao, B., Gan, H., Yang, Z., Liao, L., Chen, X. (2011). Quercetin-mediated apoptosis via activation of the mitochondrial-dependent pathway in MG-63 osteosarcoma cells. *Mol. Med. Report,* 4(5), 1017-1023.

Lin, C. W., Hou, W. C., Shen, S. C., Juan, S. H., Ko, C. H., Wang, L. M., Chen, Y. C. (2008). Quercetin inhibition *Carcinogenesis,* 29(9),1807-1815.

Lin, J., Zhang, S. M., Wu, K., Willett, W. C., Fuchs, C. S., Giovannucci, E. (2006). Flavonoid intake and colorectal cancer risk in men and women. *Am. J. Epidemiol.,* 164, 644–651.

Mackraj, I., Govender, T., Ramesar, S. (2008). The antihypertensive effects of quercetin in a salt-sensitive model of hypertension. *J. Cardiovasc. Pharmacol.,* 51, 239–245.

Manach, C., Morand, C., Texier, O., Favier, M. L., Agullo, G., Demigne, C., Regerat, F., Remesy, C. (1995). Quercetin metabolites in plasma of rats fed diets containing rutin or quercetin. *J. Nutr.,* 125, 1911–1922.

McAnlis, G. T., Mceneny, J., Pearce, J., Young, I. S. (1999). Absorption and antioxidant effects of quercetin from onions, in man. *Eur. J. Clin. Nutr.,* 53, 92–96.

Mertens-Talcott, S. U., Percival, S. S. (2005). Ellagic acid and quercetin interact synergistically with resveratrol in the induction of apoptosis and cause transient cell cycle arrest in human leukemia cells. *Cancer Lett.,* 218, 141-151.

Middleton, E. J., Kandaswami, C. (1993). The impact of plant flavonoids on mammalian biology: implications for immunity, inflammation and cancer. In: Harborne, J. B. (Ed.), *The flavonoids: advances in research since* 1986. Chapman and Hall, London, pp. 619–652.

Mu, C., Jia, P., Yan, Z., Liu, X., Li, X., Liu, H. (2007). Quercetin induces cell cycle G1 arrest through elevating Cdk inhibitors p21 and p27 in human hepatoma cell line (HepG2). *Methods Find Exp. Clin. Pharmacol.,* 29(3), 179-183.

Mukhtar, H., Ahmad, N. (1999). Cancer chemoprevention: future holds in multiple agents: contemporary issues in toxicology. *Toxicol. Appl. Pharmacol.,* 158, 207–210.

Murakami, A., Ashida, H., Terao, J. (2008). Multitargeted cancer prevention by quercetin. *Cancer Letters,* 269, 315–325.

Murota, K., Shimizu, S., Chujo, H., Moon, J. H., Terao, J. (2000). Efficiency of absorption and metabolic conversion of quercetin and its glucosides in human intestinal cell line Caco-2. *Arch. Biochem. Biophys.*, 384, 391–397.

Murota K., Terao J. (2005). Quercetin appears in the lymph of unsaturated rats at its phase II metabolites after administered into the stomach. *FEBS Lett.,* 579, 5343– 5346.

Murota, K., Terao, J. (2003). Antioxidative flavonoid quercetin: implication of its intestinal absorption and metabolism. *Arch. Biochem. Biophys.,* 417 (1), 12–17.

Nakamura, Y., Ishimitsu, S., Tonogai, Y. (2000). Effects of quercetin and rutin on serum and hepatic lipid concentrations, fecal steroid excretion and serum antioxidant properties. *J. Health. Sci.,* 46, 229–240.

Niu, G., Yin, S., Xie, S., Li, Y., Nie, D., Ma, L., Wang, X., Wu, Y. (2011). Quercetin induces apoptosis by activating caspase-3 and regulating Bcl-2 and cyclooxygenase-2 pathways in human HL-60 cells. *Acta Biochim. Biophys.,* 43(1*)*, 30-37.

Nguyen, T. T., Tran, E., Nguyen, T. H., Do, P. T., Huynh, T. H., Huynh, H. (2004). The role of activated MEK-ERK pathway in quercetin-induced growth inhibition and apoptosis in A549 lung cancer cells. *Carcinogenesis,* 25(5), 647-659.

Ogawa, S., Takita, J., Sanada, M., Hayashi, Y. (2011). Oncogenic mutations of ALK in neuroblastoma. *Cancer Sci.*, 102(2*)*, 302–308.

Okamoto, T. (2005). Safety of quercetin for clinical application. *Int. J. Mol. Med.*, 16, 275–278.

Ossola, B., Kääriäinen, T. M., Männistö, P. T. (2009). The multiple faces of quercetin in neuroprotection. *Expert Opin. Drug Saf.,* 8(4), 397-409.

Pamukcu, A. M., Yalciner, S., Hatcher, J. F., Bryan, G. T. (1980). Quercetin, a rat intestinal and bladder carcinogen present in bracken fern (Pteridium aquilinum). *Cancer Res.,* 40, 3468-3472.

Psahoulia, F. H., Moumtzi, S., Roberts, M. L., Sasazuki, T., Shirasawa, S., Pintzas, A. (2007). Quercetin mediates preferential degradation of oncogenic Ras and causes autophagy in Ha-RAS–transformed human colon cells. *Carcinogenesis,* 28, 1021-1031.

Park, M. H., Min, D. S. (2011). Quercetin-induced downregulation of phospholipase D1 inhibits proliferation *Biochem. Biophys. Res. Commun.,* 412, 710–715.

Perez-Vizcaino, F., Duarte, J., Jimenez, R., Santos-Buelga, C., Osuna, A. (2009). Antihypertensive effects of the flavonoid quercetin. *Pharmacol. Rep.,* 61(1), 67-75.

Ramos, S. (2008). Cancer chemoprevention and chemotherapy: dietary polyphenols and signaling pathways. *Mol. Nutr. Food Res.,* 52, 507-526.

Reddy, L., Odhav, B., Bhoola, K. D. (2003). Natural products for cancer prevention: a global perspective. *Pharmacol. Ther.*, 99, 1–13.

Rimm, E. C., Katan, M. B., Ascherio, A., Stampfer, M. J., Willett, W. C. (1996). Relation between intake of flavonoids and risk for coronary heart disease in male health professionals. *Ann. Int.Med.,* 125, 384-389.

Rivera, L., Moron, R., Sanchez, M., Zarzuelo, A., Galisteo, M.. (2008). Quercetin ameliorates metabolic syndrome and improves the inflammatory status in obese Zucker rats. *Obesity,* 16, 2081–2087.

Rosner, K., Röpke, C., Pless, V., Skovgaard, G. L. (2006). Late type apoptosis and apoptosis free lethal effect of quercetin in human melanoma. *Biosci. Biotechnol. Biochem.* 70(9*)*, 2169-2177.

Rouzaire-Dubois, B., Gérard, V., Dubois, J. M. (1993). Involvement of K+ channels in the quercetin-induced inhibition of neuroblastoma cell growth. *Pflugers. Arch.,* 423(3-4), 202-205.

Roy Choudhury, S., Karmakar, S., Banik, N. L., Ray, S. K. (2012). Targeting angiogenesis for controlling neuroblastoma. *J. Oncol.,* [Epub ahead of print].

Russo, G. L. (2007). Ins and outs of dietary phytochemicals in cancer chemoprevention. *Biochem. Pharmacol.,* 74, 533–544.

Russo, M., Spagnuolo, C., Tedesco, I., Bilotto, S., Russo, G. L. (2011). The flavonoid quercetin in disease prevention and therapy: Facts and fancies. *Biochem. Pharmacol.* [Epub ahead of print].

Rusznyak, S., Szent-Györgyi, A. (1936). Vitamin P: flavonols as vitamins. *Nature,* 138, 27–29.

Russell, D. S., Rubinstein, L. J. Pathology of Tumours of the Nervous System. Baltimore: Williams and Wilkins, 1989.

Sarkar, C., Jain, A., Suri, V. (2009). Current concepts in the pathology *Indian J. Cancer,* 46(2), 108-119.

Scalbert, A., Williamson, G. (2000). Dietary intake and bioavailability of polyphenols. *J. Nutr.,* 130, 2073S–2085S.

Schlachterman, A., Valle, F., Wall, K. M., Azios, N. G., Castillo, L., Morell, L., Washington, A. V., Cubano, L. A., Dharmawardhane, S. F. (2008). Combined resveratrol *Transl. Oncol.,* 1(1), 19-27.

Seibert, H., Maser, E., Schweda, K., Seibert, S., Gülden, M. (2011). Cytoprotective activity against peroxide-induced oxidative damage and cytotoxicity of flavonoids in C6 rat glioma cells. *Food Chem. Toxicol.* 49(9), 2398-2407.

Sengupta, B., Sengupta, P. K. (2003). Binding of quercetin with human serum albumin: A critical spectroscopic study. *Biopolymers,* 72, 427– 434.

Senthilkumar, K., Arunkumar, R., Elumalai, P., Sharmila, G., Gunadharini, D. N., Banudevi, S., Krishnamoorthy, G., Benson, C. S., Arunakaran, J. (2011). Quercetin inhibits invasion, migration and signalling molecules involved in cell survival and proliferation of prostate cancer cell line (PC-3). *Cell Biochem. Funct.,* 29(2*),* 87-95.

Senthilkumar, K., Elumalai, P., Arunkumar, R., Banudevi, S., Gunadharini, N. D., Sharmila, G., Selvakumar, K., Arunakaran, J. (2010). Quercetin regulates insulin like growth factor signaling and induces intrinsic and extrinsic pathway mediated apoptosis in androgen independent prostate cancer cells (PC-3). *Mol. Cell Biochem.,* 344(1-2),173-184.

Seo, H. S., Ju, J. H., Jang, K., Shin, I. (2011). Induction of apoptotic cell death by phytoestrogens by up-regulating the levels of phospho-p53 and p21 in normal and malignant estrogen receptor α-negative breast cells. *Nutr. Res.,* 31(2), 139-146.

Shan, B. E., Wang, M. X., Li, R. Q. (2009). Quercetin inhibit human SW480 colon cancer growth in association with inhibition of cyclin D1 and surviving expression through Wnt/beta-catenin signaling pathway. *Cancer Invest.,* 27, 604-612.

Sharaf, M., El-Ansari, M. A., Saleh, N. A. M. (2000) Quercetin triglycoside from Capparis. *Fitoterapia,* 71, 46–49.

Sharaf, M., El-Ansari, M. A., Saleh, N. A. M. (1997). Flavonoids of four cleome and three Capparis species. *Biochem. Syst. Ecol.,* 25, 161–166.

Shimada H., Umehara S., Monobe Y., Hachitanda Y., Nakagawa A., Goto S., Gerbing R. B., Stram D. O., Lukens J. N., Matthay K. K., (2001). International neuroblastoma pathology classification for prognostic evaluation of patients with peripheral neuroblastic tumors: a report from the Children's Cancer Group. *Cancer,* 92, 2451–2461.

Siegelin, M. D., Reuss, D. E., Habel, A., Rami, A., Von Deimling, A. (2009). Quercetin promotes degradation of survivin and thereby enhances death-receptor-mediated apoptosis in glioma cells. *Neuro Oncol.*, 11(2), 122-131.

Singh, B., Mense, S.M., Bhat, N.K., Putty, S., Guthiel, W.A., Remotti, F., Bhat, H. K. (2010). Dietary quercetin exacerbates the development of estrogen-induced breast tumors in female ACI rats. *Toxicol Appl. Pharmacol., 247(2)*, 83-90.

Spanos, G. A., Wrolstad, R. E. (1992). Phenolics of apple, pear and white grape juices and their changes with processing and storage. *J. A. Food Chem.,* 40, 1478-1487.

Soobrattee, M. A., Bahorun, T., Aruoma, O. I. (2006). Chemopreventive actions of polyphenolic compounds in cancer. *Biofactors, 27,* 19-35.

Suh, D. K., Lee, E. J., Kim, H. C., Kim, J. H. (2010). Induction of G(1)/S phase arrest and apoptosis by quercetin in human osteosarcoma cells. *Arch. Pharm. Res.,* 33(5), 781-785.

Surco-Laos, F., Cabello, J., Gómez-Orte, E., González-Manzano, S., González-Paramás, A. M., Santos-Buelga, C., Dueñas, M. (2011). Effects of O-methylated metabolites of quercetin on oxidative stress, thermotolerance, lifespan and bioavailability on Caenorhabditis elegans. *Food Funct.,* 2(8), 445-456.

Surh, Y. J. (2003). Cancer chemoprevention with dietary phytochemicals. *Nat. Rev. Cancer.,* 3, 768–380.

Tanigawa, S., Fujii, M., Hou, D. X. (2008). Stabilization of p53 is involved in quercetin-induced cell cycle arrest and apoptosis in HepG2 cells. *Biosci. Biotechnol. Biochem.,* 72(3*)*, 797-804.

Thangasamy, T., Sittadjody, S., Mitchell, G. C., Mendoza, E. E., Radhakrishnan, V. M., Limesand, K. H., Burd, R. (2010). Quercetin abrogates chemoresistance in melanoma cells by modulating deltaNp73. *BMC Cancer,* 10, 282.

Theoharides, T. C., Alexandris, M., Kempuraj, D., Lytinas, M. (2001). Anti-inflammatory actions of flavonoids and structural requirements for new design. *Int. J. Immunopathol. Pharmacol.,* 14 (3), 119–127.

Tonn, J. C., Goldbrunner, R. (2003). Mechanisms of glioma cell invasion. *Acta Neurochir. Suppl.,* 88, 163–167.

Ueno, I., Kohno, M., Haraikawa, K., Hirono, I. (1984). Interaction between quercetin and superoxide radicals. Reduction of the quercetin mutagenicity. *J. Pharmacobiodyn., 7,* 798–803.

USDA, 2000. 1994-1996, 1998 Continuing Survey of Food Intakes by Individuals (CSFII) and Diet and Health Knowledge Survey (DHKS) (On CD-ROM). US Department of Agriculture (USDA), Riverdale, Maryland. [PB2000-500027]. Cited in MacRae and Mefferd (2006).

USDA Database for the Flavonoid Content of Selected Foods http://www.nal.usda.gov/fnic/ foodcomp/Data/Flav/ flav.pdf [Accessed on September, 12 2011].

Van der Woude, H., Boersma, M. G., Vervoort, J., Rietjens, I. M. (2004). Identification of 14 quercetin phase II mono- and mixed conjugates and their formation by rat and human phase II in vitro model systems. *Chem. Res. Toxicol.,* 17, 1520-1530.

Van der Woude, H., Gliszczynska-Swiglo, A., Struijs, K., Smeets, A., Alink, G. M., Rietjens, I. M. (2003). Biphasic modulation of cell proliferation by quercetin at concentrations physiologically relevant in humans. *Cancer Lett.,* 200, 41-47.

Van Erk, M. J., Roepman, P., Van der Lende, T. R., Stierum, R. H., Aarts, J. M., Van Bladeren, P. J, Van Ommen, B. (2005). Integrated assessment by multiple gene expression analysis of quercetin bioactivity on anticancer-related mechanisms in colon cancer cells in vitro. *Eur. J. Nutr.,* 44, 143-156.

Vargas, A. D., Soto, H. M., Gonzalez, H. V. A., Engleman, E. M., Martinez, G. A. (2006). Kinetics of accumulation and distribution of flavonoids in guava (Psiduim guajava). *Agrociencia,* 40, 109–115.

Vlahos, C. J., Matter, W. F., Hui, K. Y., and Brown, R. F. (1994). A specific inhibitor of phosphatidylinositol 3-kinase, 2-(4-Morpholinyl)-8- phenyl-4H-1-benzopyran-4-one (LY294002). *J. Biol. Chem.,* 269, 5241–5248.

Verschoyle, R. D., Steward, W. P., Gescher, A. J. (2007). Putative cancer chemopreventive agents of dietary origin-how safe are they? *Nutr. Cancer* 59(2),152-162.

Vidya Priyadarsini, R., Senthil Murugan, R., Maitreyi, S., Ramalingam, K., Karunagaran, D., Nagini, S. (2010). The flavonoid quercetin induces cell cycle arrest and mitochondria-mediated apoptosis in human cervical cancer (HeLa) cells through p53 induction and NF-κB inhibition. *Eur. J. Pharmacol.,* 649(1-3), 84-91.

Xavier, C. P., Lima, C. F., Rohde, M., Pereira-Wilson, C. (2011). Quercetin enhances 5-fluorouracil-induced apoptosis in MSI colorectal cancer cells through p53 modulation. *Cancer Chemother. Pharmacol.* [Epub ahead of print]

Xiao, X., Shi, D., Liu, L., Wang, J., Xie, X., Kang, T., Deng, W. (2011). Quercetin Suppresses Cyclooxygenase-2 Expression and Angiogenesis through Inactivation of P300 Signaling. *PLoS One,* 6(8), e22934.

Xie, X., Yin, J., Jia, Q., Wang, J., Zou, C., Brewer, K. J., Colombo, C., Wang, Y., Huang, G., Shen, J. (2011). Quercetin induces apoptosis in the methotrexate-resistant osteosarcoma cell line U2-OS/MTX300 via mitochondrial dysfunction and dephosphorylation of Akt. *Oncol. Rep.,* 26(3), 687-693.

Yang, K., Lamprecht, S. A., Liu, Y., Shinozaki, H., Fan, K., Leung, D., Newmark, H., Steele, V. E., Kelloff, G. J., Lipkin, M. (2000). Chemoprevention studies of the flavonoids quercetin and rutin in normal and azoxymethane-treated mouse colon. *Carcinogenesis,* 21, 1655-1660.

Yang, J. H., Hsia, T. C., Kuo, H. M., Chao, P. D., Chou, C. C., Wei, Y. H., Chung, J. G. (2006). Inhibition of lung cancer cell growth by quercetin glucuronides via G2/M arrest and induction of apoptosis. *Drug. Metab. Dispos.,* 34(2), 296-304.

Yang, L., Li, X. F., Gao, L., Zhang, Y. O., Cai, G. P. (2011) Suppressive Effects of Quercetin-3-O-(6″-Feruloyl)-β-D-Galactopyranoside on Adipogenesis in 3T3-L1 Preadipocytes Through Down-regulation of PPARγ and C/EBPα Expression. *Phytother. Res*. [Epub ahead of print].

Yeh, S. L., Yeh, C. L., Chan, S. T., Chuang, C. H. (2011). Plasma rich in quercetin metabolites induces G2/M arrest by upregulating PPAR-γ expression in human A549 lung cancer cells. *Planta Med.,* 77(10), 992-998.

Walle, T., Walle, U. K., Halushka, P. V. (2001). Carbon dioxide is the major metabolite of quercetin in humans. *J. Nutr.,* 131, 2648–2652.

Wang, F. M., Yao, T. W., Zeng, S. (2003). Determination of quercetin and kaempferol in human urine after orally administrated tablet of Ginkgo biloba extract by HPLC. *J. Pharm. Biomed. Anal.*, 33, 317–321.

Wiczkowski, W., Nemeth, K., Bucinski, A., Piskula, M. K. (2003). Bioavailability of quercetin from flesh scales and dry skin of onion in rats. *Pol. J. Food Nutr. Sci.,* 12, 95–99.

Williamson, G., Manach, C. (2005). Bioavailability and bioefficacy of polyphenols in humans. II. Review of 93 intervention studies. *Am. J. Clin. Nutr.*, 81, S243–S255.

Zamin, L. L., Filippi-Chiela, E. C., Dillenburg-Pilla, P., Horn, F., Salbego, C., and Lenz, G. (2009). Resveratrol and quercetin cooperate to induce senescence-like growth arrest in C6 rat glioma cells. *Cancer Sci., 100*, 1655-1662.

Zhang, L., Angst, E., Park, J. L., Moro, A., Dawson, D. W., Reber, H. A., Eibl, G., Hines, O. J., Go, V. L., Lu, Q. Y. (2010). Quercetin aglycone is bioavailable in murine pancreas and pancreatic xenografts. *J. Agric. Food Chem.,* 58(12*)*, 7252-7257.

Zhang, X. M., Chen, J., Xia, Y. G., Xu, Q. (2005). Apoptosis of murine melanoma B16-BL6 cells induced by quercetin targeting mitochondria, inhibiting expression of PKC-alpha and translocating PKC-delta. *Cancer Chemother. Pharmacol.,* 55(3), 251-262.

Zhou, W., Kallifatidis, G., Baumann, B., Rausch, V., Mattern, J., Gladkich, J., Giese, N., Moldenhauer, G., Wirth, T., Büchler, M. W., Salnikov, A. V., Herr, I. (2010). Dietary polyphenol quercetin targets pancreatic cancer stem cells. *Int. J. Oncol.,* 37(3*),* 551-561.

In: Quercetin
Editors: Taiki Chikamatsu and Yuudai Hida
ISBN: 978-1 61942- 057-1

Chapter 4

MULTIPOTENT BIOFLAVONOID QUERCETIN: MOLECULAR TARGETS AND MECHANISM OF ACTION AND NANOTECHNOLOGY APPLICATIONS IN CANCER, METABOLIC DISEASES AND AGING

***S. Bhaskaran*[1], *S. Sathyaseelan*[2] *and H. B. Nair*[1,*]**
[1]Southwest National Primate Research Center, Texas Biomedical Research Institute, San Antonio TX, US
[2]Barshop Institute, UT-Health Science Center at San Antonio TX, US

ABSTRACT

Quercetin, a plant-based secondary metabolite widely present in fruits and vegetables, is a polyphenol belonging to the class of flavonoids. Studies for the past several decades have identified the great potential of this bioflavonoid in the prevention and treatment of a wide range of diseases. The biological effects of quercetin includes antimicrobial properties; antioxidative capacity; anti-allergic and anti-inflammatory activities; blood vessel protection; antitumor properties; antidiabetic and antiaging effects, anticataract and antineurodegenerative capacity; and protection against hypertension and cardiovascular diseases. Quercetin exerts this wide spectrum of effects by targeting several proteins/enzymes that are implicated in disease progression. Because of its outstanding safety profile and its availability in highly purified forms, the clinical implications for quercetin are growing rapidly. Even though quercetin is the major bioflavonoid in the human diet, its bioavailability has been debated. Recent studies to improve its bioavailability by combining it with vitamins or encapsulating it as nanoparticles are promising. This review mainly focuses on the molecular targets of quercetin and the mechanisms by which quercetin exerts its biological effects in the prevention and treatment of cancer, metabolic diseases and aging.

* Author for correspondence: Hareesh B. Nair, Southwest National Primate Research Center, Texas Biomedical Research Institute, San Antonio TX 78227. Email: hnair@txbiomedgenetics.org,. Ph: 210-258-9515.

Introduction

Quercetin is a plant-based secondary metabolite that is abundant in fruits, leaves, vegetables and grains. The richest sources of quercetin are summarized in Table.1. Fruits and vegetables, particularly onions and apples, are the primary sources of naturally occurring dietary quercetin in the typical Western diet (Hertog et al. 1992, Day and Williamson 1999; Harnly et al. 2006). Black tea is also a rich dietary source of quercetin (Hertog et al. 1993, Sampson et al. 2002). In the United States, the average daily intake of all flavonoids from a normal mixed diet was estimated to be approximately 1g/day (Kuhnau 1976, Brown 1980), with flavonol glycosides, expressed as quercetin equivalents, consumed at levels of up to 100 mg/day (Brown 1980, Jones and Hughes 1982, Rimm et al. 1996, Sampson et al. 2002). Daily intake levels of quercetin as high as 200 to 500 mg have been reported in high-end consumers of fruits and vegetables (Jones and Hughes 1982). Numerous studies have demonstrated that quercetin protects against several diseases. The present review discusses the available data on quercetin that has an appreciable role in imminent therapy against cancer, diabetes, obesity and aging.

I. Quercetin and Cancer

Natural products have played a very significant role as recognized cancer chemotherapeutic agents, either in their naturally occurring or synthetically modified forms. The anticancer effects of quercetin are broad and different, targeting several levels of regulation in the processes of cellular growth and apoptosis. *In vitro* and *in vivo* studies have attempted to reveal quercetin's effect in cancer.

A. Quercetin (QT) has antiproliferative effect against cancer cells in vitro.

In vitro studies have demonstrated the antiproliferative effect QT has against multiple cancer cell lines by targeting different molecules. This effect has been demonstrated in the following: human bladder cancer cells (Larocca 1995, Ma 2006); estrogen receptor (ER) and progesterone receptor (PR) negative breast cancer cell line MDA-MB435 (Singhal 1995, So 1996); ER-PR-positive MCF-7 cell line (Miodini 1999, So 1997); HT29 and Caco-2 colon cancer cells (Agullo 1994, Kuo 1996); head and neck cancer cell line HTB43 (Kandaswami 1991); acute myeloid and lymphoid leukemia progenitor cells (Larocca 1991); ovarian cancer cell line OVCAR-3 (Luo 2008); and HeLa cells (Vidya Priyadarsini 2010)

QT targets different proteins/enzymes in these cell lines that are responsible for cell survival and proliferation. In MDA-MB435 cells, QT inhibits 1phosphatidylinositol-4-phosphate 5-kinase (PIP kinase), an enzyme crucial for the signal transduction pathway in cancer cells (Sighal 1994, Singhal 1995, So 1996). In the MCF-7 cell line QT down-regulates ER target genes (Miodini 1999, So 1997), while in ovarian cancer cell line OVCAR-3 QT inhibits expression of vascular endothelial growth factor (VEGF) (Luo 2008). In HeLa cells QT mediates activation of AMPK, down-regulates expression of heat shock protein 70 (HSP70) and increases the activity of caspase 3 (Jung 2010). In addition, QT mediates sustained epidermal growthfactorreceptor (EGFR) activation, increases the interaction between EGFR and Cbl, and induces the tyrosine phosphorylation of Cbl in HeLa cells (Jung 2010). QT also inhibits insulin-modulated phosphatidylinositol 3-kinase-Akt kinase activity to prevent thyroid cell growth (Giuliani 2008).

QT has potential uses in adjuvant chemotherapy in combination with other drugs because QT exhibits lower toxicity. QT sensitizes primary cells from chronic lymphocytic leukemia (CLL) to death receptor (DR) agonists (recombinant TNF-related-apoptosis-inducing ligand [rTRAIL] and anti-CD95) and to fludarabine, a widely used chemotherapeutic drug against CLL (Russo et al. 2010). Thangasamy et al. (2010) reported that QT abrogates the chemoresistance of dacarbazine analogue temozolomide (TMZ) in melanoma by modulating a p53 family member protein, deltaNp73. In addition, QT sensitizes melanoma cells to hyperthermia (Piantelli 1995) and enhances the antiproliferative activity of buslphan in K562 cells (Hoffman 1989).

Table 1. Rich source of Quercetin in different fruits and vegetables

Source	Quantity	Reference
Capers (Capparis spinosa) Lovage (Levisticum officinatle) Green tea (Camellia sinensis) Black tea (Camellia sinensis) Raw Onion	1800mg/Kg 1700mg/Kg 2000–2500mg/Kg 204.66mg/100g13.27mg/100g 0.84 mg/100ml 83mg/Kg 158mg/Kg	http://www.nal.usda.gov/fnic/foodcomp (2003) Crystal Smith et al (2003) Bentz A B (2009) Bentz A B (2009) Bentz A B (2009) Bentz A B (2009)

B. Chemopreventive activity of Quercetin

Cancer chemoprevention is defined as the use of natural, synthetic, or biologic chemical agents to reverse, suppress or prevent carcinogenic progression to invasive cancer (Sporn 1976). Natural products from dietary sources have gained increased attention in the area of cancer chemoprevention. In many studies QT has interfered with the initiation, promotion and progression of cancer, leading to the modulation of proteins in diverse pathways and integration of different signals for the final chemopreventive effect. QT acts on multiple key elements in signal transduction pathways related to cellular proliferation, differentiation, apoptosis and inflammation.

In hamsters, QT inhibited 7,12-dimethylbenz[a]anthracene (DMBA)-induced buccal pouch carcinogenesis (Baasubramoniam 1996); in female Sprague-Dawley rats it abrogated the development of mammary tumors induced by DMBA (So 1996); and in swiss albino mice QT inhibited 20 methyl cholantherene-induced fibrosarcoma (Elangovan 1994b). In 9,10-dimethyl-1,2-benzanthracene-initiated and TPA-promoted two-stage mouse skin cancer models, QT exerted the strongest anticarcinogenic effects (Elangovan 1994a) by inhibiting MEK1 and Raf1 activities (KiWon Lee 2009). QT also inhibited polyp formation in the intestines of APC(Min-/+) mice (Murphy et al. 2011).

C. Quercetin and chromatin remodeling

Growing evidence implies that flavonoids may contribute to chromatin remodeling and thus impede epigenetic alterations that are important in cancer progression. The p16INK4a gene promoter, which is hypermethylated in human colon cancer cells, has been demethylated by QT (Tan 2009). Quercetin also activates histone deacetylase enzymatic activity, thus reducing the acetylation of histone H3 in human prostate cancer cells. The deacetylation of H3 could be responsible for the inhibition of survivin expression, and for the ensuing sensitization to TRAIL-induced apoptosis. QT treatment has also decreased DNA methylation levels of ERbeta, P16INK4a and RASSF1A in bladder cancer cell lines EJ, T24 and J82DNA (Ma 2006).

D. Quercetin and cell cycle

The cell cycle consists of a controlled collection of events, resulting in the creation of two daughter cells. Numerous factors control the cell cycle and ensure that a cell divides accurately. In cancer cells there is a fault in the regulation of the cell cycle, which leads to uncontrolled cell division. Quercetin treatment in different cancer cells modulates several molecular targets that regulate the cell cycle. Depending on the cell type and tumor origin, QT is able to block the cell cycle at G2/M or at the G1/S transition. QT increases the expression of p21/WAF, a cyclin dependent kinase (CDK) inhibitor in different human breast cancer cells (SKBr3, MDA-453 and MDA-MB-231, A549) and in androgen-independent prostate cancer cell line PC3 (Pao-Chen Kuo 2004, Vijyababu 2005); p21 inhibits the cell cycle progression at the G1 phase by binding to CDK2 or CDK4. In human liver cancer cell HepG2, QT modulates the expression of p27 Kip1; p27 binds to the catalytic site of CDK4 or Cyclin D1or CDK4/Cyclin D1 complex and prevents the cell cycle progression from G1 to S phase. Quercetin has also been reported to cause G2/M arrest in the human esophageal squamous cell carcinoma cell line through up-regulation of p73 and p21wafl and down-regulation of cyclin B1 (Zhang et al. 2009). Quercetin glucuronides cause cell-cycle arrest in human lung cancer cells NCI-H209 at G2/M phase by increasing expression of proteins cyclin B, Cdc25c-ser-216-p and Wee1 (Yang et al. 2006). QT also inhibits Topoisomerase II enzyme (TopII), which is essential for DNA replication (Bandele 2008, Jang 2011, López-Lázaro 2010).

E. QT induces apoptosis

The proapoptotic effect of QT is achieved through modulation of different signaling pathways. In MDA-MB-231 breast cancer cells QT treatment increases cytosolic Ca2+ levels and reduces the mitochondrial membrane potential (MMP), thus promoting activation of caspase-3, -8 and -9 (Chien 2009). In the U937 cell line, QT disrupts MMP (Ferraresi et al. 2005, Lugli et al. 2005) causing cytochrome *c release* in the cytoplasm, leading to the activation of caspase-3 and -7. Quercetin inhibits cell growth and apoptosis by down-regulating the transcriptional activity of β-catenin/Tcf signaling, with subsequent down-regulation of cyclin D1 and survivin in SW480 colon cancer cells (Shan 2009). In glioma and lung cancer cells, QT exposure results in proteasomal degradation of survivin (Siegelin 2009), while in SKBR3 breast cancer cells QT induces ubiquitination of Her-2/Neu (EGFR) and its down-regulation (Jeong 2008). In some cancer cells, QT acts as a pro-oxidant, thereby triggering apoptosis through generation of ROS and the subsequent activation of AMPKα1 and ASK1 accompanied by p38 activation and recruitment of caspases (Lee 2010). In prostate cancer cells, QT is a potent enhancer of TRAIL-induced apoptosis, through the induction of the expression of death receptor (DR)-5 (Jung 2010). The up-regulation of DR5, together with the down-regulation of c-FLIP (which is an inhibitor of caspase-8), are two mechanisms involved in QT-induced recovery of TRAIL sensitivity in hepatocellular carcinoma cells (Kim 2008). Interestingly, the enhancement of TRAIL-induced apoptosis by QT also occurs through inhibition of the expression of survivin in the ERK-MSK1 signal pathway (Kim 2008). Finally, the antiproliferative and pro-apoptotic effects could be related to the capability of QT to directly bind tubulin, provoking the depolymerization of cellular microtubules (Gupta 2002). Thus, the capability of QT to induce apoptosis in cancer cells (via both the intrinsic and extrinsic pathways) strongly renders this molecule an interesting tool in the oncology field.

F. Quercetin and p53

Several studies indicate that quercetin modifies the expression of p53 and thereby inhibits the proliferation of cancer cell lines and induces apoptosis: 1) in Xavier 2011 QT enhanced 5-fluorouracil-induced apoptosis in colorectal cancer cells through p53 modulation; 2) in Tanigawa 2008 quercetin inhibited the proliferation of HepG2 cells by inducing cell cycle arrest and apoptosis through the induction of p53 phosphorylation and stabilization of p53 protein by inhibiting ubiquitination and p53 mRNA degradation; 3) in Thangasamy 2008 QT sensitized SKMEL-5 melanoma cells to dacarbazine through tyrosinase overexpression that promotes an ATM-dependent p53 phosphorylation; and 4) in Ma 2006, quercetin induced apoptosis in bladder cancer cells (EJ, T24 and J82) through down-regulation of mutated p53 and survivin proteins. In HCT116 colon carcinoma cells, p53 contributes to QT-mediated higher expression of ***N***onsteroidal ***A***nti-inflammatory drug-activated ***G***ene-1 (NAG-1), which in turn triggers apoptosis (Park 2008). Reports suggest that cancer cells harboring wild type p53 elevates the p21 level, which may attenuate the proapoptotic effects of QT (Kuo 2004). Whereas cancer cells have mutated p53, the H1299 lung carcinoma cell line is more susceptible to QT-induced cytotoxicity than the A549 lung carcinoma cell line, which expresses wild-type p53 (Kuo 2004). In A549 cells, QT-induced cytotoxicity and apoptosis are augmented when an inhibitor of p53 or an antisense oligonucleotide targeting p53 is used

(Kuo 2004). The effect of the presence or absence of p53 on QT-induced cytotoxicity and apoptosis is steady with the contribution of QT in the oxidative cell balance. Quercetin induces gadd45 expression through a p53-independent pathway in HeLa cells, and gadd45 is known to be a downstream target of p53 (Yoshida 2005). QT also arrests S phase by decreasing the protein expression of CDK2, cyclins A and B, while increasing the p53 and p57 proteins (Chou 2010).

II. QT and Metabolic Diseases

1. Diabetes

Changing lifestyles, reduced physical activity and the increasing incidence of obesity are major causative factors for the development of type 2 diabetes, one of the world's most common chronic diseases (Wild et al. 2004). Insulin resistance in the peripheral tissues and hyperglycemia are the major characteristics of type 2 diabetes, ultimately leading to the destruction of pancreatic beta cells that produce insulin (Guillausseau et al. 2008). The major contributing factor in the development of type 2 diabetes is insulin resistance and the major predisposing factor for the development of insulin resistance is obesity. Obesity up-regulates circulating levels of inflammatory markers and free fatty acids, contributing to the development of insulin resistance (Lois and Kumar 2009). Thus, improvement of insulin sensitivity will be the major approach to prevent and treat type 2 diabetes. Changes in lifestyles and exercise could improve insulin sensitivity but could be difficult to maintain over the long term. The unwanted side effects of the current medication for diabetes turn the attention to herbal remedies because they can be applied to a general population with the least side effects and greatest preventive outcome (Matsui T et al. 2006). Naturally occurring flavonoids of plant origin are an appropriate option because dietary flavonoids are reported to delay and prevent the onset of diabetes. QT is one of the most common flavonoids in foods that shows anti-diabetic effects (Jung et al. 2011). The manner in which quercetin exerts its antidiabetic effects and the molecular targets of quercetin for this effect will be discussed in the following sections.

A. Quercetin Ameliorates Oxidative Stress

Oxidative stress plays a critical role in the development and progression of diabetes mellitus as well as other complications associated with this disease (Phillips et al. 2004). Mitochondrial released reactive oxygen species (ROS) is the major source of oxidative stress in tissues and this occurs when there is excess production of ROS from mitochondria that exceeds the capacity of cells' antioxidant defense systems to handle the situation (Knight JA, 1999). An increase in ROS causes apoptosis, leading to the onset of type 1 diabetes, and insulin resistance, leading to the development of type 2 diabetes (Bonnefont-Rousselot et al. 2000). Controlling oxidative stress associated with hyperglycemia and thereby maintaining optimal glycemic control will be the ideal approach to treat diabetes.

In streptozotocin-induced diabetic rat models, onion peel extract rich in quercetin and its derivatives improved glucose tolerance. Administration of 0.1% onion peel extract improved insulin sensitivity in peripheral tissues through multiple mechanisms: suppressing oxidative stress, improving metabolic dysregulation of free fatty acids, up-regulating glucose uptake at peripheral tissues, and/or down-regulating inflammatory gene expression in the liver (Jung et al. 2011, Mahesh and Menon 2004). The dosage of quercetin is also important in improving oxidative stress. When two different doses of quercetin (50 and 80 mg/kg body weight) were administered for 45 days in rats with streptozotocin-induced diabetes, the lower dose was more effective in ameliorating oxidative stress (Mahesh and Menon 2004). Oxidative stress is one of the major causes of diabetic nephropathy. Oral administration of quercetin for 4 weeks in diabetic rats significantly attenuated renal dysfunction and oxidative stress, suggesting that an antioxidative mechanism is responsible for the nephroprotective action of quercetin (Anjaneyulu and Chopra 2004).

Oxidative stress is also involved in the pathogenesis and progression of diabetic tissue damage. Quercetin prevented up-regulation of hepatic thiobarbituric acid-reactive substances (TBARS) concentration, hydroperoxide-initiated chemiluminescence, and SOD and catalase activities induced by streptozotocin administration in rats. In addition, QT abolished streptozotocin-mediated activation of NF-kappaB, induction of IKKalpha and iNOS protein levels, and increased degradation of IkappaBalpha. This suggests that by targeting the NF-kappa pathway, quercetin may block the production of deleterious mediators involved in the development of early diabetes tissue injury and in the evolution of late complications (Dias et al. 2005). In addition to oxidative status, quercetin also modulated carbohydrate metabolism in diabetic conditions. Quercetin administration (30 mg/kg) to diabetic rats decreased plasma glucose, increased insulin levels and restored glycogen content and the activities of carbohydrate metabolic enzymes, hexokinase, glucose 6-phosphatase and fructose 1,6-bisphosphatase (Babujanarthanam et al. 2010).

A study by Azuma et al. (2007) pointed out that diabetes-induced oxidative stress was more effectively suppressed by the intake of onion, which is rich in quercetin, than by intake of the same amount of QT aglycone alone. However, a methylated quercetin derivative, pentamethylquercetin (PMQ), exhibits great potential as an antidiabetic agent by improving hyperglycemia and reducing the incidence of peripheral complications in neonatally streptozotocin (STZ)-induced diabetic rats (Wang et al. 2011).

Onion peel extract also exhibited insulin-sensitizing and hypoglycemic effects on streptozotocin-induced diabetic rats fed a high-fat diet. Administration of 1% onion peel extract improved glucose tolerance and increased glycogen levels in the liver and skeletal muscle. This is achieved through multiple mechanisms: down-regulation of plasma FFAs, suppression of inflammation by down-regulation of IL-6 hepatic expression, inhibition of oxidative stress as assessed by decreased formation of superoxide dismutase activity and malondialdehyde formation, and up-regulating glucose uptake at peripheral tissues through up-regulation of insulin receptor and GLUT4 in muscle cells (Jung et al. 2011).

B. Quercetin Targets Pancreas

Quercetin treatment preserved pancreatic beta cell integrity by reducing oxidative stress in rats with streptozotocin-induced diabetes. Islet cell degeneration and weak insulin immunohistochemical staining was also observed. Interestingly, quercetin was able to induce regeneration of the pancreatic islets, thereby increasing insulin release in streptozocin-induced diabetic rats (Coskun et al. 2005, Vessal et al. 2003). This protective effect of quercetin occurs through decreased lipid peroxidation, NO production and increased antioxidant enzyme activity in the pancreatic cells (Coskun et al. 2005). Quercetin recovered cell proliferation in pancrease by inhibiting the expression of cyclin-dependent kinase inhibitor p21(WAF1/Cip1) (Cdkn1a) and quercetin-mediated ERK1/2 phosphorylation restored glucose-induced insulin secretion (Kobori et al. 2009, Youl et al. 2010). Quercetin administration also decreased fat infiltration in the islets of diabetic rats (Babujanarthanam et al. 2010).

C. AMPK: A Newly Identified Target of Quercetin against Diabetes

AMP-activated protein kinase (AMPK) is a cellular energy sensor that is activated by an increase in cellular AMP:ATP ratio. Once activated, AMPK switches off ATP-consuming, anabolic pathways and switches on catabolic pathways that generate ATP. AMPK exhibits both acute effects on metabolism by phosphorylating metabolic enzymes and long-term effects through regulation of transcription. These effects of AMPK make it an ideal drug target in the treatment of metabolic disorders such as insulin resistance and type 2 diabetes. The widely used antidiabetic drug metformin, derived from herbs, works in part through AMPK activation (Hardie 2011). Quercetin and quercetin-3-O-glycosides treatment increased AMPK activation in C2C12 cells, leading to increased basal glucose uptake. AMPK activation was achieved through the mild inhibition of ADP-stimulated oxygen consumption in isolated mitochondria, an effect consistent with metabolic stress. This suggests that quercetin has applications for the prevention of insulin resistance and other metabolic diseases (Eid et al. 2010).

2. QT and Obesity

A. QT Ameliorates Inflammation

In the past few decades, the growing pervasiveness of obesity and the pathologies associated with it have become a major public health threat. Obesity-associated chronic inflammation is a critical factor in the development of pathological conditions such as insulin resistance, type 2 diabetes, cardiovascular disease, and other metabolic diseases (Schenk et al. 2008, Stumvoll 2005, Shoelson 2006). Under obese conditions, inflammatory response is mainly initiated by adipose tissue. Hence, controlling inflammatory responses in obese conditions may be useful in the prevention or amelioration of obesity-related pathologies (Xu et al. 2003, Weisberg et al. 2008).

QT has been proven effective in ameliorating inflammation both *in vitro* and *in vivo*. In 3T3-L1 adipocytes, QT inhibited TNF-α-induced changes in levels of monocyte chemoattractant protein-1 (MCP-1), plasminogen activator inhibitor-1, and intracellular reactive oxygen species. Furthermore, QT also up-regulated levels of superoxide dismutase, glutathione, glutathione peroxidase, and glutathione S-transferase in TNF-α-treated 3T3-L1 adipocytes. This suggests that inhibition of TNF-α-induced changes might have very important implications in preventing obesity-related pathologies (Yen et al. 2011). QT was also demonstrated to prevent inflammation in macrophages and macrophage-mediated insulin resistance in adipocytes. Treatment of macrophages with quercetin attenuated expression of tumor necrosis factor-α, interleukin (IL)-6, IL-8, IL-1β and interferon-γ inducible protein-10, and cyclooxygenase-2. Quercetin also reduced the levels of phosphorylated c-Jun N-terminal kinase (JNK) and c-Jun, and IκBα degradation in macrophages. In addition, conditioned media from macrophages treated with quercetin attenuated the capacity of condition media to induce inflammatory response in adipocytes that causes insulin resistance (Overman et al. 2011). Administration of QT (10 mg/kg bodyweight for 10 weeks) induced anti-inflammatory effects in obese Zucker rats by down-regulating TNF-alpha production in the visceral adipose tissue. This was accompanied by a reduction in body weight gain and an increase in the circulating levels of adiponectin, an insulin-sensitizing hormone secreted by the adipose tissue (Rivera et al. 2008). In C57BL/6J mice fed a high-fat diet QT decreased circulating markers of inflammation like interferon-gamma, interleukin-1alpha, and interleukin-4 compared to highfat-diet fed and QT was also able to increase energy expenditure in these mice controls (Stewart et al. 2008). Chronic dietary intake of quercetin (0.05% for 20 weeks) decreased TNFα levels in the tissues of mice fed a typical Western diet (Kobori et al. 2011).

Interestingly, QT up-regulated adiponectin secretion in both cell culture and animal models (Kobori et al. 2011; Yen et al. 2011). Adiponectin is a secreted adipokine mainly synthesized by adipose tissue (Scherer et al. 1995). Adiponectin improves insulin sensitivity, glucose tolerance and lipid profile thereby exerting its beneficial effects on metabolism (Kadowaki et al. 2007). In various clinical conditions like type 2 diabetes, obesity, insulin resistance, cardiovascular disease and hypertension, a decrease in the level of circulating adiponectin is reported (Arita et al. 1999, Hotta et al. 2001, Kumada et al. 2003, Adamczak et al. 2003). By lowering nuclear factor kappa B (NFκB) action, adiponectin exerts its anti-inflammatory effect (Xu et al. 2011). Therefore, it is possible that the anti-inflammatory property exerted by QT is due to up-regulation of adiponectin levels.

B. QT's Effect on Dyslipidemia and Hypertension

QT is able to ameliorate metabolic syndrome abnormalities, including obesity, dyslipidemia and hypertension. Administration of QT at a dose of 2 mg/kg body weight for 10 weeks could reduce systolic blood pressure, high plasma concentrations of triglycerides, total cholesterol, free fatty acid and insulin in obese Zucker rats. At high concentrations (10 mg/kg body weight) QT increased endothelial nitric oxide synthase expression and decreased inducible nitric oxide synthase in the visceral adipose tissue of obese Zucker rats (Rivera et al. 2008). Quercetin intake of 150mg/day produced blood-pressure-lowering effects in overweight-obese humans of the apo epsilon3/epsilon3 genotype (Egert et al. 2010). Chronic dietary intake of quercetin (0.05% for 20 weeks) reduced accumulation of fat in liver and visceral adipose tissue in mice fed a Western diet. This effect of QT is mediated by the down-regulation of expression of hepatic genes related to steatosis, such as peroxisome proliferator-activated receptor γ and sterol regulatory element-binding protein-1c (Kobori et al. 2011).

C. QT Inhibits Lipid Accumulation and Promotes Apoptosis in Adipocytes

In isolated primary rat adipocytes, QT increased lipolysis and inhibited glucose uptake, thereby preventing lipid accumulation (Kuppusamy and Das 1994). In 3T3-L1 preadipocytes, the anti-adipogenesis activity of quercetin is reported to be through activation of AMPK-signaling pathway (Ahn et al. 2008). A combination of quercetin with genistein and resveratrol inhibited lipid accumulation in primary human adipocytes during differentiation, and this combination decreased cell viability and induced apoptosis in mature human adipocytes. A similar effect was observed in murine 3T3-L1 adipocytes (Park et al. 2008). In maturing preadipocytes quercetin (25 microM) suppressed intracellular lipid accumulation; in mature adipocytes quercetin (100 microM) decreased viability and increased apoptosis. A combination of resveratrol and quercetin further decreased viability and increased apoptosis. This resulted from down-regulation of the expression of peroxisome proliferators-activated receptor gamma (PPAR gamma) and CCAAT/enhancer-binding protein (C/EBP)alpha, the key transcription factors involved in adipogenesis. A combination of resveratrol and quercetin at 100 microM increased cytochrome c release from mitochondria and decreased ERK 1/2 phosphorylation (Yang et al. 2008). In 3T3-L1 mature adipocytes QT also induced apoptosis by modulating ERK and JNK pathways (Ahn et al. 2008).

The role of inflammation in the pathogenesis of insulin resistance and type 2 diabetes suggests that targeting inflammation with pharmacological and dietary interventions will be an ideal approach. Unlike the pharmacological approaches that modulate inflammatory process, dietary nutraceuticals with less side effects will undoubtedly benefit the vast number of people affected by the obesity epidemic and other metabolic diseases.

III. QT and Aging

QT treatment extended by 15% the mean lifespan of *Caenorhabditis elegans* (*C. elegans*), a well-established model system for studying aging (Kampkötter et al. 2008). QT, a strong free radical scavenger, down-regulated mitochondrial manganese superoxide dismutase in *C.elegans*. In addition, it mediated nuclear translocation of *C. elegans* FOXO transcription factor (DAF-16), a state that is correlated with stress response and longevity. This suggests that the modulation of signaling pathways, in addition to its strong antioxidant capacity, might contribute to the protective and life-prolonging action of QT. However, the involvement of DAF-16 in the life-extending effects of quercetin has been disproved by the studies of Saul et al. (2008). They demonstrated that quercetin could increase the mean lifespan by 15% in a daf-16 (mgDf50) mutant strain of *C. elegans,* and quercetin-treated daf-16(mgDf50) worms exhibited enhanced resistance to thermal and oxidative stress. Pietsch et al. (2009) further dissected quercetin's mechanism of lifespan modulation in *C. elegans*. QT did not exhibit either a sirtuin (sir-2.1) dependence or caloric restriction mimetic effect. Rather, QT-derived lifespan extension required four genes: age-1, daf-2, unc-43 and sek-1. Age-1 and daf-2 are central players in IGF-1-like signaling pathway to inhibit DAF-16 activity and mutations in daf-16 results in long-lived nematodes with robust stress-resistance. The gene sek-1 is part of the MAP kinase pathway that phosphorylates the *C. elegans* p38-family MAP kinase PMK-1, which results in elevated immune response to pathogen infection (Kim et al. 2002). The gene unc-43 is CaMKII ($Ca2+$/calmodulin-dependent protein kinase II) and mutations of the this cause diverse behavioral defects by affecting locomotor activity.

Contrary to the findings in *C. elegans*, dietary supplementation with quercetin significantly reduced life span in young mice. Five-week-old male mice receiving 0.1% quercetin had decreased median lifespan, while females experienced a decrease in both median and maximum lifespan (Jones and Hughs 1982). One possible explanation for this unexpected effect could be the young age of the mice. At that age, mice are still developing, and supplementation of high doses of antioxidants may prevent proper development. Also, QT is able to form chelation compounds with certain metals such as copper (Kühnau 1976), and prolonged ingestion of quercetin could cause a chronic deficiency of one or more of the essential elements, leading to reduced lifespan. However, quercetin has been proven effective in reversing cognitive deficits in aged mice which could be attributed to its antioxidant properties (Singh et al. 2003). A reversal of age-related retention deficits in mice was achieved with the chronic administration of QT (10, 25 and 50 mg/kg) for 30 days. Remarkably, chronic administration of quercetin failed to modulate the retention performance of young mice in memory paradigms, suggesting beneficial effects of QT in aged, not young, animals. The reversal of cognitive deficits is mainly achieved through restoration of forebrain total glutathione, superoxide dismutase and catalase levels, which are associated with the antioxidant property of QT. Formulations containing QT have also been proven effective against UV radiation-induced skin damage and skin aging (Casagrande et al. 2006). Topical formulations containing quercetin inhibited UVB irradiation-induced oxidative damages through inhibition of myeloperoxidase activity increase, glutathione depletion and proteinases secretion/activity in the skin of hairless mice.

IV. Quercetin Meets Nanotechnology

Bioactives are used as therapeutic agents in many diseases such as cancer (Salim 1996), diabetes (Desco 2002), cardiovascular diseases (Mimi´c-Oka 1999), autoimmune diseases (Namazi 2009) and neurodegenerative disorders (Singh 2004). Approximately 40% of new molecular entities fail to be new drugs because of poor biopharmaceutical properties, such as solubility and permeability (Gao et al. 2009). One of the most challenging tasks in the process of drug development is to improve solubility and oral bioavailability of novel and existing drugs. Extensive research is being carried out globally on QT to develop better therapeutics, and most of it has proved that QT is pharmacologically active (Loke 2008). Even though compelling evidence gains much attention and arouses the enthusiasm of research work on QT for cancer prevention and reduction of cardiovascular diseases, QT's application in the clinics is restricted due to its very low oral bioavailability (16.2%) (Gao et al. 2009). QT has a low solubility in water (0.17–7.7μg/ml), artificial gastric juice (5.5μg/ml) and artificial intestinal juice (28.9μg/ml) (Khaled 2003, Boots 2008, Wei 2001, Azuma 2002, Fasolo, 2007). Therapeutic use of this antioxidant molecule is limited due to poor solubility, poor permeability, instability and extensive first past metabolism before reaching the systemic circulation. Researchers have attempted to increase the bioavailability of QT by complexation with cyclodextrin and liposomes, nanoemulsions and nanoparticles (Azuma 2002, Fasolo, 2007, Pralhad 2004). In this part of the review we discuss different nano-formulations of QT.

Nanoparticles

Polymeric nanoparticles have been investigated for over three decades as drug delivery systems. They have been classified diversely according to the mode of preparation. Mainly, nanoparticles are composed of a polymeric wall containing a liquid inner core or a polymeric matrix in which the drugs are dispersed. Nanoencapsulation is considered to be ideal for drugs or compounds such as QT that are difficult to formulate in aqueous media. Depending on their hydrophobicity, organosoluble polymers have been used as encapsulating material. Different methods of preparation of polymeric nanoparticles are briefly mentioned here.

In situ polymerization: This approach is based on an emulsion-polymerization process in which the cyanoacrylic monomer is dissolved in an organic solvent and dispersed in an aqueous phase containing surfactant (Labib et al. 1991). When this technique is used for the preparation of nanocapsules, an organic phase containing the monomer and the drug is emulsified in an aqueous phase (Lenaerts et al. 1995). These particles are well adapted for the encapsulation of lipophilic drugs.

Dispersion: This method is based on the formation of an emulsion in which the polymer is solubilized in an organic solvent immiscible with the external phase. Another approach in the same method called nanoprecipitation is the direct precipitation of the solubilized polymer when in contact with a non-solvent. PLA and PLGA have been described as ideal for nanoprecipitation in several studies. In most, those employing PLGA and PLA are based on the formation of an emulsion of an organic solvent-containing polymer and the drug solubilized in an aqueous phase containing a surfactant (Xiao et al. 2008, Xing et al. 2007, Zambaux et al. 1999, Zhang et al. 2008, Nair et al. 2011).

Table 2. Completed and ongoing trials of quercetin

Trials (http://clinicaltrials.gov)	Conditions
Effect of combined exercise, heat, and quercetinsupplementationon whole body stressresponse	Heat acclimation and thermotolerance
The effect of quercetinin sarcoidosis	Sarcoidosis
Investigating the use of quercetinon glucoseabsorption in obesity, and obesity with type 2 diabetes	Diabetes Mellitus, Obesity
Physiologicaleffects of grape seedextract in diastolic heart failure	Diastolic heart failure, Hypertensive heart disease, Heart failure with preserved ejection fraction, Hypertension, Oxidative stress
The occurrence of inflammationand oxidative stressi lung diseases	Interstitial lung diseases, Sarcoidosis, Idiopathic pulmonary fibrosis, COPD
Orthomolecular therapyand asthmain children	Asthma
Lipoic acidas a treatmentfor acute optic neuritis	Optic neuritis
Nasal potential studies utilizing cystic fibrosistransmembrane regulator (CFTR) modulators	Cystic Fibrosis
Therapeutic effect of quercetinand the current treatmentof erosive and atrophic oral lichenplanus	Atrophic oral lichen planus, Erosive oral lichen Planus
Efficacy of Provex CVSupplement to Reduce Markers of Inflammatory Cytokines and Blood Pressure in Subjects With MetabolicSyndrome	Blood pressure, Plasma inflammatory markers, Blood aggregation time

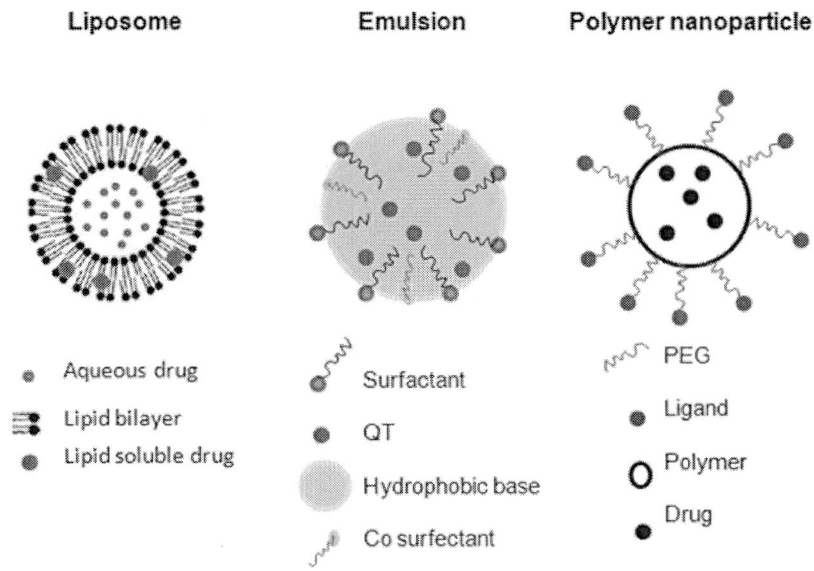

Figure 1. Different types of nanoparticle formulations.

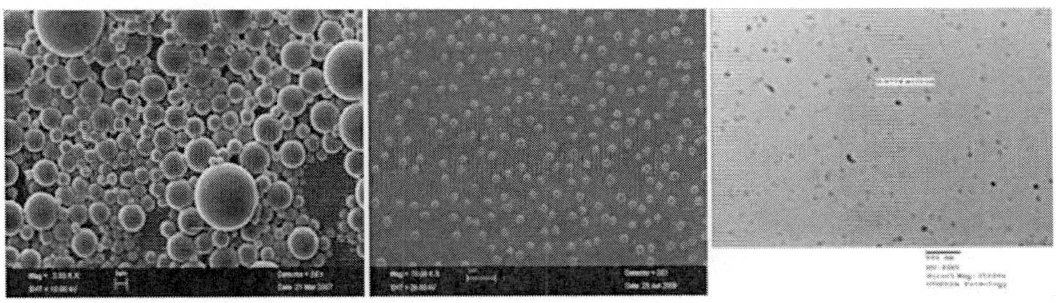

Figure 2. PLGA-PEG co-polymer nanoparticles and their size characterization: Uniform particle size is achieved by mechanical extrusion.

Emulsion diffusion: This method is used to prepare particles from a complex made of poly (sebasic anhydride) and phthalocyanine, where the drug is conjugated with the polymer before particle formation (Fu et al. 2002). Encapsulation of molecules on suitable nanocarriers is one of the promising ways to circumvent the low solubility of quercetin; poly-d,l-lactide (PLA) and poly-D,l lactide co-glycolide (PLGA) are used extensively for the encapsulation of many therapeutic agents among the biodegradable polymeric nanoparticles due to their hydrophobicity, strong mechanical strength and slow drug release. QT encapsulated on poly-d,l-lactide (PLA) nanoparticles by solvent evaporation method showed improvement in solubility, permeability and stability. The size of QT-PLA nanoparticles is 195±55 nm (Kumari et al. 2011). A cyclodextrin formulation of QT has been developed and tested; however, the use of cyclodextrin is associated with the risk of nephrotoxicity, and the problem of stability in storage remains a major concerns (Pralhad 2004, Yuan 2006, Frijlink 1991). Kumari et al. 2010 have investigated the feasibility of encapsulating synthetic QT molecule into PLA nanoparticles by a solvent evaporation method. In this study QT-loaded PLA nanoparticles were characterized and tested for bioavailability. The encapsulated QT formulation showed higher aqueous solubility and sustained release. Even though the antioxidant properties of QT were not compromised in this formulation, further *in vivo* bioavailability studies are needed to confirm the efficacy of this formulation.

Nanosuspension

The nanosuspension techniques are generally classified as bottom up and top down processes based on the differences in the production principle (Keck and Müller 2006). Generally, in the bottom up processes, a poorly water-soluble drug is dissolved in an organic solvent and then precipitated through a non-solvent addition in the presence of stabilizers, or evaporative precipitation into aqueous solution (EPAS), spray-freezing into liquid process, and emulsion-solvent evaporation (Li et al. 2007, Rabinow 2004). In top down methods the mechanical comminuting process uses larger drug particles, as in media milling, microfluidization and high press homogenization (HPH) (Van Eerdenbrugh et al. 2008). In a recent study of chemically stable nanosuspension prepared by EPAS method (Lei et al. 2011), the results of the stability studies proved that nanosuspension of QT could significantly improve the chemical- and photo-stability of QT compared with the solution stored in the same conditions.

In another study, the nanoparticles of QT-cyclodextrin complex dispersions with hydrophilic and water-soluble carriers like polyvinylpyrrolidone have been investigated using the evaporative precipitation of nanosuspension (EPN) method (Kakran et al. 2011). In this study QT nanoparticles presented enhanced dissolution. The drug was dispersed in the amorphous form and/or at the molecular level in the complexes and solid dispersions. The dissolution of the QT complexes and solid dispersions also improved significantly from the raw drug.

Nanoemulsions

Nanoemulsions are stable nanodroplets of oil dispersed in an aqueous phase, typically below 300 nm in size. Nanoemulsions have great stability for up to several months. They are used as nanocarriers for drugs or contrast agents in the applications of targeting and controlled delivery. Due to recent developments in the pharmaceutical field, solubility is easily quantifiable *in vitro* and can be manipulated by formulation strategies, such as microemulsion (ME) and self-microemulsifying drug delivery systems (SMEDDS) for its applications from drug delivery to the food industry (El-Hadidy et al. 2011).

Liposomes

Liposomes have been used as drug carriers for a long time and have a great impact in oncology. Being lipophilic, liposomes have the advantage of being able to carry drug molecules over plasma membrane. Liposomes can fuse with the plasma membrane and transfer their drug cargo into the cell. Several liposomal drug formulations are in clinical trials and many are accepted by FDA, especially for cancer indications. However, liposomes have a short half life in circulation, short *in vivo* stability and target selectivity. These drawbacks were rectified by recent innovations such as the introduction of PEG, ligand targeted techniques and antibodies (Storm et al. 1998, Klibanov et al. 1990). Pegylation increased the therapeutic efficacy of liposomal formulations by increasing the circulation time, which resulted in the approval of several liposomal formulations for clinical use (e.g., liposomal doxorubicin). Targeting with antibodies or specific ligands or tumor-associated receptors improved selectivity and reduced the rapid removal of liposomes from the blood stream by the reticulo endothelial system (RES) (Lasic 1995, Derksen 1998).

Table.3. Different applications of QT in the marketplace

Product type	Commercial source	Amount of QT
Health supplement	Puritans pride- QT+Vitamin C	500mg
Health supplement	Now foods QT	800mg
Health supplement	Jarrow formulas QT	500mg
Health supplement	Vitacost Advan-C® with Quercetin & Citrus	1000mg
Health supplement	Twinlab- QT+C	500mg
Health supplement	NSI liquid vitamin C+QT	1000mg
Health supplement	Doctor's Best -Quercetin -Bromelain	0.32Lb/bottle
Health supplement	Natrol-Quercetin	250mg
Health supplement	QBC plus	0.42lb/bottle
Health supplement	Source Naturals- Activated Quercetin™	0.47lb/bottle
Health supplement	FRS-Health Energy soft chew orange	0.38lb/bottle
Health supplement	Solgar - Quercetin Complex with Ester-C® Plus	0.63lb/bottle
Health supplement	Nature's Plus-QT + Bromelain + vitamin C	0.16 lb/bottle
Health supplement	Allergy research group- Quercetin 300	0.15lb/bottle
Health supplement	Thorne Research- Quercenase® Quercetin Chalcone and Bromelain Combination	0.14lb/bottle
Health supplement	Source Naturals-NutraDrops™-Quercetin	134mg
Skin cream	Bulk actives - Quercetin cream-gel	2%
Skin cream	Korres- Quercetin & Oak antiageing and antiwrinkle night cream	1.35oz

CONCLUSION

The use QT has been tremendously increased over the last 2 decades as a health supplement as well as numerous scientific proofs that clearly shows the potential use of QT against many disease indications including diabetes, cancer and healthy aging. It has been proved from animal studies that QT is safe and few other studies have improved the bioavailability of QT by nanoformulations. However there are unresolved doubt among the scientific community regarding the safety of QT since it is been shown to interact with cytochrome p450 enzymes and might decrease the effectiveness of some antibiotics and other drugs. Hence a *'responsible'* use of QT is warranted based on the current scientific knowledge.

ACKNOWLEDGMENT

The authors wish to thank Jennifer Meehan, Director for technical publications at Texas Biomedical Research Institute for editing this chapter.

REFERENCES

Adamczak M, Wiecek A, Funahashi T, Chudek J, Kokot F, Matsuzawa Y. *Decreased plasma adiponectin concentration in patients with essential hypertension*. Am J Hypertens. (2003) 16(1):72-5.

Agullo G, Gamet L, Besson C, Demigné C, Rémésy C. *Quercetin exerts a preferential cytotoxic effect on active dividing colon carcinoma HT29 and Caco-2 cells.* Cancer Lett. (1994) 87(1):55-63.

Ahn J, Lee H, Kim S, Park J, Ha T. *The anti-obesity effect of quercetin is mediated by the AMPK and MAPK signaling pathways.* Biochem Biophys Res Commun. (2008) 5;373(4):545-9.

Anjaneyulu M, Chopra K. *Quercetin, an anti-oxidant bioflavonoid, attenuates diabetic nephropathy in rats*. Clin Exp Pharmacol Physiol. (2004) (4):244-8.

Arita Y, Kihara S, Ouchi N, Takahashi M, Maeda K, Miyagawa J, Hotta K, Shimomura I, Nakamura T, Miyaoka K, Kuriyama H, Nishida M, Yamashita S, Okubo K, Matsubara K, Muraguchi M, Ohmoto Y, Funahashi T, Matsuzawa Y. *Paradoxical decrease of an adipose-specific protein, adiponectin, in obesity.* Biochem Biophys Res Commun. (1999) 2;257(1):79-83.

Azuma K, Ippoushi K, Ito H, Higashio H, Terao J. *Combination of lipids and emulsifiers enhances the absorption of orally administered quercetin in rats*. J Agric Food Chem. (2002) 13;50(6):1706-12.

Azuma K, Minami Y, Ippoushi K, Terao J. *Lowering effects of onion intake on oxidative stress biomarkers in streptozotocin-induced diabetic rats*. J Clin Biochem Nutr. (2007) 40(2):131-40.

Babujanarthanam R, Kavitha P, Pandian MR. *Quercitin, a bioflavonoid improves glucose homeostasis in streptozotocin-induced diabetic tissues by altering glycolytic and gluconeogenic enzymes.* Fundam Clin Pharmacol. (2010) (3):357-64.

Bandele OJ, Clawson SJ, Osheroff N. *Dietary polyphenols as topoisomerase II poisons: B ring and C ring substituents determine the mechanism of enzyme-mediated DNA cleavage enhancement.* Chem Res Toxicol. (2008) 21(6):1253-60.

Bonnefont-Rousselot D, Bastard JP, Jaudon MC, Delattre J. *Consequences of the diabetic status on the oxidant/antioxidant balance.* Diabetes Metab. (2000) (3):163-76.

Boots AW, Haenen GR, Bast A. *Health effects of quercetinfrom antioxidantto nutraceutical* Eur J Pharmacol. (2008) 585(2-3):325-37.

Brown JP. *A review of the genetic effects of naturally occurring flavonoids, anthraquinones and related compounds*. Mutat Res. (1980) 75(3):243-77.

Castillo MH, Perkins E, Campbell JH, Doerr R, Hassett JM, Kandaswami C, Middleton E Jr. *The effects of the bioflavonoid quercetin on squamous cell carcinoma of head and neck origin*. Am J Surg. (1989) 158(4):351-5.

Chien SY, Wu YC, Chung JG, Yang JS, Lu HF, Tsou MF, Wood WG, Kuo SJ, Chen DR. *Quercetin-induced apoptosis acts through mitochondrial- and caspase-3-dependent pathways in human breast cancer MDA-MB-231 cells.* Hum Exp Toxicol. (2009) (8):493-503.

Chou CC, Yang JS, Lu HF, Ip SW, Lo C, Wu CC, Lin JP, Tang NY, Chung JG, Chou MJ, Teng YH, Chen DR. *Quercetin-mediated cell cycle arrest and apoptosis involving activation of a caspase cascade through the mitochondrial pathway in human breast cancer MCF-7 cells.* Arch Pharm Res. (2010) (8):1181-91.

Coskun O, Kanter M, Korkmaz A, Oter S. *Quercetin, a flavonoid antioxidant, prevents and protects streptozotocin-induced oxidative stress and beta-cell damage in rat pancreas.* Pharmacol Res. (2005) 51(2):117-23.

Day AJ and Williamson G. 1999. *Human metabolism of dietary quercetin glycosides.* In: Gross GG, Hemingway RW, Yoshida, T (Eds.). Plant Polyphenols 2: Chemistry, Biology, Pharmacology, Ecology. Kluwer Academic / Plenum Publishers; New York. Basic LifeSciences, Vol. 66, pp. 415-34.

Derksen JT, Morselt HW, Scherhof GL. *Uptake and processing of immunoglobulin coated liposomes by subpopulations of rat liver microphages.* Biochem. Biophys. Acta (1998) 971:127-36.

Dias AS, Porawski M, Alonso M, Marroni N, Collado PS, González-Gallego J. *Quercetin decreases oxidative stress, NF-kappaB activation, and iNOS overexpression in liver of streptozotocin-induced diabetic rats.* J Nutr. (2005) (10):2299-304.

Egert S, Boesch-Saadatmandi C, Wolffram S, Rimbach G, Müller MJ. *Serum lipid and blood pressure responses to quercetin vary in overweight patients by apolipoprotein E genotype.* J Nutr. (2010) 140(2):278-84.

Eid HM, Martineau LC, Saleem A, Muhammad A, Vallerand D, Benhaddou-Andaloussi A, Nistor L, Afshar A, Arnason JT, Haddad PS. *Stimulation of AMP-activated protein kinase and enhancement of basal glucose uptake in muscle cells by quercetin and quercetin glycosides, active principles of the antidiabetic medicinal plant Vaccinium vitis-idaea.* Mol Nutr Food Res. (2010) 54(7):991-1003.

El-Hadidy GN, Ibrahim HK, Mohamed MI, El-Milligi MF. *Microemulsions as vehicles for topical administration of voriconazole: formulation and in vitro evaluation.* Drug Dev Ind Pharm. 23 June 2011. [Epub ahead of print]

Elangovan V, Sekar N, Govindasamy S. *Chemopreventive potential of dietary bioflavonoids against 20-methylcholanthrene-induced tumorigenesis.* Cancer Lett. (1994) 87(1):107-13.

Elangovan V., Balasubramanian S, Sekar N, Govindasamy S. *Studies on the chemopreventive potential of some naturally-occurring bioflavonoids in 7,12-dimethylbenz(a)anthracene-induced carcinogenesis in mouse skin.* Clin. Biochem. Nutr. (1994) 17:153-60.

Fasolo D, Schwingel L, Holzschuh M, Bassani V, Teixeira H. *Validation of an isocratic LC method for determination of quercetin and methylquercetin in topical nanoemulsions.* J Pharm Biomed Anal. (2007) 44(5):1174-7.

Ferraresi R, Troiano L, Roat E, Lugli E, Nemes E, Nasi M, Pinti M, *Fernandezfor the anti-oxidant effect of the flavonoid quercetin.* Free Radic Res. (2005) 11:1249-58.

Frijlink HW, Eissens AC, Hefting NR, Poelstra K, Lerk CF, Meijer DK. *The effect of parenterally administered cyclodextrins on cholesterol levels in the rat.* Pharm. Res. (1991) 8:9–16.

Fu J, Li XY, Ng DPK, Wu C. *Encapsulation of phthalocyanines in biodegradable poly (sebacic anhydryde) nanoparticles*. Langmuir (2002) 18:3843-7.

Gao Y, Wang Y, Ma Y, Yu A, Cai F, Shao W, Zhai G. *Formulation optimization and in situ absorption in rat intestinal tract of quercetin-loaded microemulsion.* Biointerfaces. (2009) 71(2):306-14.

Giuliani C, Noguchi Y, Harii N, Napolitano G, Tatone D, Bucci I, Piantelli M, Monaco F, Kohn LD. *The flavonoid quercetin regulates growth and gene expression in rat FRTL-5 thyroid cells*. Endocrinology. (2008) 149:84-92.

Guillausseau PJ, Meas T, Virally M, Laloi-Michelin M, Médeau V, Kevorkian JP. *Abnormalities in insulin secretion in type 2 diabetes mellitus* Metab. (2008) 34 Suppl 2:S43-8.

Gupta K, Panda D. *Perturbation of microtubule polymerization by quercetin through tubulin binding: a novel mechanism of its antiproliferative activity.* Biochemistry. (2002) 41(43):13029-38.

Hardie DG. *Sensing of energy and nutrients by AMP-activated protein kinase.* Am J Clin Nutr. (2011) (4):891S-6.

Harnly JM, Doherty RF, Beecher GR, Holden JM, Haytowitz DB, Bhagwat S, Gebhardt S. *Flavonoid content of U.S. fruits, vegetables, and nuts.* J Agric Food Chem. (2006) 54(26):9966-77.

Hertog MG, Hollman P., Katan M. *Content of potentially anticarcinogenic flavonoids of 28 vegetables and 9 fruits commonly consumed in The Netherlands*. J. Agric. Fd. Chem. (1992) 40:2379-83

Hertog MG, Hollman PC, Katan MB, Kromhout D. *Intake of potentially anticarcinogenic flavonoids and their determinants in adults in The Netherlands.* Nutr Cancer. (1993) 20(1):21-9.

Hoffman R, Graham L, Newlands ES. *Enhanced anti-proliferative action of busulphan by quercetin on the human leukaemia cell line K562*. Br J Cancer. (1989) 59(3):347-8.

Hotta K, Funahashi T, Bodkin NL, Ortmeyer HK, Arita Y, Hansen BC, Matsuzawa Y. *Circulating concentrations of the adipocyte protein adiponectin are decreased in parallel with reduced insulin sensitivity during the progression to type 2 diabetes in rhesus monkeys*. Diabetes. (2001) 50(5):1126-33.

Jang SY, Bae JS, Lee YH, Oh KY, Park KH, Bae YS. C*affeic acid and quercitrinpurified from Houttuynia cordata inhibit DNA topoisomerase I activity.* Nat ProdRes. (2011) 25(3):222-31.

Jeong JH, An JY, Kwon YT, Li LY, Lee YJ. *Quercetin-induced ubiquitination and down-regulation of Her-2/neu.* J Cell Biochem. (2008) 105(2):585-95.

Jones E, Hughes RE. *Quercetin, flavonoids and the life-span of mice.* ExpGerontol. (1982) 17(3):213-7.

Jones E, Hughes RE. *Quercetin, flavonoids and the life-span of mice*. Exp Gerontol. (1982). 17(3):213-7.

Jung JH, Lee JO, Kim JH, Lee SK, You GY, Park SH, Park JM, Kim EK, Suh PG, An JK, Kim HS. *Quercetin suppresses HeLa cell viability via AMPK-induced HSP70 andEGFR down-regulation*. J Cell Physiol. (2010) 223(2):408-14.

Jung YH, Heo J, Lee YJ, Kwon TK, Kim YH. *Quercetin enhances TRAIL-induced apoptosis in prostate cancer cells via increased protein stability of death receptor 5.* Life Sci. (2010) 86(9-10):351-7.

Jung JH, Lee JO, Kim JH, Lee SK, You GY, Park SH, Park JM, Kim EK, Suh PG, An JK, Kim HS. *Quercetin suppresses HeLa cell viability via AMPK-induced HSP70 and EGFR down-regulation.* J Cell Physiol. (2010) 223(2):408-14.

Jung JY, Lim Y, MoonMS, Kim JY, Kwon O. *Onion peel extracts ameliorate hyperglycemia and insulin resistance in high fat diet/streptozotocin-induced diabetic rats.* Nutr Metab (Lond). (2011) 8(1):18.

Kadowaki T, Yamauchi T, Kubota N, Hara K, Ueki K. *Adiponectin and adiponectin receptors in obesity-linked insulin resistance.* Novartis Found Symp. (2007) 286:164-76; discussion 176-82, 200-3.

Kakran M, Sahoo NG, Li L. *Dissolution enhancement of quercetin through nanofabrication, complexation and solid dispersion.* Biointerfaces. (2011) 88(1):121-30.

Kampkötter A, Timpel C, Zurawski RF, Ruhl S, Chovolou Y, Proksch P, Wätjen W. *Increase of stress resistance and lifespan of Caenorhabditis elegans by quercetin.* Comp Biochem Physiol B Biochem Mol Biol. (2008) 149(2):314-23.

Kandaswami C, Perkins E, Soloniuk DS, Drzewiecki G, Middleton E Jr. *Antiproliferative effects of citrus flavonoids on a human squamous cell carcinoma in vitro.* Cancer Lett. (1991) 56(2):147-52.

Keck, C.M., Müller, R.H. *Drug nanocrystals of poorly soluble drugs produced by high pressure homogenization.* Eur. Pharm. Biopharm. (2006) 62, 3–16.

Khaled KA, El-Sayed YM, Al-Hadiya BM. *Disposition of the flavonoid quercetin in rats after single intravenous and oral doses.* Drug Dev Ind Pharm. (2003) 29(4):397-403.

Kim JY, Kim EH, Park SS, Lim JH, Kwon TK, Choi KS. *Quercetin sensitizes human hepatoma cells to TRAIL-induced apoptosis via Sp1-mediated DR5 up-regulation and proteasome-mediated c-FLIPS down-regulation.* J Cell Biochem. (2008) Dec15;105(6):1386-98.

Kim YH, Lee DH, Jeong JH, Guo ZS, Lee YJ. *Quercetin augments TRAIL-induced apoptotic death: involvement of the ERK signal transduction pathway.* Biochem Pharmacol. (2008) 75(10):1946-58.

Klibanov Al, Maruyama K, Torchilin VP, Huang L. *Amphipathic polyethyleneglycols effectively prolong the circulation times of liposomes.* FEBS Lett. (1990), 268, 235-237.

Knight JA. *Free radicals: their history and current status in aging and disease.* Ann Clin Lab Sci. (1998) (6):331-46.

Kobori M, Masumoto S, Akimoto Y, Oike H. *Chronic dietary intake of quercetin alleviates hepatic fat accumulation associated with consumption of a Western-style diet in C57/BL6J mice.* Mol Nutr Food Res. (2011) 55(4):530-40.

Kobori M, Masumoto S, Akimoto Y, Takahashi Y. *Dietary quercetin alleviates diabetic symptoms and reduces streptozotocin-induced disturbance of hepatic gene expression in mice.* Mol Nutr Food Res. (2009) 53(7):859-68.

Kühnau J. *The flavonoids, a class of semi-essential food components: their role in human nutrition.* World Rev Nutr Diet. (1976); 24:117-91.

Kumada M, Kihara S, Sumitsuji S, Kawamoto T, Matsumoto S, Ouchi N, Arita Y, Okamoto Y, Shimomura I, Hiraoka H, Nakamura T, Funahashi T, Matsuzawa Y; *Osaka CADStudy Group. Coronary arterydisease. Association of hypoadiponectinemia with coronary artery disease in men.* Arterioscler Thromb Vasc Biol. (2003) 1;23(1):85-9.

Kumari A, Yadav SK, Pakade YB, Singh B, Yadav SC. *Development of biodegradable nanoparticles for delivery of quercetin* Colloids *Surf B* Biointerfaces. (2010) 15;80(2):184-92.

Kuo PC, Liu HF, Chao JI. *Survivin and p53 modulate quercetin-induced cell growth inhibition and apoptosis in human lung carcinoma cells.* J Biol Chem. (2004) 279(53):55875-85.

Kuo SM. *Antiproliferative potency of structurally distinct dietary flavonoids on human colon cancer cells.* Cancer Lett. (1996) 110(1-2):41-8.

Kuppusamy UR, Das NP. *Potentiation of beta-adrenoceptor agonist-mediated lipolysis by quercetin and fisetin in isolated rat adipocytes.* Biochem Pharmacol. (1994) 47(3):521-9.

Labib A, Lenaerts L, Chouinard F, Leroux JC, Ouellet R, Van Lier JE. *Biodegradable nanospheres containing phthalocyanines and naphthalocyanines for targeted photodynamic tumor therapy.* Pharm. Res. (1991) 8, 1027-31.

Larocca LM, Giustacchini M, Maggiano N, et al. *Growth-inhibitory effect of quercetin and presence of type II estrogen binding sites in primary human transitional cell carcinomas.* J Urol (1994) 152:1029-33.

Lasic D, Papahadjopoulos D. *Liposomes revisited.* Science. (1995) 267:1275-6.

Lee KW, Kang NJ, Heo YS, Rogozin EA, Pugliese A, Hwang MK, Bowden GT, Bode AM, Lee HJ, Dong Z. *Raf and MEK protein kinases are direct molecular targets for the chemopreventive effect of quercetin, a major flavonol in red wine.* Cancer Res. (2008) 68(3):946-55.

Lee YK, Hwang JT, Kwon DY, Surh YJ, Park OJ. *Induction of apoptosis by quercetin is mediated through AMPKalpha1/ASK1/p38 pathway.* Cancer Lett. (2010) 292(2):228-36.

Lenaerts V, Labib A, Chouinard F, Rousseau J, Ali H, Van Lier J, Van Lier JE. *Nanocapsules with a reduced liver uptake: targeting of phthalocyanines to EMT-6 mouse mammary tumor in vivo.* Eur. J. Pharm. Biopharm. (1995) 41:38-43.

Li XS, Wang JX, Shen ZG, Zhang PY, Chen JF, Yun J. *Preparation of uniform prednisolone microcrystals by a controlled microprecipitation method.* Int. J. Pharm. (2007) 342:26–32.

Lois K, Kumar S. *Obesity and diabetes.* Endocrinol Nutr. (2009) Dec;56 Suppl 4:38-42.

Loke WM, Proudfoot JM, Stewart S, McKinley AJ, Needs PW, Kroon PA, Hodgson JM, Croft KD. *Metabolic transformation has a profound effect on anti-inflammatory activity of flavonoids such as quercetin: lack of association between antioxidant and lipoxygenase inhibitory activity.* Biochem Pharmacol. (2008) 75(5):1045-53.

López-Lázaro M, Willmore E, Austin CA. *The dietary flavonoids myricetin and fisetin act as dual inhibitors of DNA topoisomerases I and II in cells.* MutatRes. (2010) 696(1):41-7.

Ma L, Feugang JM, Konarski P, Wang J, Lu J, Fu S, Ma B, Tian B, Zou C, Wang Z. *Growth inhibitory effects of quercetin on bladder cancer cell.* Front Biosci. (2006) 11:2275-85.

Mahesh T, Menon VP. *Quercetin allievates oxidative stress in streptozotocin-induced diabetic rats.* Phytother Res. (2004) (2):123-7.

Matsui T, Ogunwande IA, Abesundara KJ, Matsumoto K. *Anti-hyperglycemic potential of natural products.* Mini Rev Med Chem. (2006) 6(3):349-56.

Mimi´c-Oka J, Simi´ c DV, Simi´ c TP. *Free radicals in cardiovascular diseases. Facta Univ.* Series: Med. Biol. (1999) 6(1):11–22.

Miodini P, Fioravanti L, Di Fronzo G, Cappelletti V. *The two phyto-oestrogens genistein and quercetin exert different effects on oestrogen receptor function.* Br J Cancer. (1999) 80(8):1150-5.

Murphy EA, Davis JM, McClellan JL, Carmichael MD. *Quercetin's effects on intestinal polyp multiplicity and macrophage number in the Apc(Min/+) mouse.* NutrCancer. (2011) 63(3):421-6.

Nair HB, Huffman S, Veerapaneni P, Kirma NB, Binkley P, Perla RP, Evans DB, Tekmal RR. *Hyaluronic acidbound letrozole nanoparticlesrestore sensitivityto letrozole-resistant xenograft tumorsin mice* J Nanosci Nanotechnol. (2011) 11(5):3789-99.

Namazi M. *Cytochrome-P450 enzymes and autoimmunity: expansion of the relationship and introduction of free radicals as the link.* J. Autoimmune Dis. (2009) 6(4):1–5.

Overman A, Chuang CC, McIntosh M. *Quercetin attenuates inflammation in human macrophages and adipocytes exposed to macrophage-conditioned media.* Int J Obes (Lond). 11 Jan 2011. [Epub ahead of print].

Park HJ, Yang JY, Ambati S, Della-Fera MA, Hausman DB, Rayalam S, Baile CA. *Combined effects of genistein, quercetin, and resveratrol in human and 3T3-L1 adipocytes.* J Med Food. (2008) 11(4):773-83.

Park JY, Park KH, Bang S, Kim MH, Koh SS, Song SY. *Expression of nonsteroidal anti-inflammatory drug-activated gene-1 (NAG-1) inversely correlates with tumor progression in gastric adenomas and carcinomas.* J Cancer Res Clin Oncol. (2008) 134(9):1029-35.

Phillips M, Cataneo RN, Cheema T, Greenberg J. *Increased breath biomarkers of oxidative stress in diabetes mellitus.* Clin Chim Acta. (2004) 344(1-2):189-94.

Pietsch K, Saul N, Menzel R, Stürzenbaum SR, Steinberg CE. *Quercetin mediated lifespan extension in Caenorhabditis elegans is modulated by age-1, daf-2, sek-1 and unc-43.* Biogerontology. (2009) 10(5):565-78.

Pralhad T, Rajendrakumar K. *Study of freeze-dried quercetin-cyclodextrin binary systems by DSC, FT-IR, X-ray diffraction and SEM analysis.* J. Pharm. Biomed. Anal. (2004) 34(2): 333–9.

Rabinow BE. *Nanosuspension in drug delivery.* Nat. Rev. Drug Discov. (2004) 3:785–96.

Rimm EB, Katan MB, Ascherio A, Stampfer MJ, Willett WC. *Relation between intake of flavonoids and risk for coronary heart disease in male health professionals.* Ann Intern Med. (1996) 1;125(5):384-9.

Rivera L, Morón R, Sánchez M, Zarzuelo A, Galisteo M. *Quercetin ameliorates metabolic syndrome and improves the inflammatory status in obese Zucker rats.* Obesity (Silver Spring (2008) 16(9):2081-7.

Russo M, Spagnuolo C, Volpe S, Mupo A, Tedesco I, Russo GL. *Quercetin induced apoptosis in association with death receptors and fludarabine in cells isolated from chronic lymphocytic leukaemia patients.* Br J Cancer. (2010) 24;103(5):642-8.

Salim AS. *Role of free radicals in gastrointestinal cancer.* Singapore Med. J. (1996) 37(3): 295–298.

Sampson L, Rimm E, Hollman PC, de Vries JH, Katan MB. *Flavonol and flavone intakes in US health professionals.* J Am Diet Assoc. (2002) 102(10):1414-20.

Saul N, Pietsch K, Menzel R, Steinberg CE. *Quercetin-mediated longevity in Caenorhabditis elegans: is DAF-16 involved?* Mech Ageing Dev. (2008) 129(10):611-3.

Scambia G, Ranelletti FO, Benedetti Panici P, Bonanno G, De Vincenzo R, Piantelli M, Mancuso S. *Synergistic antiproliferative activity of quercetin and cisplatin on ovarian cancer cell growth.* Anticancer Drugs. (1990) 1(1):45-8.

Scambia G, Ranelletti FO, Panici PB, Piantelli M, Bonanno G, De Vincenzo R, Ferrandina G, Rumi C, Larocca LM, Mancuso S. *Inhibitory effect of quercetin on OVCA 433 cells and presence of type II oestrogen binding sites in primary ovarian tumours and cultured cells.* Br J Cancer. (1990) 62(6):942-6.

Schenk S, Saberi M, Olefsky JM. *Insulin sensitivity: modulation by nutrients and inflammation.* J Clin Invest. (2008) Sep;118(9):2992-3002.

Scherer PE, Williams S, Fogliano M, Baldini G, Lodish HF. *A novel serum protein similar to C1q, produced exclusively in adipocytes.* J Biol Chem. (1995) 270(45):26746-9.

Shan BE, Wang MX, Li RQ. *Quercetin inhibit human SW480 colon cancer growth in association with inhibition of cyclin D1 and survivin expression through Wnt/beta-catenin signaling pathway*. Cancer Invest. (2009) 27(6):604-12.

Shoelson SE, Lee J, Goldfine AB. *Inflammation and insulin resistance.* J Clin Invest. (2006) Jul:116(7):1793-801.

Singhal RL, Prajda N, Yeh YA, Weber G. *1-Phosphatidylinositol 4-phosphate5-kinase (EC 2.7.1.68): a proliferation- and malignancy-linked signal transduction enzyme.* Cancer Res. (1994) 1;54(21):5574-8.

Singh A, Naidu PS, Kulkarni SK. *Reversal of aging and chronic ethanol-induced cognitive dysfunction by quercetin a bioflavonoid.* (2003) 37(11):1245-52.

Singh RP, Sharad S, Kapur S. *Free radicals and oxidative stress in neurodegenerative diseases: relevance of dietary antioxidants*. J. Indian Acad. Clin. Med. (2004) 5:(3)218–25.

Singhal RL, Yeh YA, Prajda N, et al. *Quercetin down-regulates signal transduction in human breast carcinoma cells*. Biochem Biophys Res Commun. (1995) 208:425-431.

So FV, Guthrie N, Chambers AF, Moussa M, Carroll KK. *Inhibition of human breast cancer cell proliferation and delay of mammary tumorigenesis by flavonoids and citrus juices.* Nutr Cancer. (1996) 26(2):167-81.

Sporn MB. *Approaches to prevention of epithelial cancer during the preneoplastic period.* Cancer Res. (1976) (7 PT 2):2699-702.

Stewart LK, Soileau JL, Ribnicky D, Wang ZQ, Raskin I, Poulev A, Majewski M, Cefalu WT, Gettys TW. *Quercetin transiently increases energy expenditure but persistently decreases circulating markers of inflammation in C57BL/6J mice fed a high-fat diet.* Metabolism. (2008) 57(7 Suppl 1):S39-46.

Storm G, Ten Kate MT, Working PK, Bakker-Woudenberg IA. *Doxorubicin entraped in sterically stabilized liposomes: Effects of bacterial blood clearance capacity of the mononuclear phagocyte system.* Clin Can. Res. (1998) 4:111-15.

Stumvoll M, Goldstein BJ, van Haeften TW. *Type 2 diabetes: principles of pathogenesis and therapy.* Lancet. (2005) 365(9467):1333-46.

Tan S, Wang C, Lu C, Zhao B, Cui Y, Shi X, Ma X. *Quercetin is able todemethylate the p16INK4a gene promoter.* Chemotherapy. (2009) 55(1):6-10.

Tanigawa S, Fujii M, Hou DX. *Stabilization of p53 is involved in quercetin-induced cell cycle arrest and apoptosis in HepG2 cells. Biosci Biotechnol Biochem. (2008) 72(3):797-804.*

Thangasamy T, Sittadjody S, Limesand KH, Burd R. *Tyrosinase overexpression promotes ATM-dependent p53 phosphorylation by quercetin and sensitizes melanoma cells to dacarbazine*. Cell Oncol. (2008) 30(5):371-87.

Thangasamy T, Sittadjody S, Mitchell GC, Mendoza EE, Radhakrishnan VM, Limesand KH, Burd R. *Quercetin abrogates chemoresistance in melanoma cells by modulating deltaNp73*. BMC Cancer. (2010) ;10:282.

Van Eerdenbrugh, B., Van den Mooter, G., Augustijns, P. *Top-down production of drug nanocrystals: nanosuspension stabilization, miniaturization and transformation into solid products*. Int. J. Pharm. (2008) 364, 64–75.

Vessal M, Hemmati M, Vasei M. *Antidiabetic effects of quercetin in streptozocin-induced diabetic rats*. Comp Biochem Physiol C Toxicol Pharmacol. (2003) 135C(3):357-64.

Vidya Priyadarsini R, Senthil Murugan R, Maitreyi S, Ramalingam K, Karunagaran D, Nagini S. *The flavonoid quercetin induces cell cycle arrest and mitochondria-mediated apoptosis in human cervical cancer (HeLa) cells through p53 induction and NF-κB inhibition*. Eur J Pharmacol. (2010) 649(1-3):84-91.

Wang Y, Xin X, Jin Z, Hu Y, Li X, Wu J, Jin M. *Anti-diabetic effects of pentamethyl quercetin in neonatally streptozotocin-induced diabetic rats*. Eur J Pharmacol. (2011) 668(1-2):347-53.

Wei BL, Lu CM, Tsao LT, Wang JP, Lin CN. *In vitro anti-inflammatory effects of quercetinO-methyl ether and other constituentsfrom Rhamnus species* Planta Med. (2001) 67(8):745-47.

Weisberg SP, McCann D, Desai M, Rosenbaum M, Leibel RL, *Ferrante AW Jr. Obesity is associated with macrophage accumulation in adipose tissue*. J Clin Invest. (2003) 112(12):1796-808.

Wild S, Roglic G, Green A, Sicree R, King H. *Global prevalence of diabetes: estimates for the year 2000 and projections for 2030*. Diabetes Care. (2004) (5):1047-53.

Xavier CP, Lima CF, Rohde M, Pereira-Wilson C. *Quercetin enhances 5-fluorouracil-induced apoptosis in MSI colorectal cancer cells through p53 modulation*. Cancer Chemother Pharmacol. 11 Apr 2011. [Epub ahead of print] PMID: 21479885.

Xiao JB, Chen XQ, Jiang XY, Hilczer M, Tachiya M. *Probing the interaction of trans-resveratrol with bovine serum albumin: a fluorescence quenching study with Tachiya model*. J. Fluoresc. (2008) 18(3–4) 671–8.

Xing J, Zhang D, Tan T. *Studies on the oridonin-loaded poly (d,l-lactic acid) nanoparticles in vitro and in vivo*. Int. J. Biol. Macromol. (2007) 40(2):153–8.

Xu H, Barnes GT, Yang Q, Tan G, Yang D, Chou CJ, Sole J, Nichols A, Ross JS, Tartaglia LA, Chen H. *Chronic inflammation in fat plays a crucial role in the development of obesity-related insulin resistance*. J Clin Invest. (2003) 112(12):1821-30.

Xu Y, Zhang C, Wang N, Ling F, Li P, Gao Y, Hua W. *Adiponectin inhibits lymphotoxin-β receptor-mediated NF-κB signaling in human umbilical vein endothelial cells*. Biochem Biophys Res Commun. (2011) 404(4):1060-4.

Yang JH, Hsia TC, Kuo HM, Chao PD, Chou CC, Wei YH, Chung JG. *Inhibition of lung cancer cell growth by quercetin glucuronides via G2/M arrest and induction of apoptosis*. Drug Metab Dispos. (2006) 34(2):296-304.

Yang JY, Della-Fera MA, Rayalam S, Ambati S, Hartzell DL, Park HJ, Baile CA. *Enhanced inhibition of adipogenesis and induction of apoptosis in 3T3-L1 adipocytes with combinations of resveratrol and quercetin*. Life Sci. (2008) 82(19-20):1032-9.

Yen GC, Chen YC, Chang WT, Hsu CL. *Effects of polyphenolic compounds on tumor necrosis factor-α (TNF-α)-induced changes of adipokines and oxidative stress in 3T3-L1 adipocytes*. J Agric Food Chem. (2011) 59(2):546-51.

Yoshida T, Maeda A, Horinaka M, Shiraishi T, Nakata S, Wakada M, Yogosawa S, Sakai T. *Quercetin induces gadd45 expression through a p53-independent pathway.* Oncol Rep. (2005) (5):1299-303.

Youl E, Bardy G, Magous R, Cros G, Sejalon F, Virsolvy A, Richard S, Quignard JF, Gross R, Petit P, Bataille D, Oiry C. *Quercetin potentiates insulin secretion and protects INS-1 pancreatic β-cells against oxidative damage via the ERK1/2 pathway.* Br J Pharmacol. (2010) 161(4):799-814.

Yuan ZP, Chen LJ, Fan LY, Tang MH, Yang GL, Yang HS, Du XB, Wang GQ, Yao WX, Zhao QM, Ye B, Wang R, Diao P, Zhang W, Wu HB, Zhao X, Wei YQ, *Liposomal quercetin efficiently suppresses growth of solid tumors in murine models*, Clin. Cancer Res. (2006) 12 (10):3193–9.

Zambaux MF, Bonneaux F, Gref R, Dellacherie E, Vigneron C. *Preparation and characterization of protein C-loaded PLA nanoparticles.* J. Control. Release. (1999) 60(2-3):179–88.

Zhang Q, Zhao XH, Wang ZJ. *Cytotoxicity of flavones and flavonols to a human esophageal squamous cell carcinoma cell line (KYSE-510) by induction of G2/Marrest and apoptosis*. Toxicol In Vitro. (2009) (5):797-807.

Zhang Y, Yang Y, Tang K, Hu, X, Zou G. *Physicochemical characterization and antioxidant activity of quercetin-loaded chitosan nanoparticles.* J. Appl. Polym. Sci. (2008) 107:891–7.

Zhou J, Huang W, Tao R, Ibaragi S, Lan F, Ido Y, Wu X, Alekseyev YO, Lenburg ME, Hu GF, Luo Z. *Inactivation of AMPK alters gene expression and promotes growth of prostate cancer cells*. Oncogene. (2009) (18):1993-2002.

In: Quercetin
Editors: Taiki Chikamatsu and Yuudai Hida
ISBN: 978-1 61942- 057-1

Chapter 5

The Health Benefits of Quercetin: Potential Mechanisms of Action

Jun Yang*
Frito-Lay North America R&D, Plano, TX, US

Abstract

Quercetin, a major bioflavonoid, is one of the most prominent antioxidants in the human diet. It is ubiquitously present in fruits, vegetables, teas and wines as well as dietary supplements. Although some research has reported quercetin acting as potentially carcinogenic agent, many studies have documented the chemopreventive, cardioprotective, and neuroprotective effects of quercetin. Beyond antioxidant, antiproliferative, and antiinflammatory activities, quercetin possesses antibacterial, antiatherogenic, antihypertensive, antifibrotic, and anticoagulative properties. Even though the precise mechanisms by which quercetin exert their beneficial remain unclear, it may be involved in reducing capacities through its possible influences on intracellular redox status, modulating the gene expression of enzymes associated with biotransformation such as phase I and phase II metabolism, suppressing cell proliferation by interacting with type II estrogen binding sites, inhibiting chromosomal alterations and tyrosine kinase, modulating several signal transduction pathways through actions at MEK/ERK and Nrf2/keap1, and stabilizing p53 at both the mRNA and protein levels to reactivate p53-dependent cell cycle arrest and apoptosis. The target of this Chapter is to examine potential mechanisms of action in order to elucidate the possible health-beneficial effects of quercetin.

Introduction

As a member of the flavonoid family, Quercetin is a naturally-occurring flavonol which has a long history of consumption as part of human diet. Flavonols possess numerous biological and pharmacological effects, including antioxidant, chelation, anticarcinogenic,

* Email: junyang97@gmail.com.

cardioprotective properties (Middleton et al., 2000). Dietary quercetin has attracted much attention because of its potentially beneficial effects in preventing various chronic diseases such as cancer and cardiovascular disease (CVD). Understanding the mechanism of quercetin will contribute to the development of more specific preventive strategies against cancer and CVD. A wide array of *in vitro* and *in vivo* studies have revealed diverse biological activities of quercetin, including antioxidant, anticarcinogenic, antiinflammatory, antithrombotic and vasodilatory actions, antimutagenesis, protein kinase C (PKC) inhibition, modulation of cell cycle, apoptosis induction as demonstrated in numerous cellular systems, lipoxygenase inhibition, histamine-release inhibition, superoxide dismutase (SOD) activity, angiogenesis inhibition, and inhibition of phase I and induction of phase II enzymes (Erdman et al., 2007). However, quercetin intervention trials in humans have exhibited inconclusive and even conflict results (Erdman et al., 2005; Williamson and Manach, 2005). The aim of this Chapter is to provide insights into the molecular basis of the potential biological activities of quercetin, with emphasis on capacity of antioxidant and anticancer.

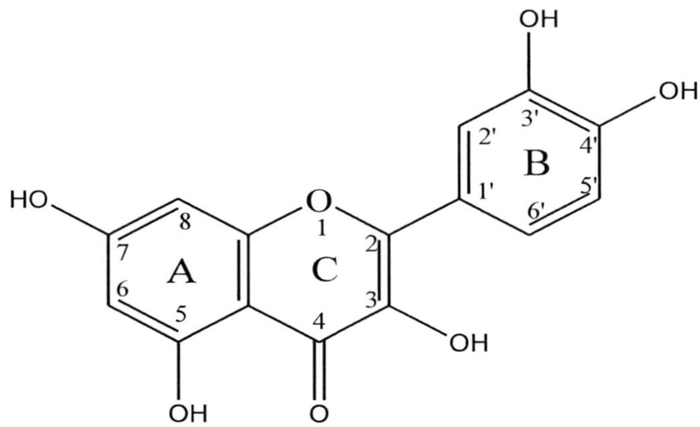

Quercetin aglycone (a)

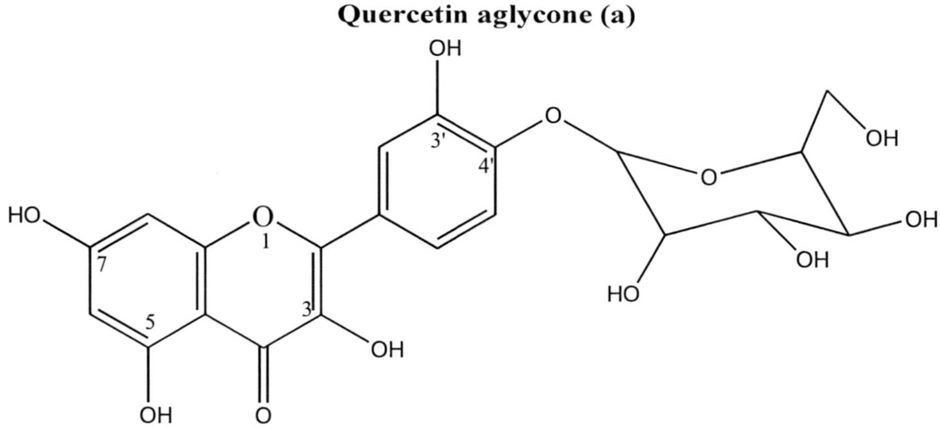

Quercetin-4'-*O*-β-D-Glucoside (b)

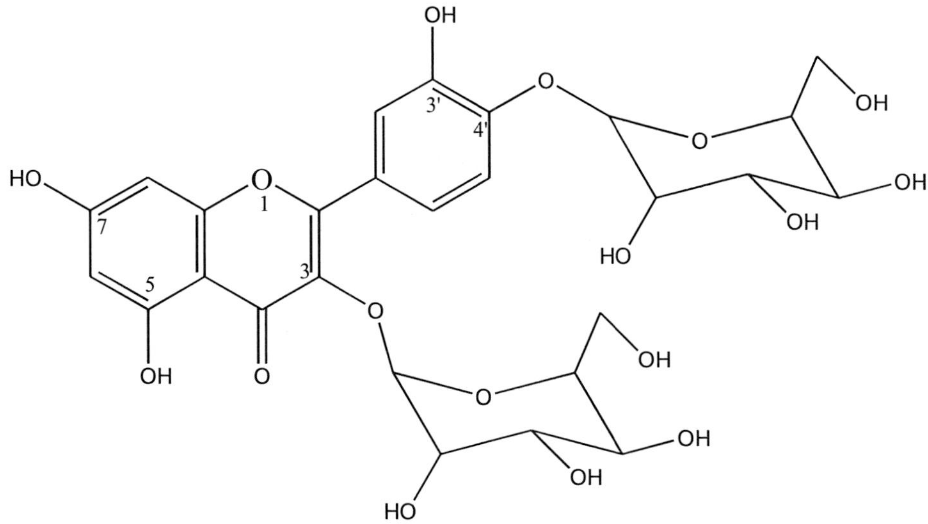

Quercetin-3,4'-*O*-bis-β-D-Glucoside (c)

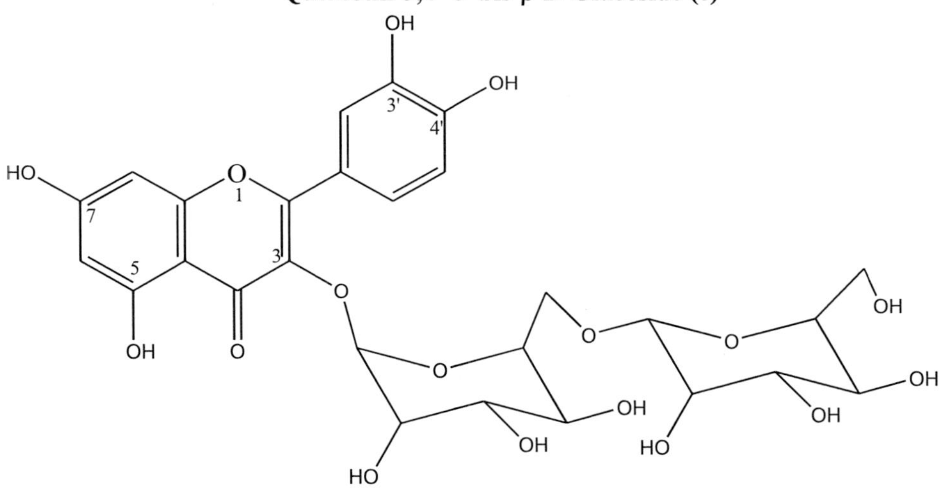

Quercetin-3-*O*-β-Rutinoside (d)

Figure 1. Chemical structure of the flavonol quercetin aglycone and glycosides.

Chemical Structure

Flavonoids are polyphenolic compounds that occur ubiquitously in foods of plant origin. There are thousands of plant-derived flavonoid compounds sharing a common skeleton of phenylchromane. Flavonoids are categorized into flavonols, flavones, flavanones, catechins, anthocyanidins, isoflavones, dihydroflavonols and chalcones. Quercetin (3,3',4',5,7-pentahydroxyflavone) is a naturally-occurring dietary flavonol compound belonging to a broad group of flavonoids, which are characterized by a phenyl benzo(c)pyrone-derived structure consisting of two (A and B) benzene rings linked by a heterocyclic pyran or pyrone C-ring [Figure 1 (a)].

The most important feature associated with antioxidant is the catechol or dihydroxylated B-ring. Other important properties include the presence of unsaturaion in the C-ring, and the presence of a 4-oxo function in the C-ring. For sugarless form, quercetin is termed the aglycone. Commonly, quercetin occurs as glycosides [Figure 1 (b)], for instance, rutin in which the hydrogen of the 3 position hydroxyl group is replaced by a disaccharide.

DIETARY SOURCES

Quercetin, widely distributed in the plant kingdom, is present in variable amounts in dietary fruits, vegetables, nuts, seeds, herbs, spices, tea and red wine. Fruits and vegetables, especially in apples, cranberries, onions, and tomatoes, are the major sources of naturally-occurring dietary quercetin in Western diet (Harnly et al., 2006). In addition, black tea, red wine and various fruit and vegetable juices, are indicated as good sources of dietary quercetin (Sampson et al., 2002). Quercetin-4'-*O*-β-D-glucoside and quercetin-3,4'-*O*-bis-β-D-glucoside majorly exist in onions (Kiviranta et al., 1988) [Figure 1 (c)]. Quercetin-3-*O*-β-rutinoside is the main component in tea (Bailey et al., 1990) [Figure 1 (d)]. Humans absorb appreciable amounts of quercetin and that absorption is enhanced by conjugation with glucose. Quercetin glycosides accounts for 60-75% of the total dietary flavonols intake.

The daily intake of quercetin with a typical Western diet ranges from 0 to 30 mg, with a median of 10 mg (Bohm et al., 1998). According to the USDA database for the flavonoid content of selected foods (2007), among fruits, elderberry juice concentrate exhibited the highest quercetin content with 108.16 mg/100 g), followed by chokeberry juice concentrate (68.17), raw elderberries (*Sambucus spp.*) (42.00), blackberry juice concentrate (22.85), apple skin only (*Malus domestica*) (19.36), wild and frozen bog whortleberries (*Vaccinium*) (17.70), raw cranberry juice (16.41), raw cranberries (*Vaccinium macrocarpon*) 15.09, and raw lingonberries (cowberries) (*Vaccinium vitis-idaea*) (12.97). As for vegetables, hot, yellow wax and raw pepper (*Capsicum annuum*) had the maximum content of quercetin with 50.63 mg/100 g, followed by ancho peppers (*Capsicum annuum*) (27.60), raw okra (*Abelmoschus esculentus*) (24.26), raw asparagus (*Asparagus officinalis*) (12.40), and red leaf, raw lettuce (*Lactuca sativa var. crispa*) (11.99). Onions, commonly consumed in our diet, are rich in quercetin. For example, quercetin content is in order from high to low as: red and raw onions (*Allium cepa*) (33.43 mg/100 g), raw onion (*Allium cepa*) (21.42), sweet and raw onion (*Allium cepa*) (14.80), and white and raw onion (*Allium cepa*) (7.29). Tea is widely consumed beverage. Green, dry and decaffeinated tea leaves possess the highest amount of quercetin with 263.95 mg/100g, followed by black, dry and decaffeinated one (256.02), green and dry one (223.97), black and dry one (199.75), and dried oolong tea leaves (108.83). Quercetin may be served as a dietary supplement within a concentration range of 10 - 125 mg/serving (Harwood et al., 2007). The average daily dietary intake of quercetin in the United States is estimated to be 25 mg (NTP Technical Report, 1991).

Mechanisms of Action

Antioxidant and Pro-oxidant Activity

As an antioxidant, quercetin derives from the reactivity of phenolic compounds with free radical species to form phenoxy radicals which are considerably less reactive. The hydroxyl groups of quercetin, acting as electron donors, are responsible for the compound's free radical scavenging activity. It was indicated that the chemical structure with presence and location of the hydroxyl substitutions and the catechol-type B-ring contributes the antioxidant property of quercetin (Silva et al., 2002; Rietjens et al., 2005; Wang et al., 2006), being related to (1) catechol group or an ortho-dihydroxy in the B-ring, (2) a 2, 3-double bond, and (3) hydroxyl substitution at positions 3 and 5. Quercetin has antioxidant structural elements characterized by a hydroxylation pattern of 3, 5, 7, 30, and 40 and a catechol B-ring. Boots et al (2003) have found that quercetin may be converted into reactive products if it exerts antioxidant activity. The antioxidant activity of quercetin can be also explained by its chelating action. On the other hand, quercetin can be oxidized to a quinoid form, which is further involved in the redox cycle.

As an anti-oxidant, quercetin protects cells against oxidative stress-mediated apoptosis when mouse thymocytes incubated with 50 μM of quercetin (Lee et al., 2003). An a pro-oxidant agent, quercetin induced cytotoxicity in umbilical vein endothelial cells, and was moderately cytotoxic in lung embryonic fibroblasts in human cells tested at concentrations of up to 300 μM (Matsuo et al., 2005). Galati et al (2002) reported that quercetin oxidizes erythrocyte oxy-hemoglobin by formation of methemoglobin, while an increase in activity was monitored in the presence of extracellular horseradish peroxidase and H_2O_2. Quercetin can be oxidized and degraded down to form a free radical ortho-semiquinone intermediate *in vitro*, which may subsequently lead to the production of reactive oxygen species (ROS) including superoxide and H_2O_2 (Metodiewa et al., 1999; Boots et al., 2003). Furthermore, quercetin was observed to co-oxidize ascorbate in rat hepatocytes with added peroxidase and H_2O_2, which may be mediated by the semiquinone radical.

Some *in vivo* studies performed in mice and rats assess quercetin-associated effect on anti-oxidant/pro-oxidant activity by using indicators of glutathione (reduced) (GSH), enzymatic activity, and markers of lipid peroxidation. Choi et al. (2005) examined quercetin-linked pro-oxidant activity with around 78 mg quercetin/kg body weight/day for 4- to 6-week oral treatments in male Sprague-Dawley rats. It was observed that quercetin significantly lowered hepatic levels of GSH, while concomitantly increasing the activity of glutathione peroxidase (GPx) and decreasing GR activity compared to controls. Moreover, this flavonol boosted serum and liver vitamin E levels and decreased hepatic malondialdehyde (MDA) levels. After consumed up to 2.6 mg quercetin/kg body weight/day through drinking water in an 8-week mouse study, the amount of GSH and glutathione-S-transferase (GST) in liver and lung significant increased in comparison with a control group (Gandhi and Khanduja, 1993). Conversely, Rangan et al (2002) reported an elevated level of renal MDA production in male Wistar rats administered quercetin in the diet for a period of 21 days at dose levels of 285 or 1133 mg/kg body weight/day. A study conducted by Duarte et al (2001) found that the level of liver GSH decreases in normotensive Wistar Kyoto rats fed by 10 mg quercetin/kg body weight/day by gavage. In the meanwhile, levels of liver and plasma MDA in quercetin-treated rats were comparable to controls. However, Fischer et al. (2002) monitored increases in GST and glutathione reductase (GR) activities in segments of the colon mucosa of Sprague Dawley rats after consuming quercetin-supplemented diets of around 500 mg/kg body weight/day. In a study of quercetin-treated rats for a period of 5 weeks at dose levels of 10 mg/kg body weight/day by gavage, it was found that plasma level of markers of oxidative liver stress such as thiobarbituric acid (TBARS) and nitrates plus nitrites (NOx) were comparable to controls (Garcı´a-Saura et al., 2005). Quercetin was found to cause DNA damage in a dose-response manner, and lipid peroxidation in isolated rat liver nuclei (Sahu and Washington, 1991) and damage in calf thymus DNA (Rahman et al., 1992) in the presence of O_2, suggesting that the oxygen radicals generated by auto-oxidation of quercetin and the pro-oxidant mechanism may be responsible for the *in vitro* mutagenicity of quercetin.

As an antioxidant, although the accurate mechanism by which quercetin influences on transcription factor complexes to target antioxidant-responsive element/electrophile-responsive element (ARE/EpRE) is not completely understood, quercetin appears to interact with cellular defense systems through the ARE/EpRE. Tanigawa et al (2007) have reported that quercetin elevated the ARE binding activity and Nrf2-mediated transcription activity in human $HepG_2$ cells by up-regulating the expression of Nrf2 mRNA and protein, and stabilizing Nrf2 protein through inhibiting the ubiquitination and proteasomal turnover of Nrf2. It was further observed that quercetin lowered the level of Keap1 protein in post-translational levels through the formation of modified Keap1 protein. It was concluded that upregulation of Nrf2 through the regulation of both transcription and post-transcription sites, and repression of Keap1 by affecting the posttranscription site are associated with the pathway of quercetin-induced ARE activity, which offers a mechanism of quercetin in cancer chemoprevention.

Anticarcinogenic Activity

Quercetin has antiproliferative effects (Wenzel et al., 2000; Van Erk et al., 2005) and performs a dose-dependent inhibitory effect on cell proliferation. It inhibits the malignant cell growth in different cell lines, including head and neck (Castillo et al., 1989), breast (Miodini et al., 1999), bladder (Larocca et al., 1994), colon (Kuo et al., 1996), leukemia (Larocca et al., 1991), gastric (Yoshida et al., 1990), melanoma (Piantelli et al., 1995), lung (Caltagirone et al., 1997), and ovarian (Scambia et al., 1990). In above i*n vitro* experiments, the concentration of quercetin in inhibiting 50% of cancer cell proliferation was from 7 nM to 100 μM (Lamson and Brignall, 2000). Although the anticarcinogenic mechanisms of quercetin are not well elucidated, several mechanisms that have been hypothesized for this effect are: 1) inhibitory effect on the cell cycle in the late G1 phase, resulting in apoptosis and blocking signal transduction pathways (Yoshida et al., 1992); 2) down-regulating the expression of oncogenes such as c-myc and k-ras (Nishioka et al., 1989); and 3) increasing DNA fragmentation and caspase-3 activity in malignant cell lines which are resistant to the CD95 (Apo1/Fas)-mediated apoptosis (Russo et al., 1999).

The potential effect of quercetin on chemical-induced carcinogenesis is involved in initiation and/or promotion stage (Matsukawa et al., 2002). Most of studies were supportive of a chemoprotective effect of quercetin (Hirose et al., 1983; Kato et al., 1985; Sato et al., 1987; Verma et al., 1988; Akagi et al., 1995; Exon et al., 1998; Tanaka et al., 1999; Devipriya et al., 2006; Dihal et al., 2006; Jin et al., 2006). On the other hand, some studies supported that quercetin promotes carcinogenesis (Pereira et al., 1996; Barotto et al., 1998; Matsukawa et al., 2002; Valentich et al., 2006). Nair et al (2004) reported that quercetin with 25 and 50 μmol/L significantly suppressed cell growth in the moderately aggressive DU145 prostate cancer cell line and highly aggressive PC-3 cell line. However, the growth inhibitory effect on LNCaP prostate cancer cells or the normal BG-9 fibroblast cell line was less. Quercetin inhibited HCT-116 and HT-29 colon cell proliferation with 30 and 80 μmol/L, respectively, while MCF-7 cell proliferation was not inhibited at concentration up to 100 μmol/L after 24 h treatment (Van der Woude et al., 2003). Xing et al (2001) demonstrated that quercetin effectively lowered the expression of androgen receptor via western blot analysis in LNCaP prostate cancer cells. It was also found that quercetin prevented the secretion of prostrate specific androgen-regulated tumor markers. Wallea et al (2003) have revealed that [^{14}C]quercetin covalently binds to macromolecules such as DNA and proteins in the intestinal Caco-2 and hepatic $HepG_2$ human cancer cells. Covalent adducts between proteins and quercetin were observed by using SDS-PAGE and liquid scintillation spectrometry after extensive purification. After incubation up to 2 hr with [^{14}C]quercetin, both cell types exhibited DNA binding with a maximum level of 5-15 pmol/mg DNA, and with a highest level of 75-125 pmol/mg protein. It was proposed that this specific binding may mediate part of the antiproliferative and other cellular actions of quercetin. Quercetin showed less toxic than drug cisplatin in treatment of the human head and neck squamous cell carcinoma in laryngeal HeP2 cells (Sharma et al., 2005). The results indicated that this flavonol suppressed the binding of survivin to caspases. The potential mechanism was associated with the inhibition of Akt/PKB phosphorylation. Interestingly, at a concentration of 10 μmol/L, it was found that quercetin protected against H_2O_2-induced cytotoxicity, DNA strand breaks, and apoptosis in H4IIIE rat hepatoma cells. However, with higher concentration with 50 μmol/L, it gave rise to cytotoxicity, oligonucleosomal DNA fragmentation and activation of caspase-2, caspase-3 and caspase-9 in the same cell line (Watjen et al., 2005). Similarly, at concentrations of 1 and 10 μmol/L, it stimulates cell growth; however, at 100 μmol/L, quercetin inhibits cell proliferation in a human squamous SCC-25 carcinoma cell line (Elattar and Virji, 2000).

Some researchers observed inhibitory activities of quercetin on colon tumorigenesis-induced by azoxymethane (AOM) (Tanaka et al., 1999; Dihal et al., 2006), by methylazoxymethanol acetate (MAM), and by DMBDD (Akagi et al., 1995). In addition, quercetin exhibited protective effects on urinary bladder neoplasms induced by *N*-Nitroso-n-butyl-(4-hydroxybutyl)amine (BBN) (Fukushima et al., 1983), on mammary gland tumors initiated by N-Nitrosomethylurea (NMU) or 9, 10- or 7,12-dimethylbenz[a]anthracene (DMBA) (Devipriya et al., 2006), and on blood lymphocyte damage and pulmonary precancerous pathologic change induced by benzo[a]pyrene (Jin et al., 2006). For some animals, quercetin did not exert effects on initiation (Sato et al., 1987) or promotion (Morino et al., 1982; Ito et al., 1988) of chemical-induced carcinogenesis. Conversely, Quercetin increased tumor formation in the renal tissues of hamsters-administered subcutaneous estradiol implants (Zhu and Liehr 1994). Moreover, enhanced incidences of pancreatic dysplastic foci were monitored in rats fed a single intraperitoneal administration of N-nitrosomethylurea (NMU) at 3 days of age, followed by quercetin treatment for 20 weeks (Valentich et al., 2006). Pereira et al. (1996) reported that quercetin boosted the formation of AOM-induced gastrointestinal tumors.

Antiinflammatory Activity

Intake of flavonols was inversely associated with subsequent coronary heart disease in both a prospective cohort study - the Zutphen Elderly Study (Hertog et al., 1993), and a cross-cultural study in the Seven Countries (Hertog et al., 1995). Dietary quercetin may lower the risk of CVD in humans (Egert et al., 2009). Quercetin exhibits potential anti-inflammatory effects demonstrated by *in vitro* and *in vivo* studies (Nair et al., 2006; Lotito and Frei, 2006; Boesch-Saadatmandi et al., 2009). This flavonol is a strong antioxidant that prevents oxidation of low-density lipoproteins (LDL) *in vitro* (de Whalley et al. 1990). It inhibits LDL oxidation and platelet aggregation (Hubbard et al., 2004), and improves of endothelial function (Lodi et al., 2009). Quercetin significantly suppressed lipid peroxidation in the rat liver (Cai et al., 1997). In addition, the quercetin derivatives may exert anti-inflammatory effects after it is glucuronidated, sulphated and methylated in intestine and liver (Tribolo et al., 2008).

Recently, the effect of quercetin and its metabolites quercetin-3-glucuronide (Q3G) and isorhamnetin on inflammatory gene expression of proinflammatory markers was investigated in murine RAW264.7 macrophages induced by lipopolysaccharide (LPS) (Boesch-Saadatmandia et al., 2011). In addition, microRNA-155 (miR-155) was examined to be modulated by quercetin and its metabolites. miR-155 is a component of the macrophage in response to different types of inflammatory mediators such as LPS. The results showed that quercetin significantly lowers mRNA levels of interleukin 1β (IL1β), interleukin 6 (IL6), macrophage inflammatory protein 1α (MIP1α) and inducible nitric oxide synthase (iNOS). Quercetin and isorhamnetin but not Q3G significantly decreased mRNA and protein levels of tumor necrosis factor alpha (TNF-α). Moreover, quercetin and isorhamnetin but not Q3G down-regulated proinflammatory miR-155. Furthermore, quercetin possessed anti-inflammatory properties in mice by fed 0.1 mg of quercetin / gram diet over 6 weeks. Finally, the researcher concluded that the NFκB signal transduction cascade and the activation of the Nrf2 pathway as well as miR-155 in response to quercetin and isorhamnetin may mediate their anti-inflammatory effects both *in vitro* and *in vivo*.

Biotransformation

Biotransformation is linked to phase I enzymes such as cytochrome P450 (CYP) mainly responsible for the activation of procarcinogen, and phase II enzymes such as NADPH:quinine oxidoreductase (NQO1) involved in the detoxification of carcinogens (Moon et al., 2006). Flavonoids modulate CYPs through binding to the aryl hydrocarbon receptor (AhR), a ligand-activated transcription factor, acting as either AhR agonists or antagonists. AhR induces tumorigenesis, teratogenesis, and tumor promotion. As a dietary ligand of the AhR, quercetin influences on CYP1A1 transcription, furthermore affects the functionality of AhR in MCF-7 cells (Ciolino et al., 1999). Jin et al (2006) also reported that quercetin enhanced the amounts of the human CYP1A1 gene in MCF-7 human breast cancer cell line, which is regulated by AhR. Quercetin also exhibited inhibitory effects on cytochrome P450 monoxygenases (Balasubramanian et al., 1996). Quercetin inhibits phenacetin *O*-deethylase activity in a recombinant CYP1A2 enzyme preparation with an IC_{50}

value of 7.5 μM (Obach 2000). Additively, quercetin as a bioactive component in St. John's wort (Hypericum perforatum) suppresses CYP1A2 (Obach, 2000) and CYP3A4 (Zou et al., 2002).

Flavonoids are proposed to interact with cellular defense systems, especially for phase II enzymes and other enzymes including NQO1, glutathione S-transferase, UDP-glucuronosyl transferase, thioredoxin heme oxygenase-1, γ-glutamylcysteine synthetase, metallothionein, inducible nitric oxide synthase, cysteine/glutamate exchange transporter, and Fra-1 (Mulcahy et al., 1995; Ren et al., 1995; Yoshioka et al., 1995; Moinova et al., 1998; Chan et al., 1999; Sasaki et al., 2002). Quercetin can activate phase II detoxifying enzymes, resulting in the detoxification of carcinogens, which represents one of mechanisms of their anticarcinogenic effects. This flavonol could stimulate phase II detoxifying systems in transcriptional level. For instance, an increase in NQO1 transcription in response to quercetin was documented (Valerio et al., 2001). It showed that quercetin induced a two-fold increase in NQO1 protein amount, and a three- to four-fold increase in NQO1 mRNA expression. Phase II enzymes possess specific nucleotide sequences in their gene promoters, which is defined as the antioxidant-responsive element/ electrophile-responsive element (ARE/EpRE), with the consensus sequence 5′-TA/CANNA/GTGAC/TNNNGCA/G-3′ (Wasserman and Fahl, 1997). ARE/EpRE has been found to protect cells against carcinogens and oxidative stress. Several molecules, such as c-Jun, nuclear factor-E2-related factor 2 (Nrf2), ATF2, and ATF4, have been indicated as potential modulators of ARE/EpRE (Venugopal et al., 1996; Itoh et al., 1999; Nguyen et al., 2000; Hayes and McMahon, 2001). For example, Nrf-2 is a transcription factor essential to Phase II enzyme induction. It is normally localized in the cytosol, where it is linked to protein-protein interactions with the chaperone Keap1 (Itoh et al., 1999). An inducer such as quercetin disrupts the Keap1 - Nrf2 interactions, permitting Nrf2 to translocate to the nucleus and further bind to the ARE/EpRE (Hayes and McMahon, 2001). The importance of Nrf2 in induction of Phase II enzymes in prevention of cancer has been proven in Nrf2 knockout mice experiments (McMahon et al., 2001; Ramos-Gomez et al., 2001). Quercetin induced Nrf2-ARE-mediated NQO1 transactivation through enhancement of the steady-state level of Nrf2 at both transcriptional and posttranslational stages, and reduction of the steady-state level of Keap1 through 26S proteasome-independent degradation (Tanigawa et al., 2007). It exhibited that ARE activity induced by quercetin was markedly affected through silencing Nrf2 or Keap1 with their siRNA, indicating that both Nrf2 up-regulation and Keap1 down-regulation activated by quercetin are essential for ARE-mediated NQO1 activation.

Signal transduction Pathway, Cell Cycle Regulation and Apoptosis

Quercetin can potentially interact with different intracellular signaling pathways to induce apoptosis, arrest cell cycle arrest and inhibit cell survival/proliferation. It has been demonstrated that, with low concentrations, this flavonol may activate the mitogen-activated protein kinase (MAPK) pathways including c-Jun N-terminal kinase (JNK), extracellular regulated kinase (ERK), and p38, which may result in the survival gene and defensive expressions such as c-fos, c-jun, and glutathione-S-transferase, giving rise to evoking survival and protective mechanisms. On the other hand, quercetin with high concentrations activates the caspase pathway, leading to apoptosis (Kong et al., 2000; Spencer et al., 2003). For examples, quercetin activated caspase-3, released cytochrome c, and decreased mitochondrial membrane potential in pancreatic BSp73AS and MiaPaCa-2 cancer cells after incubation with 100 μmol/L concentration (Mouria et al., 2002), which was in agreement with the results in HL- 60 leukemic cells with a concentration of 60 μmol/L quercetin (Wang et al., 1999). Accordingly, quercetin activated the mitochondrial pathway in colon Caco-2 cancer cells with the concentration range of 5-50 μmol/L after 48 h of incubation (Van Erk et al., 2005). On the other hand, quercetin was found to induce the cleavage of caspase-3, caspase-7, caspase-9 and PARP in a dose-dependent manner in human A549 lung cancer cells (Nguyen et al., 2004). In addition, the combination of quercetin and TNF-related apoptosis inducing ligand (TRAIL) enhanced TRAIL-induced cytotoxicity by activating caspases and suppressing phosphorylation of Akt (Kim and Lee 2007). Moreover, Murtaza et al (2006) have found that quercetin with 10 or 100 μmol/L concentration modulates genes associated with cell cycle arrest through up-regulation of p21 and down-regulation of cdk4, apoptosis through up-regulation of Bax and caspase-8, and phase I/II metabolism in CO115 colon cancer cells after 24 and 48 hr exposures.

Mutations of p53 protein are one of the most common genetic abnormalities in human cancers. Quercetin arrests the cells in different phases in cell cycle with different cell lines. In G1 phase, quercetin with 70 μM was monitored to lower DNA replication, and consequently delayed cell division in gastric cancer cells (Yoshida et al., 1990). It was observed to arrest cells in the late G1 phase of the cell cycle in human leukemic T-cells, while 64% of cells were in G0/G1 phase after treatment of 70 μM quercetin in comparison with 50% of cells in control (Yoshida et al., 1992). Additively, the suppression of p53 expression was demonstrated to arrest the cells in the G2-M phase in the cell cycle (Avila et al., 1996). Quercetin with 248 μM was reported to be down-regulation of mutant p53 protein expression in a dose-response manner in human breast cancer cell lines (Avila et al., 1994).

Quercetin can induce programmed cell death through an apoptotic mechanism in different types of tumor cells, including breast cancer (Hakimuddin et al., 2004), ovarian cancer (Chan et al., 2003), prostatic cancer (Huynh et al., 2003; Vijayababu et al., 2005), colon cancer (Van Erk et al., 2005), leukemia (Shen et al., 2003; Mertens-Talcott et al., 2005), lung cancer (Nguyen et al., 2004), murine hepatoma (Chi et al., 1997), oral cancer (Ong et al., 2004), and melanoma (Zhang et al., 2005). Generally the concentration of quercetin for induction of apoptosis ranges from 29 to 150 μmol/L in above cancer cell lines. Quercetin was observed to induce the apoptosis in squamous HSC-2 cell carcinoma, HSC-3 cells, submandibular gland HSG carcinoma cells, and promyelotic HL60 leukemia human cell cultures, but not in gingival HGF fibroblasts, pulp HPC cells and periodontal ligament HPLF fibroblasts normal human oral cells (Chowdhury et al., 2005). It was found that tumor cells are resistant to CD95-mediated apoptosis. However, treating cancer cells with quercetin could make tumor cells susceptible to apoptosis via restoration of the sensitivity to CD95 (Russo et al., 1999). On the contrary, quercetin can act as an anti-apoptotic compound, which is ascribed to its capability of inhibiting MAPK pathways and decreasing expression of genes involved in the JNK-c-Jun/AP-1 and ERK–c-Fos/AP-1 pathways (Ishikawa and Kitamura 2000).

Quercetin targets Bcl-2 family proteins by up-regulation of the proapoptotic proteins Bcl-2, Bax and caspase-3, and down-regulation of the antiapoptotic Bcl-2 proteins Bcl-x_L and Bcl-2 in prostatic PC-3 carcinoma cells at 50 and 100 μmol/L (Vijayababu et al., 2005). Kim et al (2005) revealed that Bcl-2 was significantly reduced and Bax remained unchanged in

HT-29 and SW480 colon cancer cells with 50 μmol/L quercetin after 72 h of treatment. In addition, Zhang et al (2005) have observed that 10^{-4} g/mL quercetin after 24 h of treatment enhanced caspase-3 activity, decreased Bcl-2 expression, and remained unchanged levels of Bcl-x_L.

Anti-Hypertensive Effects

High blood pressure plays an important role in developing CVDs, including stoke, coronary disease, peripheral artery disease, heart failure, and renal disease. The blood pressure-reducing effect of quercetin could be an important factor contributing to lowering risk of chronic diseases (Perez-Vizcaino et al., 2009). This flavonol has been exhibited to reduce the risk of high blood pressure in some hypertensive rat models, including spontaneously hypertensive rats (Duarte et al., 2001), L-NAME-induced rats (Duarte et al., 2002), DOCA-salt hypertensive rats (Galisteo et al., 2004), Dahl salt-sensitive hypertensive rats (Aoi et al., 2004), two-kidney one-clip Goldblatt rats (García-Saura et al., 2005), rats with aortic constriction (Carlstrom et al., 2007), and Obese Zucker rats (Rivera et al., 2008). Blood pressure was measured directly *via* arterial canulation at the end of the treatment period in most studies and quercetin reduced the systolic, the diastolic and the mean blood pressure. The effect of quercetin on antihypertensive activity was reported in spontaneously hypertensive rats (SHRs) by Duarte et al (2001). What a single oral daily dose of 10 mg of quercetin/kg was given to 14-week-old SHRs for five weeks led to a significant reduction in systolic (-18%), diastolic (-23%), mean arterial blood pressure (-21%), and heart rate (-12%). On the contrary, after a diet containing an approximately 130 mg of quercetin/kg was given to 5 week-old SHRs for 5 or 11 weeks, Carlstrom et al (2007) found that arterial blood pressure was similar in quercetin-administrated SHRs compared to the untreated animals. Dahl rats are genetically predisposed to develop hypertension upon receiving NaCl. Quercetin lowered elevated systolic blood pressure in Dahl salt-sensitive rats (Mackraj et al., 2008). Similarly, the development of hypertension in deoxycorticosterone acetate (DOCA)-salt-induced rats was suppressed by quercetin with 10 mg/kg, which showed a similar effect to that of verapamil with 20 mg/kg (Galisteo et al., 2004). Oral quercetin administration with 10 mg/kg/day decreased systolic blood pressure in two-kidney, one-clip (2K1C) Goldblatt hypertensive rats (García-Saura et al., 2005).

Other Biological Activities

The central nervous disorders such as a decline of cognitive function, dementia, and Alzheimer's disease have been linked to oxidative stress existing in nerve cells (Perkins et al., 1999; Smith et al., 2000). Youdim and Joseph (2001) reported that quercetin and its glycosides showed a neuroprotective effect, giving rise to a reduced risk of central nervous disorders. Furthermore, Wang and Joseph (1999) observed that quercetin and its glycosides serve as antioxidants against exposure to ROS in cultured rat pheochromocytoma PC-12 cells. Conjugated quercetin metabolites were evaluated to attenuate ROS produced by 13-hydroperoxyoctadecadienoic acid (13-HPODE) for the central nervous system in pheochromocytoma PC-12 cells (Shirai et al., 2006). It is concluded that antioxidative metabolites of quercetin have protective effect on nerve cells from attack of lipid hydroperoxides.

Heat shock proteins combine with mutant p53, which permits tumor cells to bypass normal mechanisms of cell cycle arrest. Quercetin was observed to suppress production of heat shock proteins in leukemia (Elia et al., 1996), colon cancer (Koishi et al., 1992), and breast cancer (Hansen et al., 1997).

Tyrosine kinases are related to the transduction of growth factor signals to the nucleus. Quercetin suppresses tyrosine kinase, which has been observed both in rat mammary tumor cells (Levy et al., 1984) and in non-malignant cells (Yokoo et al., 1997). As a chemopreventive agent, quercetin was reported as a tyrosine kinase inhibitor in a human phase I trial (Ferry et al., 1996). The study showed that an intravenous administration of quercetin resulted in inhibition of lymphocyte tyrosine kinase at one hour among nine of eleven cases in patients with cancers.

Type II estrogen receptors (ER II) are found in normal tissue and human tumor types such as breast, ovarian, leukemic, melanoma, and colorectal. Quercetin performed to modulate ER II expression in both type I estrogen receptor positive (ER+) and type I estrogen receptor negative (ER-) human breast cancer cells (Scambia et al., 1993). Quercetin was also reported to combine ER II sites with an affinity similar to tamoxifen and diethylstilbestrol in cultured human melanoma cells, as indicated by 7 nM of quercetin was required to inhibit 50% cell growth (Piantelli et al., 1995).

Ranelletti et al (1999) have found that 10 μM of quercetin inhibit the p21-Ras oncogene expression in colon cancer cell line. It was reported that quercetin was specifically inhibiting p21-Ras expression in human colon cancer cell lines and in primary colorectal cancers (Cruz-Correa et al., 2006).

Quercetin has also been exhibited to induce morphological alterations and DNA fragmentation in leukemia (Csokay et al., 1997). Moreover, it shows DNA damaging by generating ROS and endogenous reductants. It also prevents topoisomerase II and functions as a potent anti-tumor agent causing cleavage of DNA fragments to 1-2 Mb in HL-60 cells (Kawanishi et al., 2005).

Ortho-quinone/quinone methide intermediates formed in the oxidative degradation of quercetin are capable of covalently binding to DNA and protein, which is very likely a main contributor in quercetin-associated mutagenicity (Walle et al., 2003, Rietjens et al., 2005). It was also reported the binding of the quercetin aglycone to DNA in intact cultured human cell lines such as intestinal Caco-2 and hepatic HepG2 cells (Walle et al., 2003; van der Woude et al., 2006).

Conclusion and Future Study

In this Chapter, the potential mechanisms of action for quercetin associated with biological effects are discussed, although the exact mechanisms are not well understood so far. Quercetin as a bioactive molecule possesses antioxidant, anticarcinogenic, and anti-inflammatory properties. It interferes with the initiation, development and progression of cancer, modulates cellular proliferation, differentiation, angiogenesis and metastasis, inhibits growth factor and cyclooxygenase-2, induces apoptosis, interacts with NF-κB, AP-1 etc.

signaling pathways, regulates expression of anti-apoptotic proteins, and modulates phase I and phase II enzymes. Particularly, as a chemopreventive agent, quercetin functions through multiple action mechanisms, including inhibition of cell survival, cell proliferation, apoptosis induction through cell cycle control, and interaction with various signal transduction pathways. However, the existed results reveal that some of the contradictory data have been found in different studies due mainly to different cell lines and experimental conditions such as test dose, culture conditions, exposure length, and toxicity. Thus, data still need to be filled in order to determine whether quercetin plays an appreciable role in treatment of cancer and CVD. Although some *in vitro* and *in vivo* studies of quercetin have elucidated and identified several action mechanisms, clinical studies are required. The ongoing investigations on quercetin could target a diverse range of cellular functions and molecular pathways to ameliorate chronicle diseases.

References

Akagi, K., Hirose, M., Hoshiya, T., Mizoguchi, Y., Ito, N., Shirai, T. Modulating effects of ellagic acid, vanillin and quercetin in a rat medium term multi-organ carcinogenesis model. *Cancer Lett.,* 1995, 94, 113-121.

Aoi, W., Niisato, N., Miyazaki, H., Marunaka, Y. Flavonoidinduced reduction of ENaC expression in the kidney of Dahl salt-sensitive hypertensive rat. *Biochem. Biophys. Res. Commun*, 2004, 315, 892-896.

Avila, M. A., Velasco, J. A., Cansado, J., Notario, V. Quercetin mediates the down-regulation of mutant p53 in the human breast cancer cell line MDA-MB468. *Cancer Res.,* 1994, 54, 2424-2428.

Avila, M. A., Velasco, J. A., Harter, K. W., et al. Quercetin as a modulator of the cellular neoplastic phenotype. *Adv. Expl. Med. Biol.,* 1996, 401, 101-110.

Bailey, R. G., McDowell, I., Nursten, H. E. Use of an HPLC photodiode-array detector in a study of the nature of a black tea liuoe. *J. Sci. Food Agric.*, 1990, 52, 509-525.

Balasubramanian, S., Govindasamy, S. Inhibitory effect of dietary flavonol quercetin on 7, 12-dimethylbenz[a]anthracene-induced hamster buccal pouch carcinogenesis. *Carcinogenesis,* 1996, 17, 877-879.

Barotto, N. N., Lopez, C. B., Eynard, A. R., Zapico, M. E., Valentich, M. A. Quercetin enhances pretumorous lesions in the nmu model of rat pancreatic carcinogenesis. *Cancer Lett.,* 1998, 129, 1-6.

Boesch-Saadatmandia, C., Lobodab, A., Wagnera, A. E., Stachurskab, A. et al. Effect of quercetin and its metabolites isorhamnetin and quercetin-3-glucuronide on inflammatory gene expression: role of miR-155. *J. Nutri. Biochem.,* 2011, 22, 293-299.

Boesch-Saadatmandi, C., Wolffram, S., Minihane, A. M., Rimbach, G. Effect of apoE genotype and dietary quercetin on blood lipids and TNF-alpha levels in apoE3 and apoE4 targeted gene replacement mice. *Br. J. Nutr.,* 2009, 101, 1440-1443.

Bohm, H., Boeing, H., Hempel, J., Raab, B., Kroke, A. Flavonols, flavone and anthocyanins as natural antioxidants of food and their possible role in the prevention of chronic diseases. *Z. Ernahrungswiss.* 1998, 37, 147-163.

Boots, A.W., Kubben, N., Haenen, G. R. M. M., Bast, A. Oxidized quercetin reacts with thiols rather than with ascorbate: Implication for quercetin supplementation. *Biochem. Biophys. Res. Commun.,* 2003, 308, 560-565.

Cai, Q., Rahn, R. O., Zhang, R. Dietary flavonoids, quercetin, luteolin and genistein, reduce oxidative DNA damage and lipid peroxidation and quench free radicals. *Cancer Lett.,* 1997, 119, 99-107.

Caltagirone, S., Ranelletti, F. O., Rinelli, A., et al. Interaction with type II estrogen binding sites and antiproliferative activity of tamoxifen and quercetin in human non-small-cell lung cancer. *Am. J. Respir. Cell Mol. Biol.,* 1997, 17, 51-59.

Carlstrom, J., Symons, J. D., Wu, T. C., Bruno, R. S., Litwin, S. E., Jalili, T. A quercetin supplemented diet does not prevent cardiovascular complications in spontaneously hypertensive rats. *J. Nutr.,* 2007, 137, 628–633.

Castillo, M. H., Perkins, E., Campbell, J. H., et al. The effects of the bioflavonoid quercetin on squamous cell carcinoma of head and neck origin. *Am. J. Surg.,* 1989, 158, 351-355.

Chan, K., Kan, Y. W. Nrf2 is essential for protection against acute pulmonary injury in mice. *Proc. Natl. Acad. Sci. USA,* 1999, 96, 12731-12736.

Chan, M., Fong, D., Soprano, K., Holmes, W., Heverling, H. Inhibition of growth and sensitization to cisplatin-mediated killing of ovarian cancer cells by polyphenolic chemopreventive agents. *J. Cell Physiol.,* 2003, 194, 63-70.

Chi, C., Chang, Y., Ou, Y., Hsieh, C., Lui, Y., Peng, F., et al. Effect of quercetin on the in vitro and in vivo growth of mouse hepatoma cells. *Oncol. Res.,* 1997, 4, 1021-1024.

Choi, E. J., Lee, B. H., Lee, K., Chee, K.-M. Long-term combined administration of quercetin and daidzein inhibits quercetin-induced suppression of glutathione antioxidant defenses. *Food Chem. Toxicol.,* 2005, 43, 793-798.

Chowdhury, S., Kishino, K., Satoh, R., Hashimoto, K., Kikuchi, H., Nishikawa, H., et al. Tumor-specificity and apoptosis-inducing activity of stilbenes and flavonoids. *Anticancer Res.,* 2005, 25, 2055-2063.

Ciolino, H. P., Daschner, P. J., Yeh, G. C. Dietary flavonols quercetin and kaempferol are ligands of the aryl hydrocarbon receptor that affect CYP1A1 transcription differentially. *Biochem. J.,* 1999, 340(Pt 3), 715-722.

Cruz-Correa, M., Shoskes, D. A., Sanchez, P., Zhao, R., Hylind, L. M., et al., Combination treatment with curcumin and quercetin of adenomas in familial adenomatous polyposis. *Clin. Gastroenterol. Hepatol.,* 2006, 4, 1035-1038.

Csokay, B., Prajda, N., Weber, G., Olah, E. Molecular mechanisms in the antiproliferative action of quercetin. *Life Sci.,* 1997, 60, 2157-2163.

de Whalley, C. V., Rankin, S. M., Hoult, J. R., Jessup, W., Leake, D. S. Flavonoids inhibit the oxidative modification of low density lipoproteins by macrophages. *Biochem. Pharmacol.,* 1990, 39, 1743-1750.

Devipriya, S., Ganapathy, V., Shyamaladevi, C. S. Suppression of tumor growth and invasion in 9,10 dimethyl benz(a) anthracene induced mammary carcinoma by the plant bioflavonoid quercetin. *Chem. Biol. Interact.*, 2006, 162, 106-113.

Dihal, A. A., de Boer, V. C., van der Woude, H., Tilburgs, C., et al. Quercetin, but not its glycosidated conjugate rutin, inhibits azoxymethane-induced colorectal carcinogenesis in F344 rats. *J. Nutr.,* 2006, 136, 2862-2867.

Duarte, J., Jimenez, R., O'Valle, F., Galisteo, M., Perez-Palencia, R. et al. Protective effects of the flavonoid quercetin in chronic nitric oxide deficient rats. *J. Hypertens.,* 2002, 20, 1843-1854.

Duarte, J., Pérez-Palencia, R., Vargas, F., Ocete, M. A., et al. Antihypertensive effects of the flavonoid quercetin in spontaneously hypertensive rats. *Br. J. Pharmacol.*, 2001, 133, 117-124.

Egert, S., Bosy-Westphal, A., Seiberl, J., Kurbitz, C., Settler, U., et al. Quercetin reduces systolic blood pressure and plasma oxidised low-density lipoprotein concentrations in overweight subjects with a high-cardiovascular disease risk phenotype: a double-blinded, placebo-controlled cross-over study. *Br. J. Nutr.,* 2009, 102, 1065-1074.

Elattar, T., Virji, A. The inhibitory effect of curcumin, genistein, quercetin and cisplatin on the growth of oral cancer cells in vitro. *Anticancer Res.,* 2000, 20, 1733-1738.

Elia, G., Amici, C., Rossi, A., Santoro, M. G. Modulation of prostaglandin A1-induced thermotolerance by quercetin in human leukemic cells: role of heat shock protein 70. *Cancer Res.,* 1996, 56, 210-217.

Erdman, J. W. Jr, Balentine, D., Arab, L., Beecher, G., Dwyer, J. T., et al. Flavonoids and heart health: proceedings of the ILSI North America Flavonoids Workshop, May 31-June 1, 2005, Washington, DC. *J. Nutr.*, 2007, 137, S718-737.

Exon, J. H., Magnuson, B. A., South, E. H., Hendrix, K. Dietary quercetin, immune functions and colonic carcinogenesis in rats. *Immunopharmacol. Immunotoxicol.*, 1998, 20, 173-190.

Ferry, D. R., Smith, A., Malkhandi, J., et al. Phase I clinical trial of the flavonoid quercetin: pharmacokinetics and evidence for in vivo tyrosine kinase inhibition. *Clin. Cancer Res.,* 1996, 2, 659-668.

Fischer, J. G., Mikulcik, E., Power, J., Effect of dietary quercetin on glutathione-S-transferase and glutathione reductase activities. *FASEB J.,* 2002, 16, A1002 (Abstract no. 735.6).

Fukushima, S., Hagiwara, A., Ogiso, T., Shibata, M., Ito, N. Promoting effects of various chemicals in rat urinary bladder carcinogenesis initiated by N-nitroso-n-butyl-(4-hydroxybutyl) amine. *Food Chem. Toxicol.*, 1983, 21, 59-68.

Galati, G., Sabzevari, O., Wilson, J. X., O'Brien, P. J. Prooxidant activity and cellular effects of the phenoxyl radicals of dietary flavonoids and other polyphenolics. *Toxicology*, 2002, 177, 91-104.

Galisteo, M., García-Saura, M. F., Jiménez, R., Villar, I. C., et al. Effects of quercetin treatment on vascular function in deoxycorticosterone acetate-salt hypertensive rats. Comparative study with verapamil. *Planta. Med*,, 2004, 70, 334-341.

Gandhi, R. K., Khanduja, K. L. Impact of quercetin consumption on phase-I and phase-II drug-metabolizing enzymes in mice. *J. Clin. Biochem. Nutr.,* 1993, 14, 107-112.

García-Saura, M. F., Galisteo, M., Villar, I. C., Bermejo, A., et al. Effects of chronic quercetin treatment in experimental renovascular hypertension. *Mol. Cell Biochem.*, 2005, 270, 147-155.

Hakimuddin, F., Paliyath, G., Meckling, K. Selective cytotoxicity of a red grape wine flavonoid fraction against MCF-7 cells. *Breast Cancer Res. Treat.,* 2004, 85, 65-79.

Hansen, R. K., Oesterreich, S., Lemieux, P., et al. Quercetin inhibits heat shock protein induction but not heat shock factor DNA-binding in human breast carcinoma cells. *Biochem. Biophys. Res. Commun.,* 1997, 239, 851-856.

Harnly, J. M., Doherty, R. F., Beecher, G. R., Holden, J. M., et al. Flavonoid content of US fruits, vegetables, and nuts. *J. Agric. Food. Chem.,* 2006, 54, 9966-9977.

Harwood, M., Danielewska-Nikiel, B., Borzelleca, J. F., Flamm, G. W., Williams, G. M., Lines, T. C. A critical review of the data related to the safety of quercetin and lack of evidence of in vivo toxicity, including lack of genotoxic/carcinogenic properties. *Food and Chem. Toxicology*, 2007, 45, 2179-2205.

Hayes, J. D., McMahon, M. Molecular basis for the contribution of the antioxidant responsive element to cancer chemoprevention. *Cancer Lett.*, 2001, 174, 103-113.

Hertog, M. G. L., Feskens, E. l. M., Hollman, P. C. H., Katan, M. B., Kromhout, D. Dietary antioxidant flavonoids and risk of coronary heart disease: the Zutphen Elderly Study. *Lancet,* 1993, 342, 1007-1011.

Hertog, M. G. L., Kromhout, D., Aravanis, C., et al. Flavonoid intake and long-term risk of coronary heart disease and cancer in the Seven Countries Study. *Arch. Intern. Med.*,1995, 155, 381-386.

Hirose, M., Fukushima, S., Sakata, T., Inui, M., Ito, N. Effect of quercetin on two-stage carcinogenesis of the rat urinary bladder. *Cancer Lett.* 1983, 21, 23-27.

Hubbard, G. P., Wolffram, S., Lovegrove, J. A., Gibbins, J. M. Ingestion of quercetin inhibits platelet aggregation and essential components of the collagen-stimulated platelet activation pathway in humans. *J. Thromb. Haemost.,* 2004, 2, 2138-2145.

Huynh, H., Nguyen, T., Chan, E., Tran, E.. Inhibition of ErbB-2 and ErbB-3 expression by quercetin prevents transforming growth factor alpha (TGF-alpha)- and epidermal growth factor (EGF)-induced human PC-3 prostate cancer cell proliferation. *Int. J. Oncol.,* 2003, 23, 821-829.

Ishikawa, Y., Kitamura, M. Anti-apoptotic effect of quercetin: intervention in the JNK- and ERK-mediated apoptotic pathways. *Kidney Int.,* 2000, 58, 1078-1087.

Ito, N., Tsuda, H., Tatematsu, M., Inoue, T., Tagawa, Y., Aoki, T., et al. Enhancing effect of various hepatocarcinogens on induction of preneoplastic glutathione S-transferase placental form positive foci in rats – An approach for a new medium-term bioassay system. *Carcinogenesis,* 1988, 9, 387-394.

Itoh, K., Wakabayashi, N., Katoh, Y., Ishii, T., et al. Keapl represses nuclear activation of antioxidant responsive elements by Nrf2 through binding to the amino-terminal Neh2 domain. *Genes. Dev.,* 1999, 13, 76-86.

Jin, N. Z., Zhu, Y. P., Zhou, J. W., Mao, L., Zhao, R. C., Fang, T. H., Wang, X. R. Preventive effects of quercetin against benzo[a]pyrene- induced DNA damages and pulmonary precancerous pathologic changes in mice. *Basic Clin. Pharmacol. Toxicol.,* 2006, 98, 593-598.

Kato, K., Mori, H., Tanaka, T., Fujii, M., Kawai, T., et al. Absence of initiating activity by quercetin in the rat liver. *Ecotoxicol. Environ. Saf.,* 1985, 10, 63-69.

Kawanishi, S., Oikawa, S., Murata, M. Evaluation for safety of antioxidant chemopreventive agents. *Antioxid. Redox. Signal.,* 2005, 7, 1728-1739.

Kim, Y. H., Lee, Y. J. TRAIL apoptosis is enhanced by quercetin through Akt dephosphorylation. *J. Cell Biochem.,* 2007, 100, 998-1009.

Kim, W., Bang, M., Kim, E., Kang, N. et al. Quercetin decreases the expression of ErbB2 and ErbB3 proteins in HT-29 human colon cancer cells. *J. Nutr. Biochem.,* 2005, 16, 155-162.

Kiviranta, J., Huovinen, K., Hiltunen, R. Variation of phenolic substances in onion. *Acta Pharm. Fenn.*, 1988, 97, 67-72.

Koishi, M., Hosokawa, N., Sato, M., et al. Quercetin, an inhibitor of heat shock protein synthesis, inhibits the acquisition of thermotolerance in a human colon carcinoma cell line. *Jpn. J. Cancer Res.*, 1992, 83, 1216-1222.

Kong, A., Yu, R., Chen, C., Mandlekar, S., Primiano, T. Signal transduction events elicited by natural products: role of MAPK and caspase pathways in homeostatic response and induction of apoptosis. *Arch. Pharm. Res.*, 2000, 23, 1-16.

Kuo, P. C., Abe, K., Schroeder, R. A. Superoxide enhances interleukin 1beta-mediated transcription of the hepatocyte-inducible nitric oxide synthase gene. *Gastroenterology*, 2000, 118, 608-618.

Kuo, S. M. Antiproliferative potency of structurally distinct dietary flavonoids on human colon cancer cells. *Cancer Lett.*, 1996, 110, 41-48.

Lamson, D. W., Brignall, M. S. Antioxidants and Cancer III: Quercetin. *Altern. Med. Rev.*, 2000, 5, 196-208.

Larocca, L. M., Giustacchini, M., Maggiano, N., et al. Growth-inhibitory effect of quercetin and presence of type II estrogen binding sites in primary human transitional cell carcinomas. *J. Urol.*, 1994, 152, 1029-1033.

Larocca, L. M., Teofili, L., Leone G., et al. Antiproliferative activity of quercetin on normal bone marrow and leukaemic progenitors. *Br. J. Haematol.*, 1991, 79, 562-566.

Lee, J.-C., Kim, J., Park, J.-K., Chung, G.-H., Jang, Y.-S. The antioxidant, rather than prooxidant, activities of quercetin on normal cells: Quercetin protects mouse thymocytes from glucose oxidasemediated apoptosis. *Exp. Cell Res.*, 2003, 291, 386-397.

Levy, J., Teuerstein, I., Marbach, M., et al. Tyrosine protein kinase activity in the DMBAinduced rat mammary tumor: inhibition by quercetin. *Biochem. Biophys. Res. Commun.*, 1984, 123, 1227-1233.

Lodi, F., Jimenez, R., Moreno, L., Kroon, P. A., et al. Glucuronidated and sulfated metabolites of the flavonoid quercetin prevent endothelial dysfunction but lack direct vasorelaxant effects in rat aorta. *Atherosclerosis*, 2009, 204, 34-39.

Lotito, S. B., Frei, B. Dietary flavonoids attenuate tumor necrosis factor alpha-induced adhesion molecule expression in human aortic endothelial cells. Structurefunction relationships and activity after first pass metabolism. *J. Biol. Chem.*, 2006, 281, 37102-37110.

Mackraj, I., Govender, T., Ramesar, S. The antihypertensive effects of quercetin in a salt-sensitive model of hypertension. *J. Cardiovasc. Pharmacol.*, 2008, 51, 239-245.

Matsukawa, Y., Nishino, H., Yoshida, M., Sugihara, H., et al. Quercetin enhances tumorigenicity induced by Nethyl-N-nitro-N-nitrosoguanidine in the duodenum of mice. Environ. *Health Prevent. Med.*, 2002, 6, 235-239.

Matsuo, M., Sasaki, N., Saga, K., Kaneko, T. Cytotoxicity of flavonoids toward cultured normal human cells. *Biol. Pharm. Bull.*, 2005, 28, 253-259.

McMahon, M., Itoh, K., Yamamoto, M., Chanas, S. A. et al. The Cap_n_Collar basic leucine zipper transcription factor Nrf2 (NF-E2 p45-related factor 2) controls both constitutive and inducible expression of intestinal detoxification and glutathione biosynthetic enzymes. *Cancer Res.*, 2001, 61, 3299-3307.

Mertens-Talcott, S., Percival, S. Ellagic acid and quercetin interact synergistically with resveratrol in the induction of apoptosis and cause transient cell cycle arrest in human leukemia cells. *Cancer Lett.,* 2005, 218, 141-151.

Metodiewa, D., Jaiswal, A.K., Cenas, N., Dickancaite, E., Segura-Aguilar, J. Quercetin may act as a cytotoxic prooxidant after its metabolic activation to semiquinone and quinoidal product. *Free Radic. Biol. Med.,* 1999, 26, 107-116.

Middleton Jr., E., Kandaswami, C., Theoharides, T. C. The effects of plant flavonoids on mammalian cells: implications for inflammation, heart disease and cancer. *Pharmacol. Rev.,* 2000, 42, 673-751.

Miodini, P., Fioravanti, L., Di Fronzo, G., Cappelletti, V. The two phyto-oestrogens genistein and quercetin exert different effects on oestrogen receptor function. *Br. J. Cancer,* 1999, 80, 1150-1155.

Moinova, H. R., Mulcahy, R. T. An electrophile responsive element (EpRE) regulates beta-naphthoflavone induction of the human gammaglutamylcysteine synthetase regulatory subunit gene: constitutive expression is mediated by an adjacent AP-1 site. *J. Biol. Chem.,* 1998, 273, 14683-14689.

Moon, Y-J., Wang, X. D., Morris, M. E. Dietary flavonoids: Effects on xenobiotic and carcinogen metabolism. *Toxicology in Vitro*, 2006, 20, 187-210.

Morino, K., Matsukara, N., Kawachi, T., Ohgaki, H., Sugimura, T., Hirono, I. Carcinogenicity test of quercetin and rutin in golden hamsters by oral administration. *Carcinogenesis,* 1982, 3, 93-97.

Mouria, M., Gukovskaya, A., Jung, Y., Buechler, P., et al. Food-derived polyphenols inhibit pancreatic cancer growth through mitochondrial cytochrome c release and apoptosis. *Int. J. Cancer,* 2002, 98, 761-769.

Mulcahy, R. T., Gipp, J. J. Identification of a putative antioxidant response element in the 5′-flanking region of the human gammaglutamylcysteine synthetase heavy subunit gene. *Biochem. Biophys. Res. Commun.,* 1995, 209, 227-233.

Murtaza, I., Marra, G., Schlapbach, R., Patrignani, A., et al. A preliminary investigation demonstrating the effect of quercetin on the expression of genes related to cell-cycle arrest, apoptosis and xenobiotic metabolism in human CO115 colonadenocarcinoma cells using DNA microarray. *Biotechnol. Appl. Biochem.,* 2006, 45, 29-36.

Nair, H., Rao, K., Aalinkeel, R., Mahajan, S., Chawda, R., Schwartz, S. Inhibition of prostate cancer cell colony formation by the flavonoid quercetin correlates with modulation of specific regulatory genes. *Clin. Diagnostic. Lab. Immunol.,* 2004, 11, 63-69.

Nair, M. P., Mahajan, S., Reynolds, J. L., Aalinkeel, R., et al. The flavonoid quercetin inhibits proinflammatory cytokine (tumor necrosis factor alpha) gene expression in normal peripheral blood mononuclear cells via modulation of the NF-kappa beta system. *Clin. Vaccine. Immunol.,* 2006, 13, 319-328.

Nguyen, T., Huang, H. C., Pickett, C. B. Transcriptional regulation of the antioxidant response element: activation by Nrf2 and repression by MafK. *J. Biol. Chem.,* 2000, 275, 15466-15473.

Nguyen, T., Tran, E., Nguyen, T., Do, P., et al. The role of activated MEK–ERK pathway in quercetin-induced growth inhibition and apoptosis in A549 lung cancer cells. *Carcinogenesis,* 2004, 25, 647-659.

Nishioka, H., Imoto, M., Sawa, T., Hamada, M., Naganawa, H., et al. Screening of phosphatidylinositol kinase inhibitors from Streptomyces. *J. Antibiot., (Tokyo),* 1989, 42, 823-825.

NTP Technical Report (no.409) on the toxicology and carcinogenesis studies of quercetin in F344/N rats. NIH Publication No. 91-3140 (1991). U.S. Department of Health and Human Services, Public Health Service, National Toxicology Program, Research Triangle Park, NC.

Pereira, M. A., Grubbs, C. J., Barnes, L. H., Li, H., Olson, G.R., et al. Effects of the phytochemicals, curcumin and quercetin, upon azoxymethane-induced colon cancer and 7,12-dimethylbenz[a]anthacene-induced mammary cancer in rats. *Carcinogenesis,* 1996, 17, 1305-1311.

Perez-Vizcaino, F., Duarte, j., Jimenez, R., Santos-Buelga, C., Osuna, A. Antihypertensive effects of the flavonoid quercetin. *Pharmacological, Reports*, 2009, 61, 67-75.

Perkins, A. J., Hendrie, H. C., Callahan, C. M., Gao, S., et al. Association of antioxidant with the memory in a multiethnic elderly sample using the Third National Health and Nutrition Examination survey. *Am. J. Epidemiol.,* 1999, 50, 37-44.

Piantelli, M., Maggiano, N., Ricci, R., et al. Tamoxifen and quercetin interact with type II estrogen binding sites and inhibit the growth of human melanoma cells. *J. Invest. Dermatol.,* 1995, 105, 248-253.

Obach, R. S. Inhibition of human cytochrome P450 enzymes by constituents of St. John_s Wort, an herbal preparation used in the treatment of depression. *J. Pharmacol. Exp. Ther.,* 2000, 294, 88-95.

Ong, C., Tran, E., Nguyen, T., Ong, C., et al. Quercetin induced growth inhibition and cell death in nasopharyngeal carcinoma cells are associated with increase in Bad and hypophosphorylated retinoblastoma expressions. *Oncol. Rep.,* 2004, 11, 727-733.

Rahman, A., Fazal, F., Greensill, J., Ainley, K., Parish, J. H., Hadi, S. M. Strand scission in DNA induced by dietary flavonoids: role of Cu(I) and oxygen free radicals and biological consequences of scission. *Mol. Cell Biochem*., 1992, 111, 3-9.

Ramos-Gomez, M., Kwak, M. K., Dolan, P. M., Itoh, K., Yamamoto, M., Talalay, P., Kensler, T. W. Sensitivity to carcinogenesis is increased and chemoprotective efficacy of enzyme inducers is lost in NRF2 transcription factor-deficient mice. *Proc. Natl. Acad. Sci., USA* 2001, 98, 3410-3415.

Ranelletti, F. O., Maggiano, N., Serra, F. G., et al. Quercetin inhibits p21-ras expression in human colon cancer cell lines and in primary colorectal tumors. *Int. J. Cancer.,* 1999, 85, 438-445.

Rangan, G. K., Wang, Y., Harris, D. C. H. Dietary quercetin augments activator protein-1 and does not reduce nuclear facto-κB in the renal cortex of rats with established chronic glomerular disease. *Nephron.,* 2002, 90, 313-319.

Ren, Y., Smith, A. Mechanism of metallothionein gene regulation by heme-hemopexin: roles of protein kinase C, reactive oxygen species, and cis-acting elements. *J. Biol. Chem.,* 1995, 270, 23988-23995.

Rietjens, I. M., Boersma, M. G., van der Woude, H., Jeurissen, S. M., Schutte, M. E., Alink, G. M. Flavonoids and alkenylbenzenes: Mechanisms of mutagenic action and carcinogenic risk. *Mutat. Res.,* 2005, 574, 124-138.

Rivera, L., Morón, R., Sánchez, M., Zarzuelo, A., Galisteo, M. Quercetin ameliorates metabolic syndrome and improves the inflammatory status in obese zucker rats. *Obesity,* (Silver Spring), 2008, 16, 2081-2087.

Russo, M., Palumbo, R., Tedesco, I., Mazzarella, G., Russo, P., Iacomino, G., Russo, G. L. Quercetin and anti-CD95(Fas/Apo1) enhance apoptosis in HPB-ALL cell line. *FEBS Lett.,* 1999, 462, 322-328.

Sahu, S. C., Washington, M. C. Quercetin-induced lipid peroxidation and DNA damage in isolated rat-liver nuclei. *Cancer Lett.,* 1991, 58 (1and2), 75-79.

Sampson, L., Rimm, E., Hollman, P. C., de Vries, J. H., Katan, M. B. Flavonol and flavone intakes in US health professionals. *J. Am. Diet. Assoc.,* 2002, 102, 1414-1420.

Sasaki, H., Sato, H., Kuriyama-Matsumura, K., Sato, K., et al. Electrophile response element-mediated induction of the cystine/glutamate exchange transporter gene expression. *J. Biol. Chem.,* 2002, 277, 44765-44771.

Sato, H., Takahashi, M., Furukawa, F., Miyakawa, Y., Hasegawa, R., Toyoda, K., Hayashi, Y. Initiating potential of 2-2-(furyl)-3-(5-nitro-2-furyl) acrylamide (AF- 2), butylated hydroxyanisole (BHA), butylated hydroxytoluene (BHT) and 3,3,4,5,7-pentahydroxyflavone (quercetin) in two-stage mouse skin carcinogenesis. *Cancer Lett.,* 1987, 38, 49-56.

Scambia, G., Ranelletti, F. O., Benedetti Panici P, et al. Inhibitory effect of quercetin on OVCA 433 cells and presence of type II oestrogen binding sites in primary ovarian tumours and cultured cells. *Br. J. Cancer,* 1990, 62, 942-946.

Scambia, G, Ranelletti, F. O., Benedetti Panici P, et al. Quercetin induces type-II estrogenbinding sites in estrogen-receptor-negative (MDA-MB231) and estrogen-receptor-positive (MCF-7) human breast cancer cell lines. *Int. J. Cancer,* 1993, 54, 462-466.

Sharma, H., Sen, S., Singh, N. Molecular pathways in the chemosensitization of cisplatin by quercetin in human head and neck cancer. *Cancer Biol. Ther.,* 2005, 4, 949-55.

Shen, S., Chen, Y., Hsu, F., Lee, W. Differential apoptosis-inducing effect of quercetin and its glycosides in human promyeloleukemic HL-60 cells by alternative activation of the caspase 3 cascade. *J. Cell Biochem.,* 2003, 89, 1044-1055.

Shirai, M., Kawai, Y., Yamanishi, R., Kinoshita, T., Chuman, H., Terao, J. Effect of a conjugated quercetin metabolite, quercetin 3-glucuronide, on lipid hydroperoxide-dependent formation of reactive oxygen species in differentiated PC-12 cells. *Free Radic. Res.,* 2006, 40, 1047-1053.

Silva, M. M., Santos, M. R., Caroco, G., Rocha, R., Justino, G., Mira, L. Structure-antioxidant activity relationships of flavonoids: A reexamination. *Free Radic. Res.,* 2002, 36, 1219-1227.

Smith, M. A., Rottkamp, C. A., Nunomura, A., Raina, A. K., Perry, G. Oxidative stress in Alzheimer's disease. *Biochim. Biophys. Acta.,* 2000, 1502, 139-144.

Spencer, J., Rice-Evans, C., Williams, R. Modulation of pro-survival Akt/protein kinase B and ERK1/2 signaling cascades by quercetin and its in vivo metabolites underlie their action on neuronal viability. *J. Biol. Chem.,* 2003, 278, 34783-34793.

Tanaka, T., Kawabata, K., Honjo, S., Kohno, H., et al. Inhibition of azoxymethane-induced aberrant crypt foci in rats by natural compounds, caffeine, quercetin and morin. *Oncol. Rep.,* 1999, 6, 1333-1340.

Tanigawa, S., Fujii, M., Hou, D-X. Action of Nrf2 and Keapl in ARE-mediated NQO1 expression by quercetin. *Free Radical Biology and Medicine*, 2007, 42, 1690-1703.

Tribolo, S., Lodi, F., Connor, C., Suri, S., et al. Comparative effects of quercetin and its predominant human metabolites on adhesion molecule expression in activated human vascular endothelial cells. *Atherosclerosis*,2008, 197, 50-56.

U.S. Department of Agriculture. Nutrient Data Laboratory, Food Composition Laboratory. USDA Database for the Flavonoid Content of Selected Foods. Release 2.1. 2007. Agricultural Research Service.

Valentich, M. A., Eynard, A. R., Barotto, N. N., Diaz, M. P., Bongiovanni, G. A. Effect of the co-administration of phenobarbital, quercetin and mancozeb on nitrosomethylurea-induced pancreatic tumors in rats. *Food. Chem. Toxicol.,* 2006, 44, 2101-2105.

Valerio, L. G., Jr., Kepa, J. K., Pickwell, G. V., Quattrochi, L. C. Induction of human NAD(P)H:quinone oxidoreductase (NQO1) gene expression by the flavonol quercetin. *Toxicol. Lett.,* 2001, 119, 49-57.

Van der Woude, H., Boersma, M. G., Alink, G. M., Vervoort, J., Rietjens, I. M. Consequences of quercetin methylation for its covalent glutathione and DNA adduct formation. *Chem. Biol. Interact.*, 2006, 160, 193-203.

van der Woude, H., Gliszczynska-Swiglo, A., Struijs, K., Smeets, A., Alink, G., Rietjens, I. Biphasic modulation of cell proliferation by quercetin at concentrations physiologically relevant in humans. *Cancer Lett.,* 2003, 200, 41-47.

van Erk, M., Roepman, P., van der Lende, T., Stierum, R., et al. Integrated assessment by multiple gene expression analysis of quercetin bioactivity on anticancer-related mechanisms in colon cancer cells in vitro. *Eur. J. Nutr.,* 2005, 44, 143-156.

Venugopal, R., Jaiswal, A. K. Nrfl and Nrf2 positively and c-Fos and Fral negatively regulate the human antioxidant response element-mediated expression of NAD(P)H:quinone oxidoreductase 1 gene. *Proc. Natl. Acad. Sci. USA,* 1996, 93, 14960-14965.

Verma, A. K., Johnson, J. A., Gould, M. N., Tanner, M. A. Inhibition of 7,12-dimethylbenz(a)anthracene-and N-nitrosomethylureainduced rat mammary cancer by dietary flavonol quercetin. *Cancer Res.,* 1988, 48, 5754-5758, Erratum (1989) 49, pp. 1073.

Vijayababu, M., Kanagaraj, P., Arunkumar, A., Ilangovan, R., Aruldhas, M., Arunakaran, J. Quercetin-induced growth inhibition and cell death in prostatic carcinoma cells (PC-3) are associated with increase in p21 and hypophosphorylated retinoblastoma proteins expression. *J. Cancer Res. Clin. Oncol.,* 2005, 131, 765-771.

Walle, T., Vincent, T. S., Walle, U. K. Evidence of covalent binding of the dietary flavonoid quercetin to DNA and protein in human intestinal and hepatic cells. *Biochem. Pharmacol.,* 2003, 65, 1603-1610.

Wang, H., Joseph, J. A. Structure–activity relationships of quercetin in antagonizing hydrogen peroxide-induced calcium dysregulation in PC12 cells. *Free Radic. Biol. Med.,* 1999, 27, 683-694.

Wang, L., Tu, Y. C., Lian, T. W., Hung, J. T., Yen, J. H., Wu, M. J. Distinctive antioxidant and antiinflammatory effects of flavonols. *J. Agric. Food Chem.,* 2006, 54, 9798-9804.

Wasserman, W. W., Fahl, W. E. Functional antioxidant responsive elements. *Proc. Natl. Acad. Sci. USA,* 1997, 94, 5361-5366.

Watjen, W., Michels, G., Steffan, B., Niering, P., et al. Low concentrations of flavonoids are protective in rat H4IIE cells whereas high concentrations cause DNA damage and apoptosis. *J. Nutr.,* 2005, 135, 525-531.

Wenzel, U., Kuntz, S., Brendel, M., Daniel, H. Dietary flavone is a potent apoptosis inducer in human colon carcinoma cells. *Cancer Res.,* 2000, 60, 3823-3831.

Williamson, G., Manach, C., Bioavailability and bioefficacy of polyphenols in humans. II. Review of 93 intervention studies. *Am. J. Clin. Nutr.,* 2005, 81, S243-255.

Xing, N., Chen, Y., Mitchell, S. H., Young, C. Y. Quercetin inhibits the expression and function of the androgen receptor in LNCaP prostate cancer cells. *Carcinogenesis,* 2001, 22, 409-14.

Yokoo, T., Kitamura, M. Unexpected protection of glomerular mesangial cells from oxidanttriggered apoptosis by bioflavonoid quercetin. *Am. J. Physiol.,* 1997, 273, F206-F212.

Yoshida, M., Sakai, T., Hosokawa, N., et al. The effect of quercetin on cell cycle progression and growth of human gastric cancer cells. *FEBS Lett.,* 1990, 260,10-13.

Yoshida, M., Yamamoto, M., Nikaido, T. Quercetin arrests human leukemic T-cells in late G1 phase of the cell cycle. *Cancer Res.,* 1992, 52, 6676-6681.

Yoshioka, K., Deng, T., Cavigelli, M., Karin, M. Antitumor promotion by phenolic antioxidants: inhibition of AP-1 activity through induction of Fra expression. *Proc. Natl. Acad. Sci. USA,* 1995, 92, 4972-4976.

Youdim, K. A., Joseph, J. A. A possible emerging role of phytochemicals in improvingage-related neurological dysfunctions: A multiplicity of effects. *Free Radic. Biol. Med.,* 2001, 30, 583-594.

Zhang, X-M., Chen, J., Xia, Y-G., Xu, Q. Apoptosis of murine melanoma B16-BL6 cells induced by quercetin targeting mitochondria, inhibiting expression of PKC-alfa and translocating PKC-delta. *Cancer Chemother Pharmacol.,* 2005, 55, 251-262.

Zhu, B.T., Liehr, J.G. Quercetin increases the severity of estradiol induced tumorigenesis in hamster kidney. *Toxicol. Appl. Pharmacol.*, 1994, 125, 149-158.

Zou, L., Harkey, M. R., Henderson, G. L. Effects of herbal components on cDNA-expressed cytochrome P450 enzyme catalytic activity. *Life Sci.,* 2002, 71, 1579-1589.

In: Quercetin
Editors: Taiki Chikamatsu and Yuudai Hida

ISBN: 978-1 61942- 057-1

Chapter 6

MANIÇOBA, A QUERCETIN RICH AMAZONIAN DISH: ANTIOXIDATIVE PROSPECTS

Isao Kubo, Kuniyoshi Shimizu and Ken-ichi Nihei
Department of Environmental Science, Policy and Management,
University of California, Berkeley, California, US

ABSTRACT

A large quantity of quercetin was characterized from a local dish, known as maniçoba in Pará, Brazil. The fresh leaf of *Manihot esculenta* Crantz (Euphorbiaceae), a principal ingredient for maniçoba, was found to contain a large amount of rutin or quercetin 3-*O*-rutinoside which was completely hydrolyzed to quercetin during cooking processes. Antioxidant activity of quercetin and its microfloral metabolites was examined. Quercetin inhibited the oxidation of linoleic acid catalyzed by soybean lipoxygenase-1 (EC 1.13.11.12, Type 1) with an IC_{50} of 4.5 μM, while rutin did not inhibit this oxidation up to 200 μM. The progress curves for the enzyme reaction indicate that quercetin shows slow binding kinetics. In the pseudoperoxidase activity, hydroperoxides slowly oxidize quercetin to a rather stable intermediate, 2-(3,4-dihydroxybenzoyl)-2,4,6-trihydroxy-3(2*H*)-benzofuranone. A microfloral metabolite of quercetin and rutin after ingestion, 3,4-dihydroxyphenylacetic acid, also scavenged superoxide anion generated by xanthine oxidase and inhibited uric acid formation. The antioxidant activity observed with the methanol extract of maniçoba is due mainly to multifunctional quercetin's response.

INTRODUCTION

Dietary compounds, which are capable of acting as chemical antioxidants, are likely to be of benefit by augmenting cellular defenses and helping to protect components of the cell from oxidative damage [1-4]. For example, it is now recognized that cardiovascular protective effects of fruits and vegetables may at least in part be mediated via their hypochrolesterolemic and antioxidant activities [5-9]. It is likely that flavonoids, which are found abundantly in edible plants, contribute to these protective effects [10, 11] as demonstrated by green tea and grape products that inhibit LDL oxidation in vitro [12, 13]. In the past, studies have provided compelling evidence that antioxidants play an important role in reducing the risk of cancer. The oxidation of unsaturated fatty acids in biological membranes leads to a decrease in membrane fluidity and disruption of membrane structure and function [14, 15]. Antioxidants defense normally protect against such damage.

Cassava *Manihot esculenta* Crantz (Euphorbiaceae) is an important crop plant in tropical countries such as Brazil because of its high efficiency in carbohydrate production [16]. There is no doubt that the root is the most important product of *M. esculenta*. In comparison with the root, the leaf is almost completely neglected in commercial terms, although it is available in far greater tonnage and there is considerable potential for its exploitation. The leaf of cassava is known to contain cyanogenic glycosides that can release toxic cyanide [17, 18]. Maniçoba is a unique local dish in Pará, Brazil, made from the leaves of *M. esculenta* as a principal ingredient. The slenderized fresh leaves of *M. esculenta*, locally known as maniva, is simmered with sausages, bacon and pork loin for 4 to 5 days. The long cooking time is believed to eliminate the toxic cyanogenic glycosides, and the dish cooked maniçoba changes its color to almost black. The leaves of *M. esculenta* are also consumed as a vegetable in some parts of Sub-Saharan African and Asian countries [19]. In our preliminary assay, the ethanol extracts of both maniva and maniçoba scavenged 1,1-diphenyl-2-picrylhydrazyl (DPPH) radical, and maniçoba inhibited the soybean lipoxygenase-1 (EC 1.13.11.12, Type 1) catalyzed peroxidation of linoleic acid.

ISOLATION

Fractionation was guided by scavenging activity using DPPH radical. The crude ethanol extract of maniva or maniçoba was suspended into deionized water and washed with *n*-hexane to remove nonpolar compounds. Methanol was added until this water layer was completely dissolved and, then, the resultant solution was filtrated. Further fractionation of the filtrate, using rotation locular counter-current chromatography (RLCC) using ascending method [20], gave three major compounds (*1-3*). These antioxidant compounds isolated were characterized by means of spectroscopic method as rutin or quercetin 3-*O*-rutinoside (*1*) (see Figure 1 for structures) in quantities, and quercetin (*2*) and kaempferol (*3*) in trace amounts. Similarly, two antioxidant phenolics were characterized from maniçoba; quercetin in quantities and kaempferol in trace amounts. Interestingly, rutin was not isolated from maniçoba. A dish of maniçoba for one person contains approximately 1.3 g of quercetin. The fresh cassava *M. esculenta* leaves contain rutin in quantity which was all hydrolyzed after cooking processes. Although antioxidant activity of quercetin is well documented [21-23], additional assays of quercetin and its metabolites were performed to examine their role as an antioxidant of maniçoba [24].

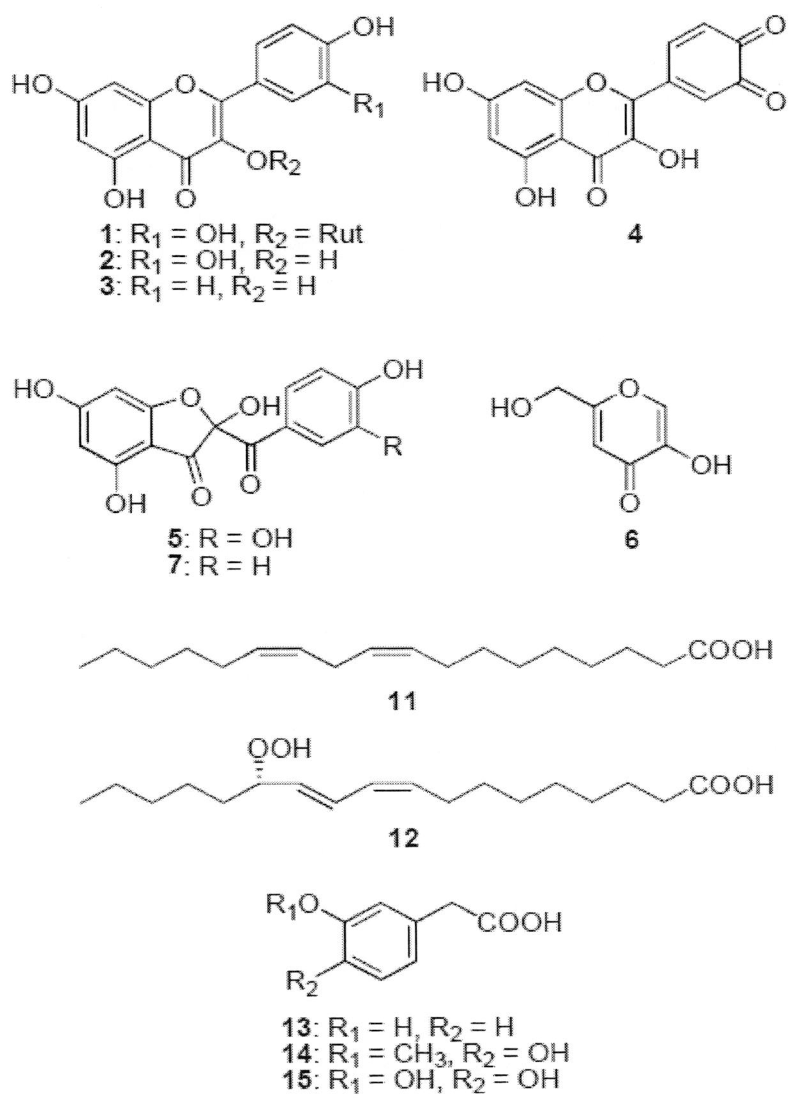

Figure 1. Chemical structures of flavonoids and related compounds.

DPPH

The radical scavenging activity on the 1,1-diphenyl-2-picrylhydrazyl (DPPH) radical, which can be measured as decolorizing activity following the trapping of the unpaired electron of DPPH, was examined first. The work was emphasized on quercetin. One molecule of quercetin scavenged nine molecules of DPPH radicals. It appears that quercetin was first oxidized to the corresponding *o*-quinone (*4*) after the abstraction of $2e^-$ and $2H^+$ from the hydroxyl groups at C-3' and C-4' [25]. This enzymatically oxidized *o*-quinone and subsequent isomerization to *p*-quinone methide type intermediate, followed by the addition of water on C-2 yielding relatively stable intermediate, 2-(3,4-dihydroxybenzoyl) -2,4,6-trihydroxy-3 (2*H*)-benzofuranone (*5*) [26]. This enzymatically generated intermediate seemed relatively stable but was gradually oxidized further, and hence, it prolongs the antioxidant activity. Recently, the same intermediate (*5*) was also characterized as the tyrosinase-catalized oxidation metabolite of quercetin [27]. Each molecule of kaempferol and rutin was found to scavenge three and six molecules of DPPH radicals, respectively. Since kojic acid (5-hydroxy-2-hydroxymethyl-4*H*-pyran-4-one) (*6*) did not show any DPPH radical scavenging activity, the γ-pyrone moiety alone is not enough to elicit the activity. It appears that the γ-pyrone moiety is required for extended conjugation between the B- and C-rings [28]. The conjugation allows extensive electron delocalization of impaired electron in the B-ring into the C-ring. It seems that kaempferol was oxidized to the similar intermediate, 2-(4-hydroxybenzoyl)-2,4,6-trihydroxy-3(2*H*)-benzofuranone (*7*) via the corresponding *p*-quinone methide type intermediate [29]. With rutin however, the only possible route is formation of the corresponding *o*-quinone.

TYROSINASE

Tyrosinase (EC 1.14.18.1), a copper-containing enzyme, catalyzes two distinct reactions of melanin synthesis, the hydroxylation of a monophenol and conversion of an *o*-diphenol to the corresponding *o*-quinone [30]. In previous cell-free experiments, the tyrosinase activity was monitored by measuring dopachrome formation at 475 nm accompanying the oxidation of L-DOPA. Dopachrome is a relatively stable intermediate but is gradually oxidized further, and hence, this spectrophotometric method measures only the very initial rate of dopachrome formation. Although tyrosinase is known to catalyze a reaction between two substrates, a phenolic compound and oxygen, the discussion previously described was based on the experiment using mainly L-DOPA as a substrate. As the need arises, L-tyrosine was also assayed to see if the inhibitors characterized were effective on monophenolase activity. In both cases, the enzyme activity was monitored by dopachrome formation at 475 nm. The assay was carried out in air-saturated aqueous solution and as a result, oxygen, which was the other substrate, was disregarded. Hence, effect of tyrosinase action on quercetin was examined by combination techniques with spectrophotometry (dopachrome formation), polarography (oxygen consumption) and HPLC analysis.

In previous papers, quercetin (*2*) was reported to inhibit the oxidation of L-DOPA catalyzed by mushroom tyrosinase [31-33]. This inhibitory activity was described to come from its ability to chelate copper in the enzyme since γ-pyrone moiety preferentially chelates copper [34]. As expected, the inhibition kinetics of quercetin was reported to be a competitive inhibitor analyzed by Lineweaver-Burk plots [35]. The chelation mechanism seems to be specific to flavonols as long as the 3-hydroxyl group is free. On the other hand, quercetin can be classified as a catechol derivative because of its B-ring structure. The catechols generally act as substrates on the tyrosinase reaction. Quercetin has recently been reported to be oxidized by polyphenol oxidase (PPO) from the chloroplast membranes of broad bean as well as mushroom tyrosinase through a complex mechanism caused by its γ-pyrone moiety [36, 37].

The oxygen consumption of quercetin (*2*) was measured in the presence of tyrosinase (1.0 μg/mL). The reaction mixture consisting 50 or 100 μM of quercetin was incubated and oxygen consumption was measured up to 20 min. The results obtained are illustrated in

Figure 2. The rate of oxygen consumption was dependent on quercetin concentrations. For example, when 50 or 100 μM of quercetin was used, 14 or 25 μM of oxygen was absorbed, respectively. Supposedly, quercetin has a catechol moiety in its B-ring, which may be affected by tyrosinase. Figure 3 represents the consecutive spectra of quercetin (50 μM) under the same conditions of the oxygen uptake experiment. Interestingly, the original yellow color was noted to fade within 10 min. This oxidation was evidently characterized by a new peak with the maxima at 342 nm. More specifically, the UV/vis absorption spectrum changed rapidly and the characteristic shift to short wave lengths (378→342 nm) was observed [35]. These observations were not contradicted by the previous report [37] and the hypsochromic shift likely indicates that quercetin was oxidized. Absorbance at 378 nm mainly comes from n→π* transition, and hence, the shift may be caused by structural changes including ketone moiety, aside from the change of catechol on the B-ring to corresponding *o*-quinone. The analysis of tyrosinase oxidation products was performed by HPLC as illustrated in Figure 4. Quercetin [retention time (t_R) 10.1 min] started being decreased and a new peak *b* (t_R 4.7 min) was gradually increased. The peak *b* was relatively stable but it seemed to be a small amount for determining the structure. On the other hand, quercetin was previously reported to be oxidized by Cu^{2+} to 2-(3,4-dihydroxybenzoyl)-2,4,6-trihydroxy-3(2*H*)-benzofuranone (*5*) in aqueous conditions [38]. The UV spectrum of *5* previously reported was similar to Figure 3 and hence, the peak ***b*** was expected to come from *5* [38]. In order to identify the peak ***b***, the synthesis of *5* was first attempted to oxidize quercetin directly using $NaIO_4$. By the HPLC experiment, the peak ***b*** was identical to that of the enzymatic oxidation product of quercetin in the reaction mixture. However, *5* was hardly purified enough for structural characterization because of the coexistence of many by-products. On the other hand, it was found that $CuCl_2$ oxidation of quercetin was run effectively and allowed to produce *5* [38, 39]. Accordingly, the peak *b* was consistent with *5* by chromatographic comparison using HPLC.

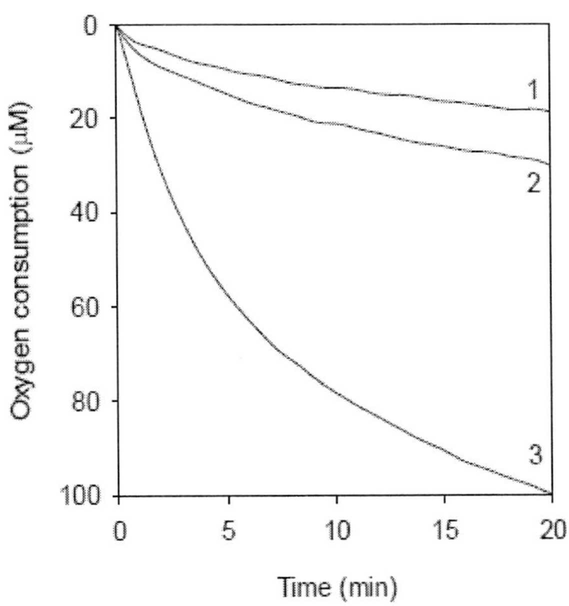

Figure 2. Oxygen consumption of L-DOPA and quercetin in the presence of mushroom tyrosinase. 100 μM L-DOPA (1), 100 μM quercetin (2), 100 μM L-DOPA and 100 μM quercetin (3).

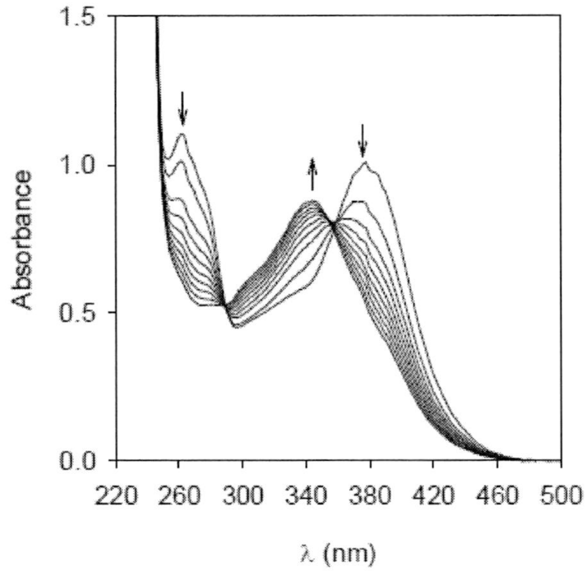

Figure 3. Consecutive spectrum obtained in the oxidation of 50 μM of quercetin by mushroom tyrosinase for 20 min. Scan speed was at 2 min intervals for 30 s. The arrows designate the evolution of the peak.

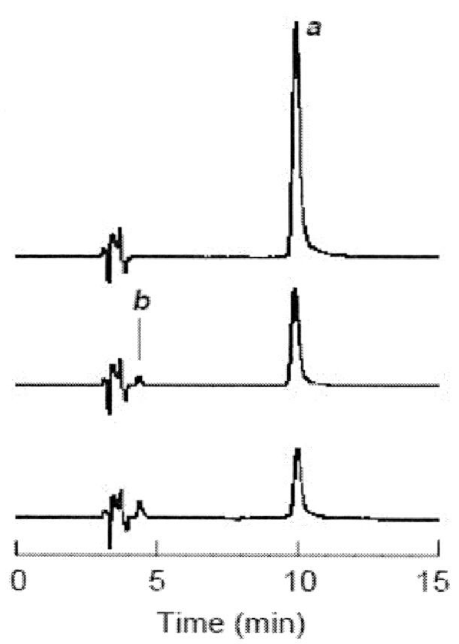

Figure 4. HPLC analysis of the reaction medium with 100 μM of quercetin (***a***) and tyrosinase. Sampling time was chosen at 0 min (upper), 20 min (middle), and 40 min (lower), respectively. The HPLC operating conditions were as follows: column; Capcell Pak C-18 (Shiseido, Tokyo, Japan), solvent; 30% $MeCN/H_2O$ containing 0.1% TFA, flow rate; 0.8 mL/min, detection; UV at 254 nm, injected amount; 20 μL from 3-mL assay system.

Proposed mechanism for the oxidative degradation of quercetin catalyzed by mushroom tyrosinase was illustrated in Scheme 1. Quercetin was rapidly oxidized to the corresponding *o*-quinone (*4*) after the abstraction of $2e^-$ and $2H^+$ from the hydroxyl groups at C-3' and -4' and subsequent isomerization to *p*-quinone methide type intermediate (*8*) [25, 40], followed by the addition of water on C-2 yielding the dione intermediate. This dione was tautomerized to the relatively stable protocatechuate intermediate (*5*) in aqueous solution via trione intermediate (*9*). In continuing spectrophotometrical experiment for 1 h, the changes in its UV/visible absorption spectrum started decreasing in absorbance at 342 nm but increasing at 270 and 400-550 nm. Although the protocatechuate intermediate (*5*) was relatively stable, it was further oxidized, presumably to the corresponding *o*-quinone (*10*) at a slow rate.

As far as the cell-free experiment using mushroom tyrosinase is concerned, the inhibition kinetics reported did not exceed 1 min [35]. In the current experiment, quercetin was found to be rapidly oxidized to *5*, followed by further oxidation presumably to the corresponding *o*-quinone. As long as the enzyme activity was monitored by dopachrome formation at 475 nm, this peak was not detectable up to 20 min. Even if L-DOPA was oxidized, the oxidized intermediates form adducts with quercetin. The amount of L-DOPA oxidized within 1 min is negligible. Hence, the inhibition kinetics previously reported with respect to the oxidation of L-DOPA is still seemingly accurate, but it is not. Apparently, quercetin acts as a tyrosinase substrate and forms adducts in part with L-DOPA or its oxidation products. Hence, the inhibition mechanism could not follow simple Michaelis-Menten kinetics.

In the preincubation experiment of tyrosinase with quercetin but without L-DOPA, the enzymatically generated intermediate was characterized as 2-(3,4-dihydroxybenzoyl)-2,4,6-trihydroxy-3(2*H*)-benzofuranone (*5*) [27]. Subsequently, the effects of rutin on the tyrosinase-catalyzed oxidation of L-DOPA were tested. Rutin was found to act as a neither inhibitor nor substrate, and hence, the hydroxyl group at the 3-position is related to the activity. The bulky hydrophilic sugar moiety likely disrupts to bind with the enzyme.

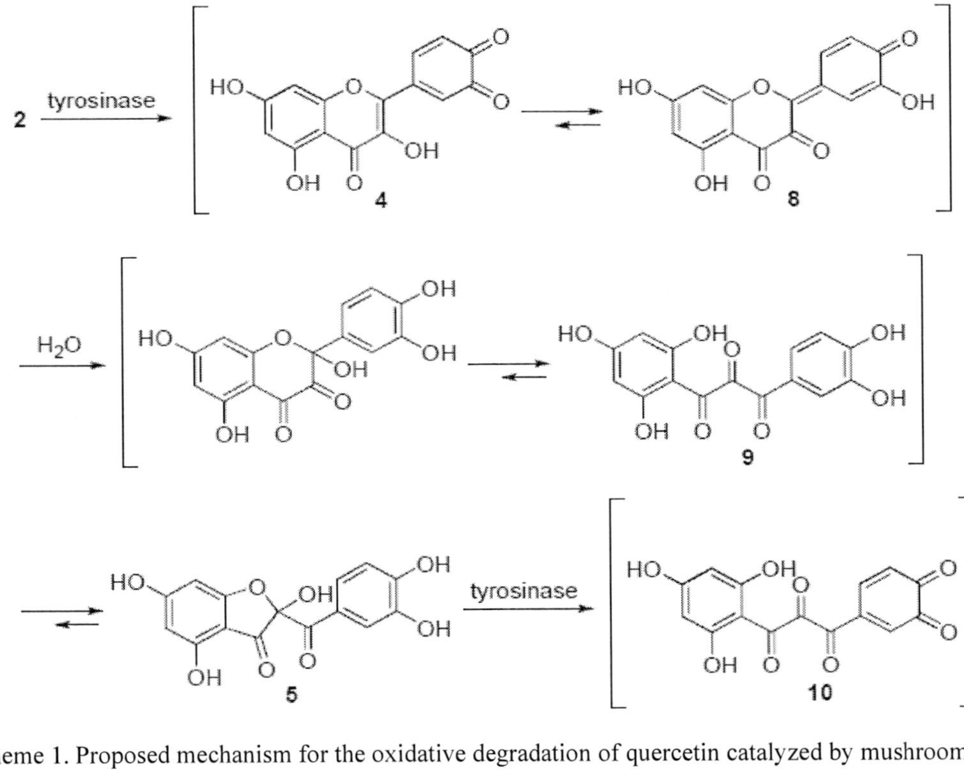

Scheme 1. Proposed mechanism for the oxidative degradation of quercetin catalyzed by mushroom tyrosinase.

The experiment was extended to examine the effect of quercetin on the tyrosinase-catalyzed oxidation of L-DOPA. Interestingly, the oxidation of quercetin catalyzed by tyrosinase was accelerated by the addition of the catalytic amount (10 μM) of L-DOPA. It has also been reported that quercetin acts as cofactor [34]. Hence, L-DOPA enhanced the oxidation of quercetin except by the accumulation of *oxy*-form tyrosinase in the reaction mixture. To clarify how L-DOPA affected oxidation, HPLC analysis was performed in the presence of 0.5 mM of L-DOPA. The experiment was monitored by HPLC analysis for 40 min (Figure 5). The result indicates that both quercetin and L-DOPA were simultaneously oxidized, presumably to the corresponding *o*-quinone (*4*) and dopaquinone, respectively. Remarkably, the decomposition rate of quercetin with L-DOPA was faster than the experiment without L-DOPA (see Figure 5). Moreover, some polar peaks around t_R 5.0 min emerged beside the peak of *5,* whereas these peaks were not observed on L-DOPA oxidation. The oxidation products are a complex mixture of polar compounds and the unstable nature of the intermediates makes their characterization difficult. Recently, glutathionyl adducts were identified in the incubation experiment with quercetin and glutathione in the presence of tyrosinase by LC/MS analysis [25]. It appears that dopaquinone accompanying the oxidation of L-DOPA is chemically highly reactive intermediate and forms adducts with quercetin. Incidentally, flavonols form adducts as long as their 3-hydroxyl group is free. The relatively stable oxidized intermediate (*5*) did not show the characteristic absorbance with maximum at around 475 nm corresponding to dopaquinone up to 10 min, seemingly indicating that quercetin inhibited the enzymatic oxidation of L-DOPA. As long as the enzyme activity is monitored by the spectrophotometric method, the inhibition kinetics previously described is seemingly valid, but does not.

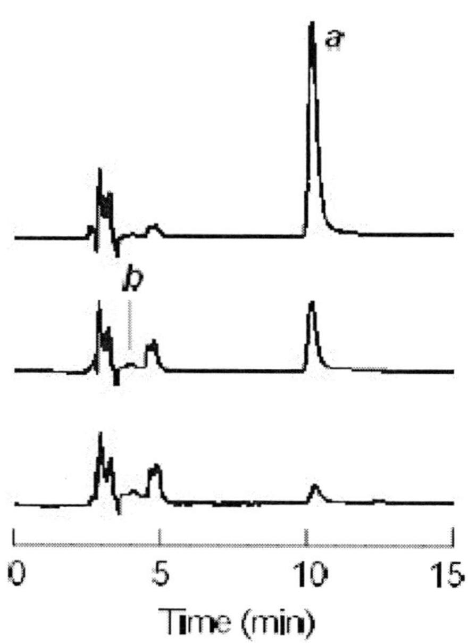

Figure 5. HPLC analysis of the reaction medium with 100 μM of quercetin (***a***) and tyrosinase in presence of 500 μM L-DOPA. Sampling time was chosen at 0 min (upper), 5 min (middle), and 20 min (lower), respectively. The HPLC operating conditions were same as Figure 4.

Melanine Formation

The oxidation of L-tyrosine catalyzed by tyrosinase to melanin is of considerable importance since melanin has many functions. Alterations in melanin synthesis occur in many disease states. Melanoma specific anticarcinogenic activity is also known to be linked with tyrosinase activity [41]. Melanins are also found in the mammalian eye and brain. Tyrosinase may play a role in neuromelanin formation in the human brain and could be central to dopamine neurotoxicity as well as contribute to the neurodegeneration associated with Parkinson's disease [42].

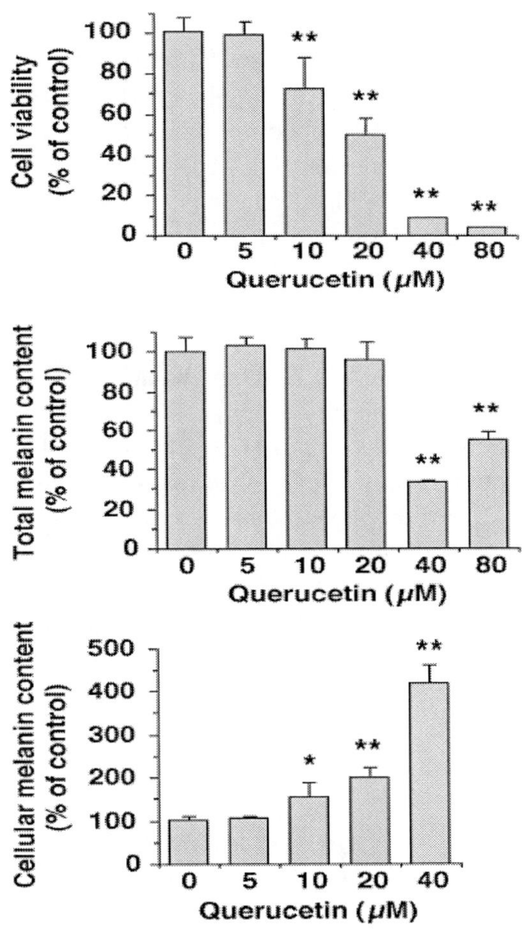

Figure 6. (a) Viabilities of B16 melanoma cells following treatment with quercetin for 72 h were measured by trypan blue exclusion as described in 'Materials and methods'. Data are expressed as a percentage of the number of viable cells observed with the control, and each column represents the mean ± S. D. of at least 6 determinations. (b) Total melanin content in B16 melanoma cells following treatment with quercetin for 72 h. Data are expressed as a percentage of melanin content per well observed with the control, and each column represents the mean ± S. D. of four determinations. (c) Cellular melanin content in B16 melanoma cells following treatment with quercetin for 72 h were measured as a percentage of melanin content per cell observed with the control, and each column represents the mean ± S. D. of four determinations. The statistical significance of differences was evaluated using Student's or Welch's t-test. Significantly different from the control value: $^{*}p<0.05$, $^{**}p<0.01$.

Tyrosinase is a key enzyme the in melanin synthetic pathway. Hence, its inhibitors are expected to inhibit melanin production, although the inhibition of mushroom tyrosinase activity was reported not to correlate with that of cellular tyrosinase or melanin production in cultured melanocytes [43]. The recent report indicates that *o*-phenylphenol, which is known as a depigmenting agent, has little depigmenting action while its metabolite, phenylhydroquinone is a potent depigmenting agent affecting melanocytes [44]. There is a gap between the simplified cell free experiments and cellular application. This prompted us to see if quercetin is oxidized to the corresponding *o*-quinone (*4*) in melanocytes and blocks melanin biosynthesis. Hence, the effects of quercetin on melanin synthesis in cultured murine B16-F10 melanoma cells were examined.

The appropriate concentrations for the preliminary assays performed were selected by microscopic observation. The highest concentration tested was 80 μM. Cell viability was determined on the third day for melanocytes using both trypan blue dye exclusion and 3-(4,5-dimethylthiazole-2-yl)-2,5-diphenyltetrazolium bromide (MTT) colorimetric assays. The specificity of melanogenesis inhibition was assessed by dividing the melanin content by the number of cells determined by trypan blue exclusion. Melanin production was not noticeably suppressed when the cells were cultured with quercetin up to 20 μM. However, quercetin became cytotoxic in a dose-dependent increase as shown in Figure 6a; indicating that the observed action at 40 μM may be due, at least in part, to its melanocytotoxicity. The concentration leading to 50% viable cells lost (IC_{50}) was established as 20 μM and almost complete lethality was observed at 80 μM. It should be noted that quercetin was highly toxic at 80 μM but the amount of melanin production was enhanced as illustrated in Figure 6b. More specifically, the number of viable cell at 80 μM is less than that of 40 μM but the amount of total melanin production was more than that of 40 μM. The melanin content per cell was higher at 80 μM, but this concentration showed a high melanocytotoxic effect. Hence, the cellular melanin content was more than that of 40 μM (Figure 6c). The result observed is similar to the previous report that quercetin enhanced melanogenesis in human melanoma cells and in normal human melanocytes by increasing the activity and synthesis of tyrosinase [45]. It should be noted that the amount of cellular melanin production was increased but the total amount was not exceeding the control up to 80 μM. Rutin showed neither cytotoxicity nor suppressed melanin formation up to 200 μM.

LIPOXYGENASE

The human body produces free radicals during the course of its normal metabolism. Free radicals are even required for several normal biochemical processes. For example, the phagocyte cells involved in the body's natural immune defenses generate free radicals in the process of destroying microbial pathogens [46]. It is well established that lipid peroxidation is one of the reactions set into motion as a consequence of the formation of free radicals in cells and tissues. Several oxidative enzymes, such as xanthine oxidase (EC 1.1.3.22), produce the $O_2^{\cdot-}$ radical as a normal product of the one-electron reduction of O_2, resulting in tissue injury [47]. If free radicals are produced during the normal cellular metabolism in sufficient amounts to overcome the normally efficient protective mechanisms, metabolic and cellular disturbances will occur in a variety of ways. Some flavonoids such as quercetin and kaempferol are known to exhibit both non-enzymatic and enzymatic inhibitory effect on xanthine oxidase [48], but the sharp distinction may not be appropriate. In addition to xanthine oxidase, superoxide is produced during mitochondrial respiration [49] and by NADPH oxidase [50], cyclooxygenase and lipoxygenase [51], nitric oxidase synthetase (NOS) [52] and cytochtome P450 [53]. Lipoxygenases (EC 1.13.11.12) are suggested to be involved in the early event of atherosclerosis by inducing plasma low-density lipoprotein (LDL) oxidation [54, 55]. On the other hand, it is well known that lipid peroxidation is one of the major factors in deterioration during the storage and processing of foods, because it can lead to the development of unpleasant rancid or off flavors as well as potentially toxic end products [56]. Hence, lipoxygenase inhibitors should have broad applications [57]. Many flavonoids have been reported to be lipoxygenase inhibitors [58].

In the current study, linoleic acid (*11*) was used as a substrate. Soybean lipoxygenase-1 (EC 1.13.11.12, Type 1) is known to catalyze the dioxygenation of the (1*Z*, 4*Z*)-diene moiety of linoleic acid. In plants, the primary dioxygenation product is 13*S* linoleic acid hydroperoxide (13-HPOD) (*12*) [59]. The enzyme assay was first performed using a UV spectrophotometer to detect the increase at 234 nm associated with the (2*Z*, 4*E*)-conjugated double bonds newly formed in the product but not the substrate. However, this spectrophotometric method was not appropriate because the absorption overlapped with that of quercetin itself. Hence, the enzyme activity was monitored by measuring oxygen consumption. The results are illustrated in Figure 7. Quercetin exhibited a dose-dependent inhibitory effect on this oxidation, indicating that the enzymatically generated oxidation of linoleic acid to 13-HPOD was inhibited. Interestingly, rutin did not show this inhibitory activity up to 200 mM. On the other hand, kaempferol exhibited the activity but much weaker compared to that of quercetin. Overall, being the major phenolic compound in maniçoba, quercetin is more likely to be responsible for the observed soybean lipoxygenase-1 inhibitory activity of the crude methanol extract of maniçoba.

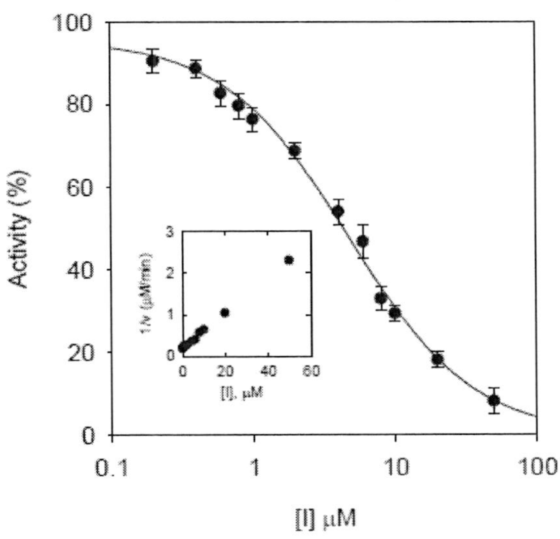

Figure 7. Effects of quercetin on the activity of soybean lipoxygenase-1 for the catalysis of linoleic acid at 25 °C. The inset shows the replots of data as $1/v$ vs [I].

Quercetin inhibited soybean lipoxygenase-1 by slow-binding inhibition mechanism as shown in Figure 8. The k_{obs} values for the quercetin inhibition of lipoxygenase-1 at different concentrations of quercetin were determined by fitting data to the slow-binding equation (eq 1). The k_{obs} values were plotted as a function of quercetin concentration. The results indicated that quercetin inhibits soybean lipoxygenase-1 by simple reversible slow binding. This was evidenced by the observation that the k_{obs} values exhibited a liner dependence on the inhibitor concentration as shown in Figure 8 inset. Thus, analysis of data according to eq 1 and 2 yielded the following values: $k_3 = 0.0325 \pm 0.01\ \mu M^{-1}\ min^{-1}$, $k_4 = 0.0345 \pm 0.02\ min^{-1}$, $K_i^{app} = 1.06 \pm 0.2\ \mu M$.

$$P = v_s t + (v_i - v_s)\,(1 - \exp(-\,k_{obs}t))/k_{obs} \qquad \text{(eq 1)}$$

$$k_{obs} = k_4\,[I]/K_i^{app} + k_4 \qquad \text{(eq 2)}$$

Most slow binding enzyme inhibitors act as competitive inhibitors, binding at the enzyme active site [60, 61], although it is possible for them to interact with the enzyme by competitive, noncompetitive, or uncompetitive inhibition patterns. To distinguish the mode of inhibition of a time-dependent inhibitor, it is convenient to analyze the effect of various substrate concentrations on k_{obs} at fixed inhibitor concentration. For a competitive type inhibitor will display a decrease of k_{obs} with increasing substrate concentration. In contrast, uncompetitive inhibitor the value of k_{obs} will increase with increasing substrate concentration, while k_{obs} is independent of substrate concentration at a noncompetitive type inhibition [62]. Figure 9 also illustrates typical progress curves of time-dependent inhibition of quercetin when the enzymatic reaction is initiated by the addition of lipoxygenase-1 but different of linoleic acid concentration. The k_{obs} values were determined by fitting data to eq 1. As a result, quercetin is a noncompetitive inhibitor because k_{obs} did not vary with substrate concentration (Figure 9 inset).

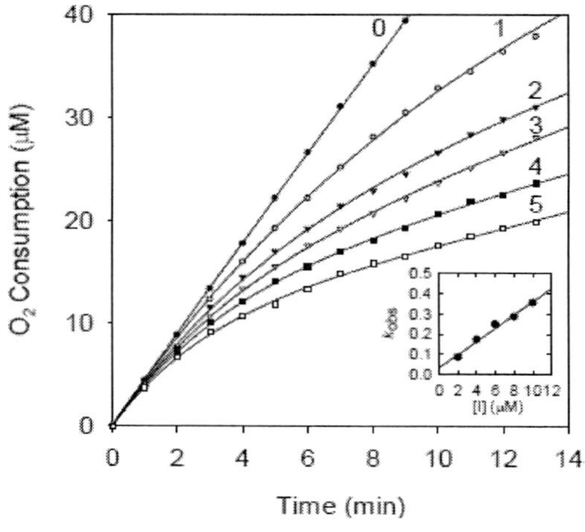

Figure 8. Time-dependent inhibition of soybean lipoxygenase-1 in the presence of quercetin. Conditions were as follows: 80 μM linoleic acid, 4.35 nM lipoxygenase-1, and concentrations of quercetin for curves 0-5 were 0, 2, 4, 6, 8, and 10 μM. (Inset) Dependence of the values for k_{obs} on the concentration of quercetin.

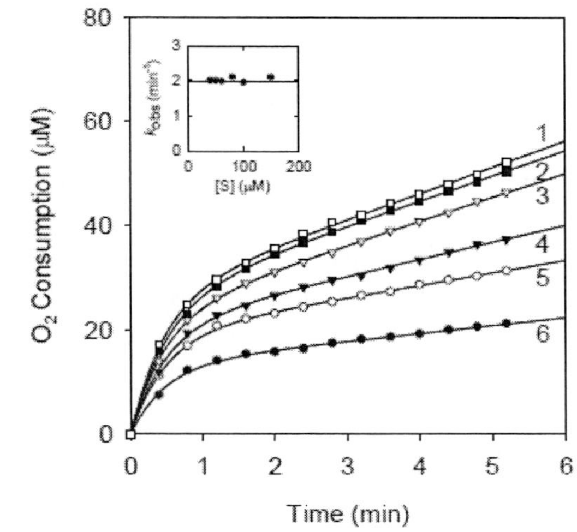

Figure 9. Progress curves for the noncompetitive behavior of quercetin. Conditions were as follows: 50 μM quercetin, 50 nM lipoxygenase-1, and concentrations of linoleic acid for curves 1-6 were 150, 100, 80, 60, 50 and 40 μM. (Inset) Dependence of the values for k_{obs} on the concentration of linoleic acid.

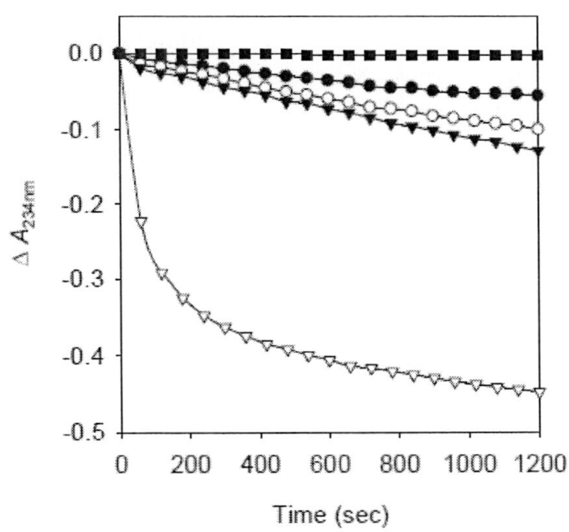

Figure 10. Effects of quercetin, kaempferol and NDGA on soybean lipoxygenase-1 catalyzed consumption of 13-HPOD. The conditions of incubation were as described for pseudoperoxidase assay using 50 μM kaempferol (■), 5 μM quercetin (•), 10 μM quercetin (○), 30 μM quercetin (▼) and 10 μM NDGA (▽) in the presence of enzyme.

Many lipoxygenase inhibitors such as flavonoids, catechols, benzofuranol, and aminopyrazolines have been reported [63-65] and act in different ways; by a chelating the iron of the active site of enzyme [66, 67] and/or by reducing the ferric form of the enzyme to an inactive ferrous form [68, 69]. This enzyme reduction mechanism is directly measurable by ESR and fluorescence. And also this mechanism indirectly observations that the inhibitor-dependent decrease in 13-HPOD concentration catalyzed by lipoxygenase-1 using the variation in A_{234}. NDGA tested as a reference compound for comparison is well known soybean lipoxygenase-1 inhibitor by reducing the catalytically active ferric enzyme to the catalytically inactive ferrous enzyme [68]. As a result, Figure 10 demonstrates that the fast decrease in A_{234} observed with addition of NDGA in the pseudoperoxidase activity assay system. And quercetin also slowly reducing the oxidized form to native reduced form. Thus, quercetin inhibit the catalyze the dioxygenation of linoleic acid to 13-HPOD by reducing ferric form to the inactive ferrous form. However, kaempferol did not cause any significant stimulation of the pseudoperoxidase activity.

Many inhibitors were also oxidized by the enzyme during the reaction in the presence of 13-HPOD. Thus, the oxidation of quercetin during pseudoperoxidase activity was studied by repetitive scans (Figure 11) and by reverse phase high performance liquid chromatography (RP-HPLC) (Figure 12). Quercetin was seemingly oxidized slowly by soybean lipoxygenase-1 in the presence 13-HPOD. This observation is consistent with the previous report [70]. As shown in Figure 6, the decrease in the absorbance of the band centered at 272 and 386 nm, the concomitant increase in the absorbance at 330 nm, and the presence of two isosbestic points at 286 and 357 nm, respectively. The observations were not contradicted by the previous report and the hypsochromic shift likely indicates that quercetin was oxidized. Absorbance at 385 nm mainly comes from n→π* transition, and hence, the shift may be caused by structural changes including ketone moiety, aside from the change of catechol on the B-ring to corresponding *o*-quinone.

Thus, quercetin was first oxidized to the corresponding *o*-quinone (*4*) after the abstraction of $2e^-$ and $2H^+$ from the hydroxyl groups at C-3' and C-4' as illustrated in Scheme 2 [38]. This enzymatically oxidized *o*-quinone and subsequent isomerization to *p*-quinone methide type intermediate, followed by the addition of water on C-2 yielding relatively stable intermediate, 2-(3,4-dihydroxybenzoyl)-2,4,6-trihydroxy-3(2*H*)-benzofuranone (*5*). This enzymatically generated intermediate seemed relatively stable but was gradually oxidized further, and hence, it prolongs the antioxidant activity.

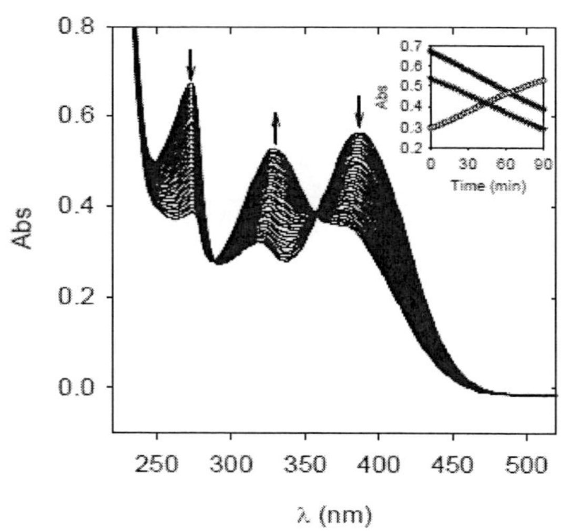

Figure 11. Repetitive scans of 30 μM quercetin by soybean lipoxygenase-1 in the presence of 13-HPOD. The reaction medium contained 0.1M Tris-HCl buffer, pH8.0, 10 μM 13-HPOD, and lipoxygenase-1 (320 nM). The elapsed time between scans was 3 min during 90 min. The inset corresponds to the time course of the absorbance measured at 272 (•), 330 (○), and 386 nm (▼).

The results indicate that the soybean lipoxygenase-1 generated intermediate of quercetin is the same as the DPPH generated intermediate, 2-(3,4-dihydroxybenzoyl)-2,4,6-trihydroxy-3(2*H*)-benzofuranone (*5*) [26]. Subsequently, RP–HPLC analysis was performed using reaction mixture with quercetin and lipoxygenase-1 under the same conditions of pseudoperoxidase experiments (Figure 12). It shows that peak ***a*** (17.4 min) identified as quercetin was rapidly decreased and peak ***b*** (7.2 min) was most visibly increased.

The same intermediate was also characterized as the relatively stable mushroom tyrosinase generated intermediate [27]. The reaction was initiated by a hydrogen atom abstraction reaction producing a linoleic acid radical. The radical is oxygenated producing a linoleic acid peroxyradical, which was subsequently reduced to form a linoleic acid hydroperoxide. It seems that quercetin scavenged 13-HPOD radical generated by soybean lipoxygenase-1.

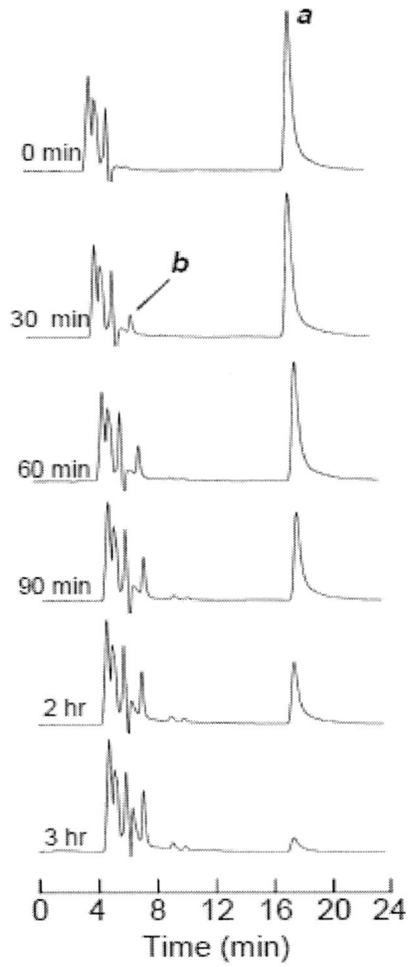

Figure 12. HPLC analysis of the reaction medium with 100 μM of quercetin and soybean lipoxygenase-1. Sampling time was chosen at 0, 30, 60, 90, 120, and 180 min, respectively. The HPLC operating conditions was as follow: column; Capcell Pak C-18, solvent; 30% MeCN/H_2O containing 0.1% TFA, flow rate; 0.5mL/min, detection; UV at 254 nm, injected amount; 10 μL from 3 mL assay system. The peak ***a*** at t_R 17.4 min, identified as quercetin, rapidly decreased and that prak ***b*** at t_R 7.2 min, identified as 2-(3,4-dihydroxybenzoyl)-2,4,6-trihydroxy-3(2*H*)-benzofuranone, increased up to 3 h.

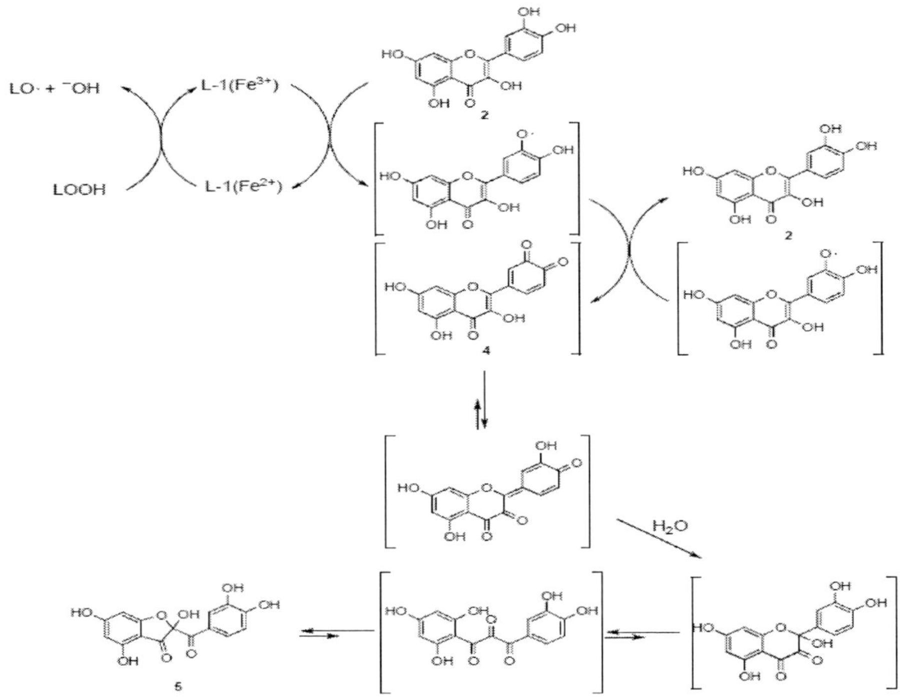

Scheme 2. Proposed mechanism for the oxidative degradation of quercetin catalyzed by soybean lipoxygenase-1.

Subsequently, the oxidation of quercetin during pseudoperoxidase activity was studied by repetitive scans and by reverse phase high performance liquid chromatography (data not illustrated). Quercetin was seemingly oxidized rapidly by soybean lipoxygenase-1 in the presence 13-HPOD. As illustrated in Figure 11, the decrease in the absorbance of the band centered at 270 and 385 nm, the concomitant increase in the absorbance at 330 nm, and the presence of two isosbestic points at 286 and 357 nm, respectively. The results indicate that the soybean lipoxygenase-1 generated intermediate of quercetin is the same as the DPPH, lipoxygenase or tyrosinase generated intermediate, 2-(3,4-dihydroxybenzoyl)-2,4,6-trihydroxy-3(2*H*)-benzofuranone (*5*) [46]. It seems that quercetin scavenged 13-HPOD radical generated by soybean lipoxygenase-1.

Metabolites

Despite their potent antioxidant activity, it is not clear if the ingested flavonols are absorbed into the biological system through the intestinal tract and delivered to the places where antioxidants are needed. The colonic microfloras convert most of these ingested flavonols into metabolites that then reach the circulation. For example, phenyl acetic acids (phenyl-C_2 metabolite) were reported as the major metabolites of quercetin and rutin in subjects with an intact colon and accounted for about half of the ingested these flavonols. More specifically, quercetin and rutin were metabolized mainly to phenyl acetic acids, i.e., 3-hydroxyphenylacetic acid (*13*), 3-methoxy-4-hydroxyphenylacetic acid (*14*) and 3,4-dihydroxyphenylacetic acid (*15*) [71, 72]. As expected, one molecule of 3,4-

dihydroxyphenylacetic acid scavenges six molecules of DPPH radical, while the other two did not show this scavenging activity (Table 1). However, none of these metabolites showed noticeable inhibitory activity of soybean lipoxygenase-1 and mushroom tyrosinase. It appears that metabolites of the ingested flavonols have lower antioxidant activity than their parent compounds, and hence, the contribution of ingested flavonols to antioxidant activity in vivo was suggested to be lower than expected from in vitro tests [71]. Interestingly, 3,4-dihydroxyphenylacetic acid scavenged superoxide anion generated by xanthine oxidase and inhibited the enzyme. The superoxide anion generated by xanthine oxidase was scavenged by 3,4-dihydroxyphenylacetic acid a dose-dependent effect with an IC_{50} of 3.5 ± 0.5 μM, which is slightly more potent compared to that of quercetin (Table 2). The inhibition kinetics of 3,4-dihydroxyphenylacetic acid analyzed by Lineweaver-Burk plots is shown in Figure 13. The result demonstrates that the plots of $1/v$ versus 1/[S] give a family of straight lines with different slope and intercept, but they were intersected one another in the second quadrant, indicating that 3,4-dihydroxyphenylacetic acid is a competitive and noncompetitive mixed type inhibitor. Mixed type inhibition with 3,4-dihydroxyphenylacetic acid is of the type partially mixed competitive and noncompetitive as 3,4-dihydroxyphenylacetic acid binds both to the catalytic site and to the substrate-induced active site. 3,4-Dihydroxyphenylacetic acid can bind not only to E, but also to ES complex, and their equilibrium constants are different.

Table 1. Scavenging activity of quercetin and related compounds for superoxide anion generated by xanthine oxidase

Compounds tested	μM		Inhibition Type
	IC_{50}	K_i	
Quercetin	4.4 ± 0.2	1.4 ± 0.1	Mixed [a]
Rutin	47 ± 7	27.5 ± 1.0	Mixed [b]
3-Hydroxyphenylacetic acid	>200	-	-
3-Methoxy-4-hydroxyphenylacetic acid	>200	-	-
3,4-Dihydroxyphenylacetic acid	3.5 ± 0.5	2.0 ± 0.4	Mixed [c]

-, Not tested, [a], K_{is} 6.4 ± 0.5 μM, [b], K_{is} 63.3 ± 2.3 μM, [c], K_{is} 3.5 ± 0.5 μM.

Table 2. Kinetics constants of quercetin and related compounds on uric acid formation by xanthine oxidase

Compounds tested	μM		Inhibition Type
	IC_{50}	K_i	
Quercetin	25.0 ± 2.0	4.0 ± 0.2	Competitive
Rutin	>200	-	-
3-Hydroxyphenylacetic acid	>200	-	-
3-Methoxy-4-hydroxyphenylacetic acid	>200	-	-
3,4-Dihydroxyphenylacetic acid	302 ± 22 [*]	173 ± 13	Mixed [a]

-, Not tested, [*], estimated, [a], K_{is} 399 ± 30μM.

3,4-Dihydroxyphenylacetic acid also inhibited uric acid formation. This oxygen-atom-transfer reaction was a dose-dependent effect with an IC_{50} of 302±22 μM. The inhibition kinetic analyzed by Lineweaver-Burk plots is shown in Figure 14. The result demonstrates that 3,4-dihydroxyphenylacetic acid is a mixed type inhibitor. In the lipid peroxidation assay generated by AAPH in liposomes, 3,4-dihydroxyphenylacetic acid was found to act as a radical scavenger and was found to be the most effective compound among the dihydroxy and trihydroxyphenolic acids that were tested [73, 74]. In addition, TEAC value of 3,4-dihydroxyphenylacetic acid (2.1 mM) was found to be comparative to that of rutin (2.4 mM). The other two metabolites (*14* and *15*) showed lower TEAC and were comparable to the values of vitamin E and C (TEAC, 1 mM) or slightly higher [75].

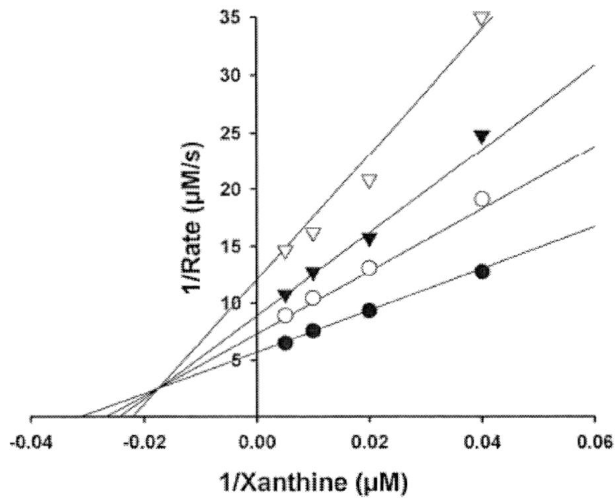

Figure 13. Lineweaver-Burk plot of superoxide anion generation by xanthine oxidase in the presence of 3,4-dihydroxyphenylacetic acid.

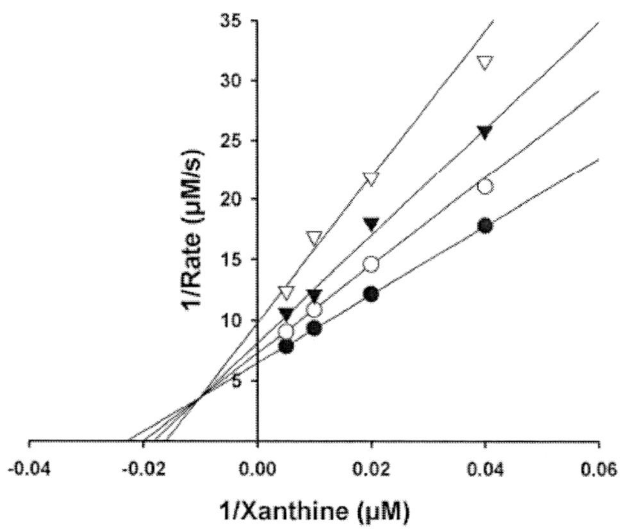

Figure 14. Lineweaver-Burk plot of uric acid formation by xanthine oxidase in the presence of 3,4-dihydroxyphenylacetic acid.

Conclusion

The protective effect of flavonoids in the diet is of much interest and the biological activity of those polyphenolic compounds is of great importance in understanding the health benefit derived from a diet rich on flavonoids [76]. Flavonoids like quercetin and kaempferol are potent antioxidants in vitro and reduce the oxidative damage [77]. For example, incubation of human lymphocytes with quercetin (10 μM) for 30 min significantly increased their resistance to oxidative damage induced by H_2O_2 [78]. Quercetin is known to protect against vascular disorders. The mechanism of this action could be related to its antioxidant function since vascular disorders may be caused by oxidative damage of cell membranes. Similarly, quercetin has nonsteroidal anti-inflammatory activity that may have applications for the treatment of inflammatory diseases [79].

Membrane lipids are particularly susceptible to oxidation not only because of their high polyunsaturated fatty acid content but also because of their association in the cell membrane with enzymatic and non-enzymatic systems capable of generating free radical species [49]. Microsomes, especially smooth surfaced endoplasmic reticulum, easily produce lipid peroxides and are thought to supply the peroxidation products to other tissues [80]. NADPH-cytochrome P-450 reductase is involved in NADPH-induced microsomal lipid peroxidation. Lipid peroxidation, which can be measured by the thiobarbituric acid (TBA) method, occurs when rat liver microsomes are incubated with Fe(III)-ADP/NADPH [81]. Malondialdehyde, a stable product of lipid peroxidation in living cells, is also a carcinogenic substance [82] and detectable as a TBA reactive material. Both quercetin and kaempferol strongly inhibited the production of the lipid peroxides induced by microsomal NADPH oxidation [83]. 3,4-Dihydroxyphenylacetic acid also inhibited this activity but to a lesser extent.

The other metabolically active compartment needs to be considered is the liver and kidneys in which biotransformation enzymes act upon absorbed flavonoids and their absorbed colonic metabolites [84]. Conjugation of the polar hydroxyl groups with glucuronic acid, sulphate or glycine has been reported for flavonoids and their colonic metabolites [85]. The presence of quercetin conjugates in humans was reported [86]. If the catechol group is not involved in conjugation reactions, antioxidant activity does not decrease significantly and the quercetin metabolites contribute to the antioxidant potential of plasma [87].

It should be noted that the majority of cancer patients who succumb to their disease die from metastasis. Metastasis is a sequential process in which tumor cells detach from the primary growth, invade through the surrounding host tissue into the circulation and subsequently disseminate to distant organs, where they arrest, extravasate and proliferate to form metastatic foci [88]. Quercetin and rutin were previously tested for the inhibition of lung metastasis induced by B16-F10 melanoma cells in mice. Oral administration of rutin at concentrations of 200 nmol/kg body weight was found to inhibit the lung tumor nodule formation but quercetin did not [89].

Safety is a primary consideration for antioxidants in food products. The radical-scavenging antioxidant traps an active radical and the antioxidant-derived radical is formed. The fate of this newly formed radical is important in determining the total potency of the antioxidant. For example, several inhibitors of lipid peroxidation have the potential to accelerate free radical damage to other biomolecules [90]. Because of this Janus-like property, scavenging antioxidants are also known as a double-edged sword. Quercetin was rapidly oxidized to the corresponding *o*-quinone after the abstraction of $2e^-$ and $2H^+$ from the hydroxyl groups at C-3' and -4' and subsequent isomerization to *p*-quinone methide type intermediate (*8*) [38], followed by the addition of water on C-2 yielding the dione intermediate. This dione was tautomerized to the relatively stable neutral protocatechuate intermediate (*5*) in aqueous solution via trione intermediate (*9*). In the continuing spectrophotometrical experiment for 1 h, the changes in its UV/visible absorption spectrum started decreasing in absorbance at 342 nm but increasing at 270 and 400-550 nm (data not illustrated). Although the protocatechuate intermediate (*5*) was relatively stable, it was further oxidized, presumably to the corresponding *o*-quinone (*10*) at an extremely slow rate. This can be supported as the measurement of oxygen consumption was extended to 1 h. Thus, the oxygen consumption was continued and the colored products started visible. The protocatechuate derivative (*5*) seems to be common as an oxidized intermediate of DPPH and AIBN and various oxidases such as tyrosinase, laccase, lipoxygese and peroxidase, and seems to be a key intermediate to understand quercetin's diverse biological activities [91, 92] together with the above mentioned microfloral metabolites, phenyl acetic acids.

In summary, quercetin characterized in a large quantity in maniçoba and its microfloral metabolite, 3,4-dihydroxyphenylacetic acid, may act as scavengers of reactive oxygen species and prevent from causing further cellular damage. Antioxidants may act in variety of ways including direct quenching of reactive oxygen species, inhibition of enzymes involved in the production of the reactive oxygen species, chelation of low valent metal ions such as Fe^{2+} or Cu^{2+}, and regeneration of membrane bound antioxidants such as α-tocopherol [77], but the sharp distinction may not be appropriate. Quercetin's antioxidant activity includes direct scavenging of superoxide anion, inhibition of various oxidases involved in the production of the reactive oxygen species, chelation of divalent metal ions such as Fe^{2+} or Cu^{2+} [93]. Quercetin is known to chelate transition metal ions, which are powerful promoters of free radical damage in both the human body [94] and foods [95]. The chelation ability, rendering the metal ions inactive to participate in free radical generating reactions, should be of considerable advantage as an antioxidant. In addition, quercetin is known as a highly efficient 148ydroxyl radical scavenger, and inhibits the development of stomach, colon, and oral cancer. However, the relevance of the in vitro experiments in simplified systems to in vivo protection from oxidative damage should be carefully considered. Further evaluation needs to be investigated from a whole and dynamic perspective.

ACKNOWLEDGMENTS

The work has involved a number of scientists. We are greatly indebted to our colleagues cited in the references, namely Dr. T. J. Ha, Dr. N. Masuoka, Ms. B. Burgheim and Dr. T. Nitoda, and special thanks to Mr. T. K. Nagano for his assistance to obtaining the raw materials of both maniva and maniçoba in Belém, Pará, Brazil.

REFERENCES

[1] Halliwell, B; Gutteridge, JMC. *Free Radicals in Biology and Medicine*. 2nd Ed. Oxford: Clarendon Press; 1989.

[2] Duthie, SJ; Ma, A; Ross, MA; Collins, AR. Antioxidant supplementation decreases oxidative DNA damage in human lymphocytes. *Cancer Res*. 1996, 56, 1291-1295.

[3] Boyle, SP; Dobson, VL; Duthie, SJ; Kyle, JAM; Collins, AR. Absorption and DNA protective effects of flavonoid glycosides from an onion meal. *Eur. J. Nutr*. 2000, 39, 213-223.

[4] Horvathova, K; Vachalkova, A; Novotny, L. Flavonoids as chemoprotective agents for civilitation diseases. *Neoplasma* 2001, 48, 435-441.

[5] Frankel, EN; Bosanek, CA; Meyer, AS; Silliman, K; Kirk, LL. Commercial grape juice inhibits the in vitro oxidation of human low-density lipoproteins. *J. Agric. Food Chem.* 1998, 46, 834-838.

[6] Kurowska, EM; Spence, JD; Jordan, J; Wetmore, S; Freeman, DJ; Piche, LA; Serratore, P. HDL-cholestrol- raising effect of orange juice in subjects with hypercholesterolemia. *Am. J. Clin. Nutr.* 2000, 130, 2200-2206.

[7] Bub, A; Watzl, B; Abrahamse, L; Delincee, H; Adam, S; Wever, J; Muller, H; Rechkemmer, G. Moderate intervention with carotenoid-rich vegetable products reduces lipid peroxidation in men. 2000, *J. Nutr.* 130, 2200-2206.

[8] Hodgson, JM; Puddey, IB; Croft, KD; Burke, V; Mori, TA; Caccetta, RA; Beilin, LJ. Acute effects of ingestion of black and green tea on lipoprotein oxidation. *Am. J. Clin. Nutr.* 2000, 71, 1103-1107.

[9] Collins, AR; Harrington, V. Antioxidants; not the only reason to eat fruit and vegetables. *Phytochem. Rev.* 2002, 1, 167-174.

[10] Cook, NC; Samman, S. Flavonoids-chemistry, metabolism, cardioprotective effects, and dietary sources. *J. Nutr. Biochem.* 1996, 7, 66-76.

[11] Collins, BH; Horská, A; Hotten, PM; Riddoch, C; Collins, AR. Kiwifruit protects against oxidative DNA damage in human cells and in vitro. *Nutr. Cancer* 2001, 39, 148-153.

[12] Leung, LK; Su, Y; Chen, R; Zhang, Z; Huang, Y; Chen, ZY. Theaflavins in black tea and catechins in green tea are equally effective antioxidants. *J. Nutr.* 2001, 131, 2248-2251.

[13] Fuhrman, B; Volkova, N; Suraski, A; Aviram, M. White wine with red wine-like properties: increased extraction of grape skin polyphenols improves the antioxidant capacity of the derived white wine. *J. Agric. Food Chem.* 2001, 49, 3164-3168.

[14] Slater, TF; Cheeseman, KH; Davies, MJ; Proudfoot, K; Xin, W. Free radical mechanisms in relation to tissue injury. *Proc. Nutr. Soc.* 1987, 46, 1-12.

[15] Machlin, L; Bendich, A. Free radical tissue damage: protective role of antioxidant nutrients. *Fed. Am. Soc. Exp. Biol. J.* 1987, 1, 441-445.

[16] Ravi, V; Aked, J. Review on tropical root and tuber crops. II. Physiological disorders in freshly stored roots and tubers. *Crit. Rev. Food. Sci. Nutr.* 1996, 36, 711-731.

[17] White, WLB; McMahon, JM; Sayre, RT. Regulation of cyanogenesis in cassava. *Acta Hort.* 1994, 375, 69-77.

[18] Ngudi, DD; Kuo, YH; Lambein, F. Cassava cyanogens and free amino acids in raw and cooked leaves. *Food Chem. Toxicol.* 2003, 41, 1193-1197.

[19] Almazan, AM; Theberge, RL. Influence of cassava mosaic virus on cassava leaf-vegetable quality. *Trop. Agric.* 1989, 66, 305-308.

[20] Kubo, I; Vieira, PC; Fukuhara, K. Efficient isolation of the insect growth inhibitory flavone glycoside rutin from two tropical medicinal plants by rotation locular countercurrent chromatography (RLCC). *J. Liq. Chromatogr.* 1990, 13, 2441-2448.

[21] Hortog, MC; Hollman, PC. Potential health effects of the dietary flavonol quercetin. *Eur. J. Clin. Nutr.* 1996, 50, 63-71.

[22] Peterson, J; Dwyer, J. Flavonoids: dietary occurrence and biochemical activity. *Nutr. Res.* 1998, 18, 1995-2018.

[23] Hollman, PC; Katan, MB. Dietary flavonoids: intake, health effects and bioavailability. *Food Chem. Toxicol.* 1999, 37, 937-942.

[24] Kubo, I; Masuoka, N; Nihei, K; Burgheim, B. Maniçoba, a quercetin rich Amazonian dish. *J. Food Compos. Anal.* 2006, 19, 579-588.

[25] Awad, HM; Boersma, MG; Vervoort, J; Rietjens, IMCM. Peroxidase-catalyzed formation of quercetin quinone methide-glutathione adducts. *Arch. Biochem. Biophys.* 2000, 378, 224-233.

[26] Krishnamachari, V; Levine, LH; Paré, PW. Flavonoid oxidation by the radical generator AIBN: a unified mechanism for quercetin radical scavenging. *J. Agric. Food Chem.* 2002, 50, 4357-4363.

[27] Kubo, I; Nihei, K; Shimizu, K. Oxidation products of quercetin by mushroom tyrosinase. *Bioorg. Med. Chem.* 2004, *12*, 5343-5347.

[28] Furuno, K; Akasako, T; Sugihara, N. The contribution of the pyrogallol moiety to superoxide radical scavenging activity of flavonoids. *Biol. Pharm. Bull.* 2002, *25*, 19-23.

[29] Tsimogiannis, DI; Oreopoulou, V. The contribution of flavonoid C-ring on the DPPH free radical scavenging efficiency. A kinetic approach for the 3',4'-hydroxy substituted members *Innov. Food Sci. Emerg. Technol.* 2006, 7, 140-146.

[30] Sánchez-Ferrer, A; Rodríguez-López, JN; Garcia-Cánovas, F; García-Carmona, F. Tyrosinase: A comprehensive review of its mechanism. *Biochem. Biophys. Acta* 1995, 1247, 1-11.

[31] Matsuda, H; Higashino, M; Chen, WZ; Tosa, H; Imura, M; Kubo, M. Studies of cuticle drugs from natural sources. III. Inhibitory effect of Myrica rubra on melanin biosynthesis. *Biol. Pharm. Bull.* 1995, 18, 1148-1150.

[32] Nagatsu, A; Zhang, HL; Mizukami, H; Sakakibara, J; Tokuda, H; Nishino, H. Tyrosinase inhibitory and ant-tumor promoting activities of compounds isolated from sanfflower (Carthamus tinctorius L.) and cotton (Gossypium hirsutum L.) oil cakes. *Nat. Prod. Lett.* 2000, 14, 153-158.

[33] Xie, LP; Chen, QY; Huang, H; Wang, HZ; Zhang, RQ. Inhibitory effects of some flavonoids on the activity of mushroom tyrosinase. *Biochemistry-Moscow* 2003, 68, 487-491.

[34] Kubo, I; Kinst-Hori, I; Chaudhuri, SK; Kubo, Y; Sánchez, Y; Ogura, T. Flavonols from *Heterotheca inuloides*: tyrosinase inhibitory activity and structural criteria. *Bioorg. Med. Chem.* 2000, 8, 1749-1755.

[35] Chen, QX; Kubo, I. Kinetics of tyrosinase inhibition by quercetin. *J. Agric. Food Chem*. 2002, 50, 4108-4112.

[36] Jiménez, M; García-Carmona, F. Oxidation of the flavonol quercetin by polyphenol oxidase *J. Agric. Food Chem.* 1999, 47, 56-60.

[37] Fenoll, LG; García-Ruiz, PA; Varón, R; García-Cánovas, F. Kinetic study of the oxidation of quercetin by mushroom tyrosinase. *J. Agric. Food Chem.* 2003, 51, 7781-7787.

[38] Jungblush, G; Rühling, I; Ternes, W. Oxidation of flavonols with Cu(II), Fe(II) and Fe(III) in aqueous media. *J. Chem. Soc., Perkin Trans. 2*, 2000, 1946-1952.

[39] Utaka, M; Takeda, A. Copper(II)-catalysed oxidation of quercetin and 3-hydroxyflavone. *J. Chem. Soc., Chem. Commun.* 1985, 1824-1826.

[40] Blois, MS. Antioxidant determinations by the use of a stable free radical. *Nature* 1959, *181*, 1199-1200.

[41] Prezioso, JA; Epperly, MW; Wang, N; Bloomer, WD. Effects of tyrosinase activity on the cytotoxicity of 4-*S*-cysteaminylphenol and *N*-acetyl-4-*S*-cysteaminylphenol in melanoma cells. *Cancer Lett.* 1992, 63, 73-79.

[42] Xu, Y; Stokes, AH; Freeman, WM; Kumer, SC; Vogt, BA; Vrana, KE. Tyrosinase mRNA is expressed in human substantia nigra. *Mol. Brain Res*. 1997, 45, 159-162.

[43] Maeda, K; Fukuda, M. Arbutin: Mechanism of its depigmenting action in human melanocyte culture. *J. Pharm. Exp. Therap*. 1996, 276, 765-769.

[44] Tayama, K; Takahama, M. Depigmenting action of phenylhydroquinone, an o-phenylphenol metabolite, on the skin of JY-4 black guinea-pigs. *Pigment Cell Res*. 2002, 15, 447-453.

[45] Nagata, H; Takekoshi, S; Takeyama, R; Homma, T. Quercetin enhances melanogenesis by increasing the activity and synthesis of tyrosinase in human melanoma cells and in normal human melanocytes. *Pigment Cell Res*. 2004, 17, 66-73.

[46] Wiswedel, I; Ulbright, O; Augustin, W. Studies of lipid peroxidation in isolated rat heart mitochondria. *Biomed. Biochim. Acta* 1989, 2, 73-76.

[47] Mayumi, T; Schiller, HJ; Bulkley, GB. Pharmaceutical intervention for the prevention of post-ischemic reperfusion injury. In: Poli, G; Albano, E; Dianzni, MU. Eds. *Free Radical: From Basic Science to Medicine*. Switzerland: Birkhäuser Verlag; 1993; 438-457.

[48] Cimanga, K; DeBruyen, T; Hu, JP; Cos, O; Apers, S; Pieters, L; Tona, L; Kambu, K; Van den Berghe, D; Vlietink, AJ. Constituents from *Morinda morindoides* leaves as inhibitors of xanthine oxidase and scavengers of superoxide anions. *Pharm. Pharmacol. Commun*. 1999, 5, 419-424.

[49] Halliwell, B; Gutteridge, JMC. Role of free-radicals and catalytic metal-ions in human-disease - an overview. In: Packer, L; Glazer, AN. Eds., *Methods in Enzymology* Vol. 186. New York: Academic Press; 1990; 1-85.

[50] Pagano, P; Ito, Y; Tomheim, K; Gallop, P; Tauber, A; Cohen, RA. An NADPH oxidase superoxide-generating system in the rabbit aorta. *Am. J. Physiol.* 1995, 268, H2274-H2280.

[51] Kukreja, RC; Kontos, HA; Hess, ML; Ellis, EF. PGH synthase and lipoxygenase generate superoxide in the presence of NADH or NADPH. *Circ. Res.* 1986, 59, 612-619.

[52] Cosentino, F; Patton, S; D'Uscio, LV; Werner, ER. Tetrahydrobiopterin alters superoxide and nitric oxide release in prehypertensive rats. *J. Clin. Invest.* 1998, 101, 1530-1537.
[53] Fleming, I; Michaelis, UR; Bredenkotter, D; Fisslthaler, B; Dehghani, F; Brandes, RP; Busse, R. Endothelium-derived hyperpolarizing factor synthase (cytochrome P450 2C9) is a functionally significant source of reactive oxygen species in coronary arteries. *Circ. Res.* 2001, 88, 44-51.
[54] Cornicelli, JA; Trivedi, BK. 15-Lipoxygenase and its inhibition: a novel therapeutic target for vascular disease. *Curr. Pharm. Des.* 1999, 5, 11-20.
[55] Kris-Etherton, PM; Keen, CL. Evidence that the antioxidant flavonoids in tea and cocoa are beneficial for cardiovascular health. *Curr. Opin. Lipidol.* 2002, 13, 41-49.
[56] Shibata, D.; Axelrod, B. Plant lipoxygenases. *J. Lipid Mediat. Cell Signal.* 1995, 12, 213-228.
[57] Richard-Forget, F; Gauillard, F; Hugues, M; Jean-Marc, T; Boivin, P; Nicolas, J. Inhibition of horse bean and germinated barley lipoxygenases by some phenolic compounds. *J. Food Sci.* 1995, 60, 1325-1329.
[58] Sadik CD; Sies, H; Schewe, T. Inhibition of 15-lipoxygenases by flavonoids; structure-activity relations abd mode of action. *Biochem. Pharmacol.* 2003, 65, 773-781.
[59] Grechkin, A. Recent developments in biochemistry of the plant lipoxygenase pathway. *Prog. Lipid Res.* 1998, 37, 317–352.
[60] Morrison, JF. The slow binding and slow, tight binding inhibition of enzyme catalyzed reaction. *Trends Biochem. Sci.* 1982, 7, 102-107.
[61] Morrison, JF; Walsh, CT. The behaviors and significance of slow binding enzyme inhibitors. *Adv. Enzymol. Relat. Areas Mol. Biol.* 1988, 61, 201-302.
[62] Copeland, RA. Enzyme: A practical introduction to structure, mechanism, and data analysis. New York: Wiley-VCH; 2000; 266-332.
[63] Yoshimoto, T; Furukawa, M; Yamamoto, S; Horie, T; Watanabe-Kohno, S. Flavonoids: potent inhibitors of arachidonate 5-lipoxygenase. *Biochem. Biophys. Res. Commun.* 1983, 116, 612-618.
[64] Jackson, WP; Islip, JP; Kneen, G; Pugh, A.; Wates, PJ. Acetohydroxamic acid as potent, selective, orally active 5-lipoxygenase inhibitors. *J. Med. Chem.* 1988, 31, 499-500.
[65] Summers, JB; Mazdiyasni, H; Holms, JH; Ratajczyk, JD; Dyer, RD; Carter, GW. Hydroxamic acid inhibitors of 5-lipoxygenase. *J. Med. Chem.* 1987, 30, 574-580.
[66] Clapp, CH; Banerjee, A; Rotenberg, SA. Inhibition of soybean lipoxygenase 1 by *N*-alkylhydroxylamines. *Biochemistry* 1985, 24, 1826-1830.
[67] Nelson, MJ. Catecholate complex of ferric soybean lipoxygenase 1. *Biochemistry* 1988, 27, 4273-4278.
[68] Kemal, C; Louis-Flamberg, P; Krupinski-Olsen, R; Shorter, A. Reductive inactivation of soybean lipoxygenase 1 by catechols: a possible mechanism for regulation of lipoxygenase activity. *Biochemistry* 1987, 26, 7064-7072.
[69] Mansuy, D; Cucurou, C; Biatry, B; Battioni, JP. Soybean lipoxygenase-catalyzed oxidations by linoleic acid hydroperoxide: different reducing substrates and dehydrogenation of phenidone and BW 755C. *Biochem. Biophys. Res. Commun.* 1988, 151, 339-346.

[70] Takahama, U. Inhibition of lipoxygenase-dependent lipid peroxydation by quercetin: mechanism of antioxidative function. *Phytochemistry* 1985, 24, 1443-1446.

[71] Olthof, MR; Hollman, PCH; Buijsman, MNCP; van Amelsvoort, JMM; Katan, MB. Chrorogenic acid, quercetin-3-rutinoside and black tea phenols are extensively metabolized in humans. *J. Nutr.* 2003, 133, 1806-1814.

[72] Konishi, Y. Transepithelial transport of microbial metabolites of quercetin in intestinal Caco-2 cell monolayers. *J. Agric. Food Chem.* 2005, 53, 601-607.

[73] Siquet, C; Paiva-Martins, F; Lima, JLFC; Reis, S; Borges, F. Antioxidant profile of dihydroxy- and trihydroxyphenolic acids- A structure-activity relationship study. *Free Radic. Res.* 2006, 40, 433-442.

[74] Raneva, V; Shimasaki, H; Ishida, Y; Ueta, N; Niki, E. Antioxidative activity of 3,4-dihydroxyphenylacetic acid and caffeic acid in rat plasma. *Lipids* 2001, 36, 1111-1116.

[75] Pietta, P; Simonetti, P; Gardana, C; Mauri, P. Trolox equivalent antioxidant capacity (TEAC) of Ginkgo biloba flavonol and Camellia sinensis catechin metabolites. *J. Pharm. Biomed. Anal.* 2000, 23, 223-226.

[76] Formica, JV; Regelson, W. Review of the Biology of quercetin and related bioflavonoids. *Food Chem. Toxicol.* 1995, 33, 1061-1080.

[77] Rice-Evans, C; Miller, NJ; Paganga, G. Antioxidant properties of phenolic compounds. *Trends Plant Sci.* 1997, 2, 152-159.

[78] Duthie, SJ; Collins, AR; Duthie, GG; Dobson, VL. Quercetin and myricetin protect against hydrogen peroxide-induced DNA damage (strand breaks and oxidized pyrimidines) in human lymphocytes. *Mutat. Res.* 1997, 393, 223-231.

[79] Donnelly, LE; Newton, R; Kennedy, GE; Fenwick, PS; Leung, RH; Ito, K; Russell, RE; Barnes, PJ. Anti-inflammatory effects of resveratrol in lung epithelial cells: molecular mechanisms. *Am. J. Physiol.* 2004, 287, L774-783.

[80] Roders, MK; Glende, EA; Recknagel, RO. NADPH-dependent microsomal lipid peroxidation and the problem of pathological action at a distance: new data on induction of red cell damage. *Biochem. Pharmacol.* 1978, 27, 437-443.

[81] Pederson, TC; Buege, JA; Aust, SD. Microsomal electron transport. *J. Biol. Chem.* 1973, 248, 7134-7141.

[82] Shamberger, RJ; Andreone, TL; Willis, CF. Antioxidants and cancer. IV. Initiating activity of malonaldehyde as a carcinogen. *J. Natl. Cancer Inst.* 1974, 53, 1771-1773.

[83] Haraguchi, H; Ishikawa, H; Sanchez, Y; Ogura, T; Kubo, Y; Kubo, I. Antioxidative constituents on *Heterotheca inuloides*. *Bioorg. Med. Chem.* 1997, 5, 865-871.

[84] Hollman, PCH. Evidence for health benefits of plant phenols: local or systemic effects. *J. Sci. Food Agric.* 2001, 81, 842-852.

[85] Hollman, PC; Katan, MB. Bioavailability and health effects of dietary flavonols in man. *Arch. Toxicol. Suppl.* 1998, 20, 237-248.

[86] Manach, C; Morand, C; Crespy, V; Demigné, C; Texier, O; Régérat, F; Rémésy, C. Quercetin is recovered in human plasma as conjugated derivatives which retain antioxidant properties. *FEBS Lett.* 1998, 426, 331-336.

[87] Justino, GC; Santos, MR; Canário, S; Borges, C; Florêncio, MH; Mira, L. Plasma quercetin metabolites: structure-antioxidant activity relationships. *Arch. Biochem. Biophys.* 2004, 432, 109-121.

[88] Poste, G; Fidler, IJ. The pathogenesis of cancer metastasis. *Nature* 1980, 283, 139-146.

[89] Menon, LG; Kuttan, R; Kuttan, G. Inhibition of lung metastasis in mice induced by B16F10 melanoma cells by polyphenolic compounds. *Cancer Lett.* 1995, 95, 221-225.

[90] Halliwell, B; Murcia, MA; Chirico, S; Aruoma, OI. Free radicals and antioxidants in food and in vivo: What they do and how they work. *Crit. Rev. Food. Sci. Nutr.* 1995, 35, 7-20.

[91] Rice-Evance, AA; Packer, L. Flavonoids in health and disease. New York: Marcel Dekker; 1998.

[92] Murota, K; Terao, J. Antioxidative flavonoid quercetin: implication of its intestinal absorption and metabolism. *Arch. Biochem. Biophys.* 2003, 417, 12-17.

[93] Mel'nikova, NB; Ioffe, ID; Tsareva, LA. Reaction of bioflavonoids with copper(II) acetate in aqueous solution. *Chem. Nat. Comp.* 2002, 39, 33-39.

[94] Henle, ES; Linn, S. Formation, prevention, and repair of DNA damage by iron/hydrogen peroxide. *J. Biol. Chem.* 1997, 272, 19095-19098.

[95] Aruoma, OI; Halliwell, B. *Free Radicals and Food Additives*. London: Taylor and Francis; 1991.

In: Quercetin
Editors: Taiki Chikamatsu and Yuudai Hida
ISBN: 978-1 61942- 057-1

Chapter 7

BENEFICIAL HEALTH EFFECTS OF QUERCETINA AND HOW TO IMPROVE

M. T. Mercader-Ros, C. Lucas-Abellán, M. I. Fortea, A. Martínez-Cachá, J. A. Gabaldón and E. Núñez-Delicado [*]

Dpto. de Tecnología de la Alimentación y Nutrición,
Universidad Católica San Antonio de Murcia, Murcia, España

ABSTRACT

Quercetin (3, 5, 7, 3′, 4′-pentahydroxy flavon), is the major flavonoid in the human diet, its daily intake in foods is estimated to be 50–500 mg and it is one of the main dietary antioxidants. It is ubiquitously present in foods including onions, apples, green and black tea, in smaller amounts in leafy green vegetables and beans as well as countless food supplements. Quercetin is typically found in plants as glycone or carbohydrate conjugates. Olive oil, grapes, dark cherries, and dark berries, such as blueberries, blackberries, and bilberries are also high in flavonoids including quercetin. It is being studied for apparent benefical effects including cardiovascular protection, anti-cancer activity, anti-ulcer effects, anti-allergy activity, cataract prevention, antiviral activity, and anti-inflammatory effects. In the body, quercetin has potent antioxidant and anti-inflammatory activity, where it can protect cellular structures and blood vessels from the damaging effects of free radicals. The biological activity of this flavonol is attributed to the presence of two antioxidants in their chemical structure, the catechol group in ring B and the OH group in position 3 of ring C.

This compound shows an optimum configuration to scavenge free radicals, which together their ability to form metal complexes (chelates), lets inhibit lipid peroxidation, a process by which unsaturated fatty acids become free radicals by the loss of hydrogen, that may trigger cardiovascular and neurodegenerative diseases. This process can be interrupted by antioxidant compounds such as quercetin, interfering with their own radical reactions of the oxidative process.

[*] Corresponding author: Estrella Núñez Delicado. Dpto. Tecnología de la Alimentación y Nutrición; Universidad Católica San Antonio de Murcia (UCAM); Avenida de los Jerónimos s/n.; 30107 Guadalupe. Murcia (Spain). E-mail: enunez@pdi.ucam.edu.

All these beneficial health effects attributed to quercetin, make this natural compound interesting for the development of functional foods. The main problem is its low water solubility and its stability against various factors such as oxygen, light and temperature.

In recent years, cyclodextrin complexation has been successfully used to improve solubility, chemical stability and bioavailability of a number of poorly soluble compounds. Cyclodextrins (CDs) are a group of naturally occurring cyclic oligosaccharides derived from starch with six, seven or eight glucose residues linked by $\alpha(1\rightarrow4)$ glycosidic bonds in a cylinder-shaped structure, denominated α-, β- and γ-CDs, respectively. The central cavity of these molecules is hydrophobic, while the rims of the surrounding walls are hydrophilic. This hydrophobic cavity forms inclusion complexes with a wide range of organic and inorganic guest molecules, altering their physicochemical behaviour and reducing their undesirable effects. It has been demonstrated that complexation can considerably increase the solubility, stability and bioavailability of the guest molecule. Quercetin can be included in CD increasing the solubility, possibly its bioavailability and beneficial health effects.

INTRODUCTION

Chemistry and Classification of Flavonoids

Flavonoids consist of 2 benzene rings (A and B), which are connected by an oxygencontaining pyrene ring (C). Flavonoids containing a hydroxyl group in position C-3 of the C ring are classified as 3-hydroxyflavonoids (flavonols, anthocyanidins, leucoanthocyanidins, and catechins), and those lacking it as 3-desoxyflavonoids (flavanones and flavones). Classification within the 2 families is based on whether and how additional hydroxyl or methyl groups have been introduced to the different positions of the molecule (Erlund, 2004).

Isoflavonoids differ from the other groups; the B ring is bound to C-3 of ring C instead of C-2. Anthocyanidins and catechins, on the other hand, lack the carbonyl group on C-4 (Kühnau, 1976).

Flavonoids are mainly present in plants as glycosides. Aglycones (the forms lacking sugar moieties) occur less frequently. At least 8 different monosaccharides or combinations of these (di- or trisaccharides) can bind to the different hydroxyl groups of the flavonoid aglycone (Williams & Harborne, 1994).

The large number of flavonoids is a result of the many different combinations of flavonoid aglycones and these sugars. The most common sugar moieties include D-glucose and L-rhamnose. The glycosides are usually O-glycosides, with the sugar moiety bound to the hydroxyl group at the C-3 or C-7 position (Erlund, 2004).

Occurrence in Food of Flavonoids

Flavonoids are widely distributed in foods and beverages of plant origin, such as fruits, vegetables, tea, cocoa, and wine. A large body of literature exists regarding their content in various foods. Within the subgroup of flavonols and flavones, the flavonol quercetin is the most frequently occurring compound in foods. Also common are kaempferol, myricetin, and the flavones apigenin and luteolin. Tea and onions are the main dietary sources of flavonols and flavones. Quercetin is the most abundant flavonol present in onions, whereas tea contains notable amounts of both quercetin and kaempferol (Ross & Kasum, 2002).

QUERCETIN

Quercetin [2-(3,4-dihydroxyphenyl)-3,5,7-trihydroxy-4H-chromen-4-one] (Figure 1) is a flavonol naturally present in onions and to a lesser extent in French beans, broad beans, apples, apricots, cherries, grapes, wine, fruit juices, black tea and green tea (Table 1).

Quercetin is present in plants in many different glycosidic forms (Kühnau, 1976), with quercetin-3-rutinoside, also called quercetin-3-rhamnoglucoside or rutin, being one of the most widespread forms. In onions, quercetin is bound to 1 or 2 glucose molecules (quercetin-4′-glucoside and quercetin-3, 4′-glucoside). Examples of other dietary quercetin glycosides are quercetin galactosides, which are found in apples, and quercetin arabinosides, which are present in berries. Other flavonols in the diet include kaempferol (broccoli), myricetin (berries), and isorhamnetin (onion) (Erlund, 2004).

The importance of different foods as quercetin sources varies between countries. Hertog et al. (1995) calculated a flavonol intake from the Seven Countries Study, which was started in the late 1950s, and reported that tea, was the predominant source of quercetin in the Netherlands and Japan. Wine was the major source of quercetin in Italy, while onion and apples contributed most in the United States, Finland, Greece. More recently, Häkkinen et al. (1999) estimated that onions, followed by tea, apples, and berries are the major sources of quercetin in Finland. It should be noted that onion is usually not consumed in high quantities, but it is an important source because of its high quercetin content. Tea and especially wine, on the other hand, contain relatively low amounts of quercetin but are consumed, at least in some countries, in rather high quantities. The daily intake of quercetin was estimated to range between 3 and 38 mg in the seven countries study (Hertog et al., 1995). In the United States, the estimated intake of flavonols and flavones was 20 to 22 mg/day, of which 73% to 76% was quercetin (Sampson et al., 2002).

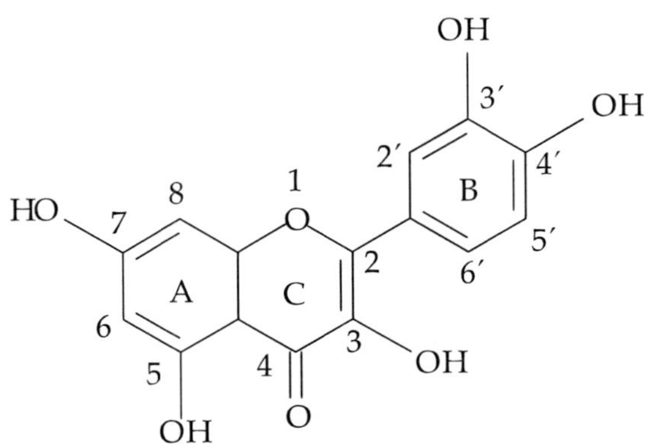

Figure 1. Chemical structure of Quercetin.

Table 1. Quercetin content in fruits and vegetables, edible porcion (mg/100g)

Food	Quercetin	
	min	max
Apples, Golden Delicious (*Malus domestica*)	1.57	4.40
Apples, Red Delicious (*Malus domestica*)	0.25	7.60
Apples, Royal Gala (*Malus domestica*)	2.73	10.10
Apricots raw (*Prunus armeniaca*)	1.15	2.60
Broad beans (*Vicia faba*)	0.55	0.55
French beans (*Phaseolus vulgaris var. vulgaris*)	3.20	4.50
Onions (*Allium cepa* L.)	1.50	118.70
Cherries (*Pronus cerasus*)	2.92	2.92
Cherries (*Pronus avium*)	0.86	3,93
Grape, Black (*Vitis vinifera*)	1,26	3,7
Grape, red (*Vitis vinifera*)	0	3,98
Grape, White or Green (*Vitis vinifera*)	0	0,45
Lettuce cos and romaine (*Lactuca sativa var. logifolia*)	1.04	8.78
Lettuce, green leaf (*Lactuca sativa var. crispa*)	0.04	20.60
Lettuce, iceberg (*Lactuca sativa var. capitata*)	0	9.40

Source: USDA http://www.ars.usda.gov/SP2UserFiles/Place/12354500/ Data/Flav/Flav02-1.pdf.

Metabolism of Quercetin

The flavonoid quercetin is metabolised in the organism to the extent that little or no free aglycone is present in the plasma. Instead, the major bioavailable forms in animals and humans are represented by quercetin conjugates, namely glucuronides, O-methylated glucuronides, and sulphated derivatives (Pollard et al., 2006). The major *in vivo* reported metabolites of this flavonol are 3′-O-methyl quercetin, 4′-Omethyl quercetin and quercetin 7-glucuronide. After consumption of onions by humans, also metabolites quercetin 3′-sulphate and quercetin 3-glucuronide were found in the plasma (Terao, 1999).

Studies carried out on the bioavailability and metabolism indicate that β-glycosides of quercetin, found in onions, can be absorbed in the small intestine, while the routines of apple, green tea and many other foods are not absorbed the small intestine, reaching the large intestine, where they are absorbed to a lesser extent when released aglycones, being degraded by the colonic flora in most cases. Terao in 1999 found that oral administration of (-)-epicatechin and quercetin enhanced the antioxidant capacity of rat plasma, although both flavonoids accumulated mainly as glucuronide and sulfate conjugates in blood plasma. This finding suggests that conjugated metabolites of flavonoids may play a role in the antioxidant defenses of blood plasma (Ross & Kasum, 2002).

Interestingly, the metabolic pattern of quercetin depends on the way of administration. Santos et al. (2008) proved that when rats were fed by the chow supplemented with 0.02% quercetin over 3 weeks, major plasma metabolites were 3′-O-methyl quercetin (isorhamnetin) glucuronide and sulphate conjugates, the most plausible conjugation positions being at the 3-, 5- and 7-hydroxyl positions. Isorhamnetin conjugates were methylated at the 3′-OH position, which decreased the high antioxidant activity of quercetin and its metabolites and their contribution to plasma antioxidant potential. On the other hand, after a single high-dose administration, where the major metabolites were quercetin conjugates at 5- and 7-hydroxyl positions, a significantly increased plasma antioxidant activity was observed (Procházková et al., 2011). Justino et al. (2004) reported that plasma antioxidant status was significantly higher in rats to which quercetin was administrated, suggesting that quercetin metabolites can retain some antioxidant activity when the *o*-catechol group does not undergo conjugation reactions.

Quercetin and Health

Quercetin is a flavonol that has attracted the most interest in relation to their biological activity, it is the one most widely distributed in foods of plant origin. This biological activity has been associated with its antioxidant capacity, because it shows *in vitro* neutralizing properties of free radicals. However, evidence on antioxidant or free radical scavengers in vivo is very low, probably due to the low bioavailability of its metabolites (Tomás-Barberán & Espín, 2001).

Quercetin has been shown to be an excellent *in vitro* antioxidant. Within the flavonoid family, quercetin is the most potent scavenger of ROS, including $O_2^{\cdot-}$ (Hanasaki et al., 1994; Cushnie & Lamb, 2005), RNS like $NO^{\cdot}$ (van Acker et al., 1995; Haenen & Bast, 1999) and $ONOO^-$ (Heijnen et al., 2001). These antioxidative capacities of quercetin are attributed to the presence of two antioxidant pharmacophores within the molecule that have the optimal configuration for free radical scavenging, i.e. the catechol group in the B ring and the OH group at position 3 of the AC ring (Heijnen et al., 2002). Moreover, quercetin is suggested to substantially empower the endogenous antioxidant shield due to its contribution to the total plasma antioxidant capacity which is 6.24 times higher than the reference antioxidant trolox, whereas for example the contribution of both vitamin C and uric acid virtually equals that of trolox (Arts et al., 2004).

Furthermore, it has been shown *in vitro* that quercetin also possesses anti-fibrotic (Lee et al., 2003), anti-coagulative (Bucki et al., 2003), anti-bacterial (Cushnie & Lamb, 2005), anti-atherogenic (de Whalley et al., 1990; Pérez-Vizcaino et al., 2006), anti-hypertensive (Perez-Vizcaino et al., 2006) and anti-proliferative properties (Kuo, 1996; Orsolic et al., 2004; Gulati et al., 2006). Furthermore, quercetin is reported to directly modulate the gene expression of enzymes involved in biotransformation (Walle et al., 1995; Pacifici, 2004; Schwarz et al., 2005; Moon et al., 2006) and to inhibit cell proliferation by interacting with estrogen binding sites (Piantelli et al., 1995; Caltagirone et al., 1997). Altogether, these studies indicate that quercetin may exert health-beneficial capacities via various damage modulating effects. However, most of these studies have been performed with immortalized or cultured cell lines only and are thus not easy to extrapolate to the *in vivo* human situation (Boots et al., 2008).

Another harmful effect caused by free radicals is the oxidation of low density lipoprotein (LDL) and may lead to the formation of atherosclerotic plaques, leading to cardiovascular disease (Hollman & Katan, 1997). Several studies in humans have shown that quercetin inhibits the oxidation of LDL (Graf et al., 2005; Chopra et al., 2000), this could be related, at least in part, to a direct effect of quercetin on LDL, to which is attached via an ether linkage (R-O-R ') (Hayek et al., 1997).

The effects that quercetin and other polyphenols have on glucose and lipid metabolism have complex and have been extensively studied in recent years. Quercetin has been shown to exert a beneficial effect on lipid homeostasis in liver and adipose tissue (Peluso, 2006), which may be reflected in a substantial improvement in lipid profile in the blood plasma of obese animals (Zang et al., 2006). It has also seen an improvement in insulin sensitivity following treatment with high doses of quercetin (50 mg/kg/day) in healthy humans and rats with streptozotocin-induced diabetes (Kato et al., 2008). The mechanisms proposed to explain these effects are focus on the power-inflammatory and antioxidant flavonol, as obesity and metabolic syndrome are seen as chronic inflammatory diseases (Hotamisligil, 2006). This anti-inflammatory effect, as seen both *in vitro* and *in vivo*, resulting in less release of fatty acids into plasma, which in turn reduces the inflammatory response and insulin resistance (Boden et al., 2005).

On the other hand, quercetin interferes with the activity of inducible nitric oxide synthase (iNOS), reducing the production of peroxynitrite (Shutenko et al., 1999). The nitric oxide synthase (NOS) is the enzyme responsible for transforming the L-arginine to nitric oxide (NO) in cells, including endothelial cells and macrophages. It is important to release NO to the dilation of blood vessels, but at high concentrations causes oxidative damage, it acts with free radicals to produce peroxynitrite, which oxidizes LDL, causing irreversible damage to the cell membrane. Quercetin has been shown to act by capturing free radicals, thus preventing that can react with NO, reducing the ischemia (cell suffering caused by reduced blood flow) (Shoskes, 1998). It also has antihypertensive activity and improves endothelial function (Romero et al., 2009). This antioxidant protection prevents vascular stroke (Knekt et al., 2000).

Inhibition of xantina-deshidrogenasa/xantina-oxidasa system is another important mechanism by which quercetin reduced the oxidative damage (Bindoli et al., 1985). Xanthine dehydrogenase (form of the enzyme in normal physiological conditions) changes to xanthine oxidase in ischemic conditions, a process that can trigger an increase in uric acid generation, since these two enzymes are involved in their metabolism. Xanthine oxidase reacts with molecular oxygen releasing superoxide radicals. There have been several studies showing that quercetin inhibits the activity of xanthine oxidase, thus reducing oxidative damage (Shoskes, 1998, Zeng et al., 1997).

For several years, quercetin has been presented as a possible anti-inflammatory active ingredient (Oršolić et al., 2004), as has been shown to be inhibiting the release of histamine and other inflammatory mediators in response to lipopolysaccharide (LPS) in macrophages isolated (Manjeet and Ghosh, 1999) and mast cells (Theoharides et al., 2001). Macrophages are key to the development of atherosclerosis and insulin resistance. Given the importance of macrophage accumulation in the onset of inflammation in tissues, has also been studied and shown anti-inflammatory effect of quercetin in organs such as liver (Dias et al., 2005), brain (Singh et al. 2008), intestine (Comala et al., 2005) and in adipose tissue cells (Rivera et al., 2008). The mechanisms involved in this anti-inflammatory process are not fully defined, but numerous studies suggest a reduction in the production of proinflammatory cytokines (messengers physiological inflammatory response) (Min et al., 2007) and inhibition of the inducible isoform of NOS (iNOS), cyclooxygenase (COX) and lipoxygenase (LOX), blocking the path of arachidonic acid and C-reactive protein and increased expression of adiponectin (a hormone synthesized by adipose tissue only involved in metabolism of glucose and fatty acids) (Rivera et al., 2008).

Another effect that has quercetin, acting as a "natural drug" is an antiallergic action, proving an effective antihistamine in the treatment and prevention of asthma and bronchitis (Chaabi et al., 2007). Several studies in animal models, previously treated with quercetin have demonstrated a dramatic reduction of adverse reactions to chemicals that trigger asthma attacks (Rogerio et al. 2007).

In addition to the anti-inflamatory and antioxidant effects atributed to quercetin, the antitumoral activity has been studied by other autors. Epidemiological studies showed that populations whose diet abundant flavonoid-rich foods such as fruits and vegetables had a lower incidence of certain cancers. Finally, studies were conducted *in vitro* (van der Waud et al., 2005) and in vivo (Schlachterman et al., 2008) confirmed this hypothesis. The proposed mechanism by which quercetin exerts its antitumor effect is based on the inhibition of DNA topoisomerases I and II, thereby inducing a DNA damage and apoptosis (Yamashita and Kawanishi, 2000). Actually there are many mechanisms by which both quercetin and other flavonoids may exert their antitumor action (Havsteen, 2002).

It has also been shown that quercetin inhibits reverse transcriptase of immunodeficiency virus (HIV) (Ono et al., 1990). However, since there are other molecules effective against this virus, it has not been used for this purpose. Instead, it has been used to treat infections caused by other viruses such as Influenza (Neznanov et al., 2008) or poliovirus (Davis et al., 2008).

Encapsulation in Food Industry

Encapsulation involves the incorporation of food ingredients, enzymes, cells or other materials in small capsules. Applications for this technique have increased in the food industry since the encapsulated materials can be protected from moisture, heat or other extreme conditions, thus enhancing their stability and maintaining viability.

In the food industry, the microencapsulation process can be applied for a variety of reasons, which have been summarized by Desai & Park (2005) as follows: (i) protection of the core material from degradation by reducing its reactivity to its outside environment; (ii) reduction of the evaporation or transfer rate of the core material to the outside environment; (iii) modification of the physical characteristics of the original material to allow easier handling; (iv) tailoring the release of the core material slowly over time, or at a particular time; (v) to mask an unwanted flavor or taste of the core material; (vi) dilution of the core material when only small amounts are required, while achieving uniform dispersion in the host material; (vii) to help separate the components of the mixture that would otherwise react with one another. Food ingredients of acidulants, flavoring agents, sweeteners, colorants, lipids, vitamins and minerals, enzymes and microorganisms, are encapsulated using different technologies.

Limitations in many of the encapsulation techniques have occurred due to high costs of production and the lack of food-grade available materials. Research is necessary to eliminate these limitations. Encapsulation currently is an art that is difficult for the food scientist to master. The food scientist does not have the information available in databases to enable him to make informed choices concerning the most appropriate material and encapsulation process. For example, the appropriate blends of starches and maltodextrins as encapsulating materials could prove highly beneficial. The development of CDs has led to new products with longer shelf-life, reduced volatility and protection of heat-labile substances. There is a great deal of research that needs to be done concerning the use of CDs in the food industry. Unlike the pharmaceutical industry, which can tolerate high costs, manufacturing costs will have to be reduced for food applications (Gibbs et al., 1999).

Cyclodextrins

After their discovery, CDs were considered important substances and its capacity for complexes formation was only considered a scientific curiosity. Later on, research on CDs proved that they are not only non-toxic but they can be helpful for protecting flavours, vitamins and natural colours (Astray et al., 2009). The preparation process of CDs consists of four principal phases: (i) culturing of the microorganism that produces the CD glucosyl transferase enzyme (CGT-ase); (ii) separation, concentration and purification of the enzyme from the fermentation medium; (iii) enzymatical conversion of prehydrolyzed starch in mixture of cyclic and acyclic dextrins; and (iv) separation of CDs from the mixture, their purification and crystallization. CGT-ase enzymes degrade the starch and produce intramolecular reactions without the water participation. In the process, cyclic and acyclic dextrins are originated, which are oligosaccharides of intermediate size. The cyclic resulting products are CDs.

Structure and Properties of CDs

CDs are cyclic oligosaccharides that consist of (α-1, 4)-linked α-D-glucopyranose units and contain a somewhat lipophilic central cavity and a hydrophilic outer surface. Due to the chair conformation of the glucopyranose units, CDs are shaped like a truncated cone rather than perfect cylinders. The hydroxyl functions are orientated to the cone exterior with the primary hydroxyl groups of the sugar residues at the narrow edge of the cone and the secondary hydroxyl groups at the wider edge. The central cavity is lined by the skeletal carbons and ethereal oxygens of the glucose residues, which gives it a lipophilic character (Figure 2). The polarity of the cavity has been estimated to be similar to that of an aqueous ethanolic solution (Loftsson et al., 2005).

The natural α-, β- and γ-CDs consist of six, seven, and eight glucopyranose units, respectively. The natural CDs, in particular β-CDs, are of limited aqueous solubility meaning that complexes resulting from interaction of apolar molecules with these CDs can be of limited solubility resulting in precipitation of solid CDs complexes from water and other aqueous systems. In fact, the aqueous solubility of the natural CDs is much lower than that of comparable acyclic saccharides. This is thought to be due to relatively strong intermolecular hydrogen bonding in the crystal state (Loftsson et al. 2005) (Table 2).

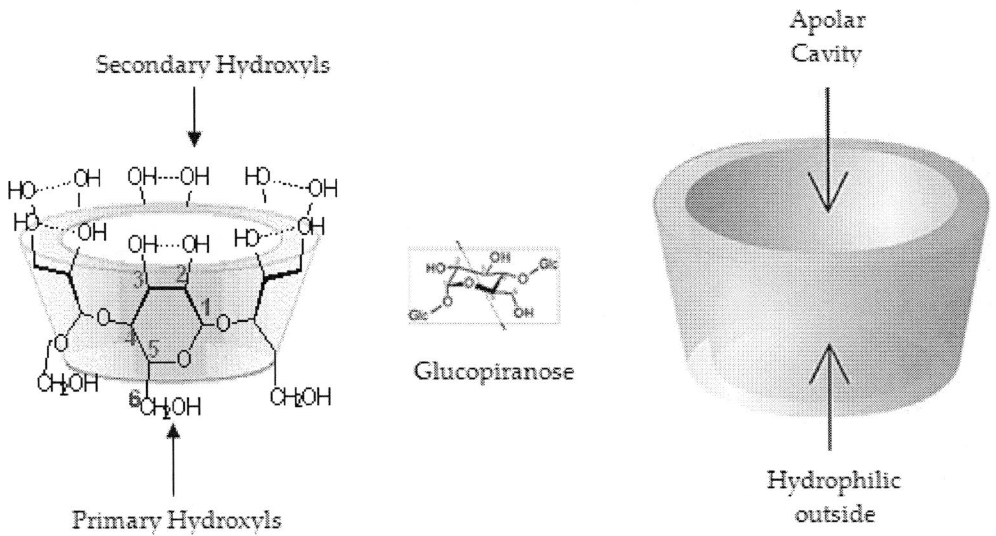

Figure 2. CD structure.

Substitution of any of the hydrogen bond forming hydroxyl groups, even by lipophilic methoxy functions, results in dramatic improvement in their aqueous solubility. CDs derivatives of pharmaceutical interest include hydroxypropyl derivatives of β- and γ-CDs, randomly methylated β-CDs, sulfobutylether β-CDs, and the so-called branched CDs such as glucosyl-β-CDs (Loftsson et al., 2005) (Figure 3).

Table 2. CDs properties

Properties	**α-CDs**	**β-CDs**	**γ-CDs**
Number of glucopyranose units	6	7	8
Molecular weight (g/mol)	972	1135	1297
Solubility in water at 25 °C (%, w/v)	14,5	1,85	23,2
Outer diameter (Å)	14,6	15,4	17,5
Cavity diameter (Å)	4,7-5,3	6,0-6,5	7,5-8,3
Height of torus (Å)	7,9	7,9	7,9
Cavity volumen ($Å^3$)	174	262	427

Martin del Valle, 2004.

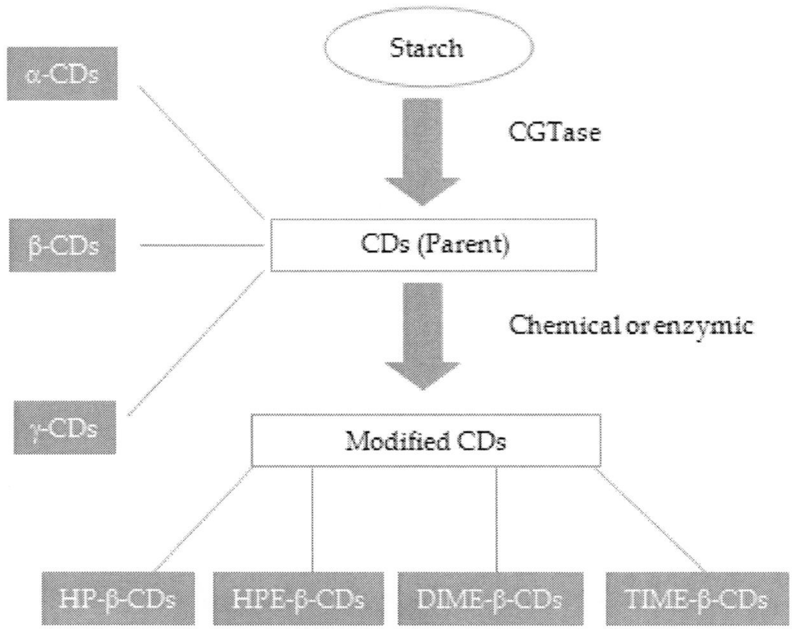

- HP-β-CDs: Hidroxypropyl-β-CDs.
- HPE-β-CDs: Hydroxyethyl-β-CDs.
- DIME-β-CDs: (2, 6-dimethyl)-β-CDs.
- TIME-β-CDs: (2, 3, 6-trimethyl)-β-CDs.

Singh et al., 2002.

Figure 3. Natural CDs and CDs derivatives formation.

The natural α- and β-CDs, unlike γ-CDs, cannot be hydrolyzed by human salivary and pancreatic amylases. However, both α- and β-CD can be fermented by the intestinal microflora. CDs are both large (MW ranging from almost 1,000 to over 2,000 Daltons) and hydrophilic with a significant number of H-donors and acceptors and, thus, are not absorbed from the gastrointestinal tract in their intact form. Hydrophilic CDs are considered non-toxic at low to moderate oral dosages. Lipophilic CD derivatives, such as the methylated CDs, are to some extent absorbed from the gastrointestinal tract into the systemic circulation and have been shown to be toxic after parenteral administration (Loftsson et al., 2005).

Actually, oral administration of methylated β-CDs is limited by its potential toxicity (Loftsson et al., 2005). About 30 different pharmaceutical products containing CDs are now on the market worldwide. In the pharmaceutical industry, CDs have mainly been used as complexing agents to increase the aqueous solubility of poorly water-soluble drugs, and to increase their bioavailability and stability. In addition, CDs can be used to reduce or prevent gastrointestinal and ocular irritation, reduce or eliminate unpleasant smells or tastes, prevent drug-drug or drug-additive interactions, or to convert oils and liquid drugs into microcrystalline or amorphous powders (Loftsson et al., 2004).

Complex Formation and Drugs

CDs can be considered as empty capsules of a certain molecular size that can include a great variety of molecules in this cavity. In this case, a complex called ''inclusion complex'' is formed. Inclusion complexes are entities comprising two or more molecules. One of the molecule, the ''host'', includes, totally or partly the ''guest'' molecules by physical forces. Therefore, CDs are considered typical host molecules (Szente et al., 1998; García-Río et al., 2006; Brewster & Loftsson, 2007). The type of bond established between the guest and the host is no covalent. **Figure 4** illustrates the approximate capsule volumes of each capsule (α-, β-, and γ-CDs).

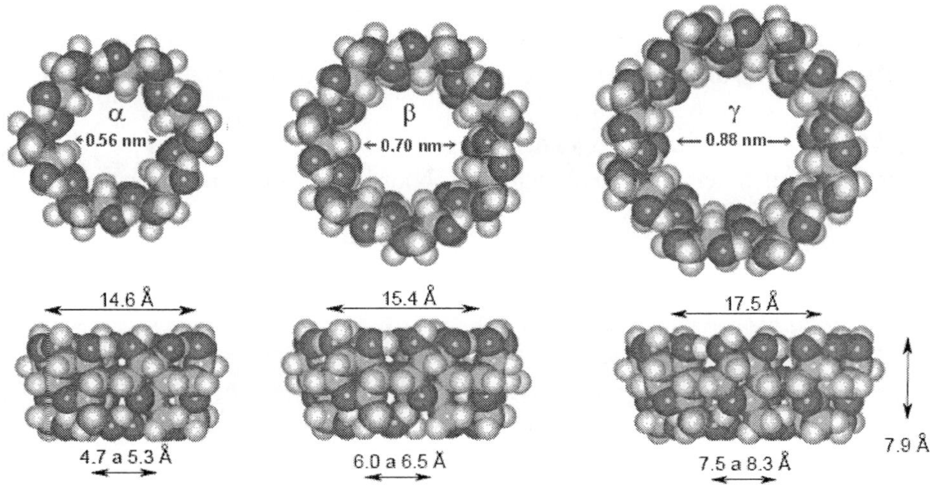

Figure 4. Outer diameter and cavity diameter of different CDs.

Complex formation in solution is a dynamic equilibrium process which can be illustrated by the equation (1), where CDs are the encapsulating agent, quercetin is the guest molecule, and CDs-quercetin is the inclusion complex. The stability of the inclusion complex can be described by the complexation constant K_c (2).

$$quercetin + CDs \xleftrightarrow{K_C} quercetin - CDs \quad (1)$$

$$K_C = \frac{quercetin - CDs}{[quercetin]_L [CDs]_L} \quad (2)$$

Energy and Inclusion Mechanisms

The inclusion of a guest in a CDs cavity consists basically of a substitution of the included water molecules by the less polar guest (Figure 5). The process is energetically favoured by the interactions of the guest molecule with the solvated hydrophobic cavity of the host. In this process entropy and enthalpy changes have an important role.

In spite of the fact that the ''driving force'' of complexation is not yet completely understood, it seems that it is the result of various effects (Astray et al. 2009):

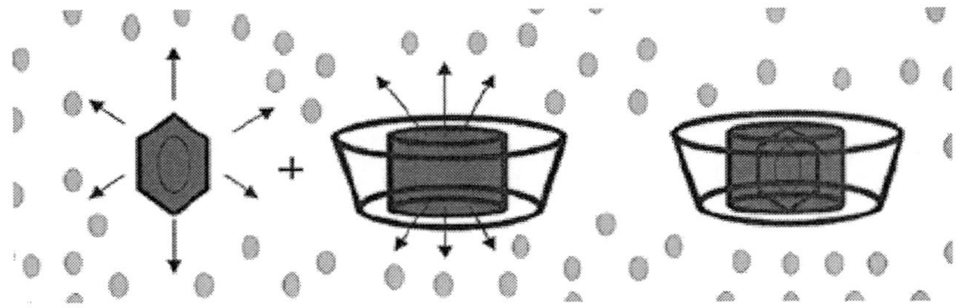

Figure 5. The inclusion complex of quercetin-CDs.

a) Substitution of the energetically unfavoured polar–apolar interactions (between the included water and the CDs cavity on the one hand, and between water and the guest on the other) by the more favoured apolar–apolar interaction (between the guest and the cavity), and the polar–polar interaction (between bulk water and the released cavity-water molecules).
b) CDs-ring strain release on complexation.
c) Van der Waals interactions and hydrogen bonds between host and guest.

Properties of CDs-Included Guests in Solution

When a more or less non-polar poorly water-soluble substance reacts with an aqueous CDs solution, the following consequences can occur (Liu et al., 1999):

1) The concentration of the guest in the dissolved phase significantly increases, and when solid complexes are simultaneously formed, the concentration of dissolved CDs decreases (except with ionized guests, or hydrogen bond establishing).
2) The spectral properties of the guest are modified.
3) The reactivity of the included molecule is modified. In most cases their reactivity decreases.
4) The formerly hydrophobic guest in complexed form becomes hydrophilic.

Use and Regulatory of CDs

The use of CDs has increased annually around 20–30%, of which 80–90% was in food products. The widespread utilization of CDs is reflected in pharmaceutical, food, chemical and other industrial areas (Szejtli, 1997). In the pharmaceutical industry, CDs and their derivatives have been used in drugs either for complexation or as auxiliary additives such as solubilizers, diluents, or tablet ingredients to improve the physical and chemical properties, or to enhance the bioavailability of poorly soluble drugs (Frömming & Szejtli, 1994). In the chemical industry, CDs and their derivatives are used as catalysts to improve the selectivity of reactions, as well as for the separation and purification of industrial-scale products (Hedges, 1998). In the food, cosmetics, toiletry, and tobacco industries, CDs have been widely used either for stabilization of flavours and fragrances or for the elimination of undesired tastes, microbiological contaminations, and other undesired compounds (Martín del Valle, 2004; Singh et al., 2002).

However, the regulatory status of CDs in foods differs between countries. In the USA α-, β-, and γ-CDs have obtained the GRAS list (FDA list of food additives that are 'generally recognized as safe') status and can be commercialized as such. In Japan α-, β-, and γ-CDs are recognized as natural products and their commercialization in the food sector is restricted only by considerations of purity. In Australia and New Zealand α- and γ-CDs are classified as Novel Foods from 2004 and 2003, respectively (Cravotto et al., 2006). The recommendation of Joint FAO/WHO Expert Committee on Food Additives (JECFA) for a maximum level of β-CDs in foods is 5 mg/kg per day. For α- anḍ γ-CDs no Acceptable Daily Intake (ADI) was defined because of their favourable toxicological profiles. Moreover, in July 2005 the U.S. Environmental Protection Agency (EPA) did away with the need to establish a maximum permissible level for residues of α-, β-, and γ-CDs in various food commodities (US Federal Register, 2005).

In Europe, α- and β-CDs has been approved by ingredients food products. The designation "α-CD" and "β-CD" must appear in the list of ingredients food products containing it.

Applications of CDs

Since each guest molecule is individually surrounded by CDs the molecule is micro-encapsulated from a microscopical point of view. This process can lead to advantageous changes in the chemical and physical properties of the guest molecules (Martín del Valle, 2004) such us:

- Stabilization of light- or oxygen-sensitive substances.
- Modification of the chemical reactivity of guest molecules.
- Fixation of very volatile substances.
- Improvement of solubility of substances.
- Modification of liquid substances to powders.
- Protections against degradation of substances by microorganisms.
- Masking of ill smell and taste.
- Masking pigments or the colour of substances.
- Catalytic activity of CDs with guest molecules.

These characteristics of CDs make them suitable for applications in analitycal chemistry, agriculture, the pharmaceutical field, in toilet articles, and food industry. (Singh et al., 2002).

The use of CDs in the food industry has increased significantly in the last years. These compounds are highly recommended for applications in food processing and as food additives. Thus, volatile compounds can be encapsulated in CDs in order to limit aroma degradation or loss during processing and storage (Lubbers et al., 1998). Moreover, the use of CDs-flavour inclusion complexes allows using minor amounts of flavours. On the other hand, CDs can also be used for deodorizing and removing undesirable components such as off flavours or bitter components present in the food in its natural form (Binello et al., 2004), or for improving the nutritional characteristics of many dairy foods such as milk (Kwak et al.,

2004), mayonnaise (Jung et al., 2008), lard (Kim et al., 2007) or cream (Shim et al., 2003) through their complexation with cholesterol molecules.

In addition, CDs can play an important role as food colour modulators due to the ability of these compounds to form complexes with the polyphenol-oxidase substrates, which are responsible of enzymatic browning in foods (Martín Del Valle, 2004; Núñez-Delicado et al., 2005). Another interesting application of CDs is their incorporation in the food packaging materials as antiseptic or conserving agents (Wood, 2001).

ENCAPSULATION OF QUERCETIN IN CYCLODEXTRINS

Research on the application of polyphenols, have recently attracted great interest in the functional foods, nutraceutical and pharmaceutical industries, due to their potential health benefits to humans. However, the effectiveness of polyphenols dependes on preserving their stability, boactivity and bioavability. Moreover, the unpleasant taste of most phenolic compounds also limits their application. The utilization of encapsulated polyphenols, insteated of free compounds, can effectively alleviate these deficiencies. One outstanding advantage of the inclusion of polyphenols in CDs is the effect in improving their water solubility, especially for the less water soluble phytochemicals.

The high hydrophobicity of quercetin and its sensitivity to external agents such us air, light and oxidative enzymes may constitute a serious problem for its bioavailability, formulation and manipulation in the elaboration of functional foods. In order to avoid this limitation, inclusion of quercetin in CDs has been widely studied (Lucas-Abellán et al., 2008; Mercader-Ros et al., 2010; Calabrò et al., 2004). The inclusion complex formation will modify physico-chemical properties such as solubility, stability and bioavailability of poorly water-soluble quercetin. In addition, its antioxidant activities increased in these encapsulated form. The improved antioxidant efficacy of the inclusion complex may come from the protection of the quercetin against rapid oxidation by free radicals (Mercader-Ros et al., 2010), which may, in part, be explained by an increase in its solubility in the biological moiety (Ding et al., 2003).

The complexation of quercetin with native (α-, β- and γ-CDs) and different types of modified β-CDs (Hydroxypropyl-β- and Maltosyl-β-CDs) has been studied in order to establish the optimum type of CDs to complex quercetin (Lucas-Abellán et al., 2008).

The *in vitro* formation of quercetin-CDs inclusion complex in acidic medium has been characterized using the enzymatic system horseradish peroxidase, which oxidizes this flavonol in the presence of H_2O_2. The study of this oxidation process permits the determination of complexation constant between flavonol and different types of CDs. The presence of CDs in the reaction medium inhibits flavonol oxidation due to the complexation of the flavonol in the hydrophobic cavity of CDs. The K_C values obtained followed the order HP-β-CDs > G_2-β-CDs > β-CDs > γ-CDs > α-CDs, reflecting the greater affinity of modified CDs for the studied flavonols than their parental β-CDs (Table 3).

Table 3. Stability constants (K_C) for complexes formed between different types of CDs and the quercetin obtained by the enzymatic method

Guest	α-CDs $K_c M^{-1}$	β-CDs $K_c M^{-1}$	γ-CDs $K_c M^{-1}$	HP-β-CDs $K_c M^{-1}$	G_2-β-CDs $K_c M^{-1}$
Quercetin	-----	426	233	1195	650

One interesting property of CDs is that they can be saturated with flavonols, increasing the total concentration of flavonol in solution, whereas the free flavonol concentration remains constant. To study this effect, Lucas-Abellán et al. (2008) have studied the solubility of quercetin in the presence of CDs at acidic pH, as described by Higuchi & Connors (1965).

Phase solubility diagrams of quercetin at pH 4.5 with HP-β-CDs or G_2-β-CDs are shown in Figure 6. In all cases phase solubility diagrams showed a linear relationship between the amounts of flavonol solubilised and the concentration of CDs in solution (A_L type), indicating that the stoichiometry of complexes were 1:1 in all cases.

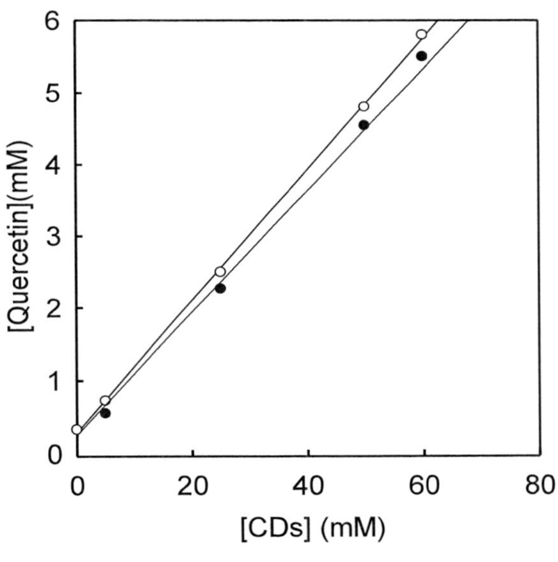

Figure 6. Phase of solubility diagram of quercetin with HP-*β*-CDs (○) and G_2-*β*-CDS (•) in sodium acetate buffer (100mM, pH 4.5) at 25°C.

Effect of CDs Complexation on the Antioxidant Activity of Quercetin

Antioxidants are chemical substances that reduce or prevent oxidation. The growing interest in free radical biology and the lack of effective therapies for most chronic diseases have meant that the usefulness of antioxidants in protection against these diseases is increasingly studied (Lucas-Abellán et al., 2011).

Many studies have shown that phenolic compounds display antioxidant activity as a result of their capacity to scavenge free radicals (Seyoum et al., 2006). They can also act as antioxidants by chelating metal ions, preventing radical formation and improving the antioxidant endogenous system (Al-Azzawie & Alhamdani, 2006).

CDs can be used as a flavonol complexation agent, since they act as a substrate reservoir in a dose-controlled manner. The effect of complexing quercetin with HP-β-CDs on its antioxidant capacity has been studied by means of the ORAC-fluorescein (ORAC-FL) assay (Mercader-Ros et al., 2010). This complexation phenomenon increased the antioxidant activity of quercetin, which reached a maximum level when quercetin has been complexed in the hydrophobic cavity of CDs (Figure 7). The antioxidant activity increased because of the flavonol was protected against rapid oxidation by free radicals.

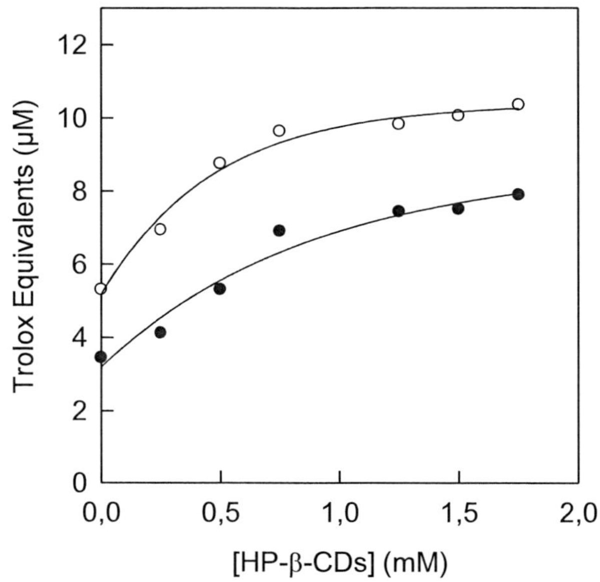

Figure 7. Effect of HP-β-CDs concentration on the μM Trolox equivalents of quercetin 0.5 μM (•), 0.75 μM (○).

Summary and Trends

It is clear that the utilization of encapsulated quercetin instead of free compound, can lead to an improvement in both, stability and bioavailability of the compound. Because there is still a lack of direct evidence for the use of polyphenols in preventing and treating of human diseases (Scalbert et al., 2005), most of polyphenols encapsulated are classified as 'functional foods' or 'nutriceuticals', which limits their potential markets. In food grade products, cost is an important factor for their industrialization. Future research of polyphenol encapsulation is likely to focus on aspects of delivery and the potential use of co-encapsulation methodologies, where two or more bioactive ingredients can be combined to have a synergistic effect. It is possible that the understanding of the health benefits of quercetin, improvement in manufacturing technology, new strategy for stabilization of fragile nutraceuticals, and the development of novel approaches to site-specific carrier targeting, encapsulated quercetin will play an important role in increasing the efficacy of functional foods or even pharmaceuticals, over the next decade.

REFERENCES

Al-Azzawie, H.F., & Alhamdani, M.S.S. (2006). Hypoglycemic and antioxidant effect of oleuropein in alleoxan-diabetic rabbits. *Life Sciences, 78*, 1371-1376.

Arts, M.J.T.J., Dallinga, J.S., Voss, H.P., Haenen, G.R.M.M., A., B. (2004). A new approach to assess the total antioxidant capacity using the TEAC assay. *Food Chemistry, 88*, 567–570.

Astray, G., Gonzalez-Barreiro, C., Mejuto, J.C., Rial-Otero, R., Simal-Gándara J. (2009). A review on the use of cyclodextrins in foods. *Food Hydrocolloids*, *23*, 1631–1640.

Bindoli, A., Valente, M., Cavallini, L. (1985). Inhibitory action of quercetin *Pharmacological research communications*, *17*, 831-839.

Binello, A., Cravotto, G., Nano, G. M., & Spagliardi, P. (2004). Synthesis of chitosancyclodextrin adducts and evaluation of their bitter-masking properties. *Flavour Fragrance Journal*, *19*, 394–400.

Boden, G., She, P., Mozzoli, M., Cheung, P., Gumireddy, K., Reddy, P., Xiang, X., Luo., Ruderman, N. (2005). Free fatty acids produce insulin resistance and activate the proinflammatory nuclear factor-kappaB pathway in rat liver. *Diabetes*, *54,* 3458-3465.

Boots, A.W., Drent, M., de Boer, V.C.J., Bast, A., Haenen, G.R.M.M. (2011). Quercetin reduces markers of oxidative stress and inflammation in sarcoidosis. *Clinical Nutrition,* 1-7.

Brewster, M. E., & Loftsson, T. (2007). Cyclodextrins as pharmaceutical solubilizers. *Advanced Drug Delivery Reviews*, *59*, 645–666.

Bucki, R., Pastore, J.J., Giraud, F., Sulpice, J.C., Janmey, P.A. (2003). Flavonoid inhibition of platelet proagulant activity and phosphoinositide synthesis. *Journal of Thrombosis and Haemostasis, 1*, 1820–1828.

Calabrò, M.L., Tommasini, S., Donato, P., Raneri, D., Stancanelli, R., Ficarra, P. et al. (2004). Effects of α- and β-cyclodextrins complexation on the physico-chemical properties and antioxidant activity of some 3-hydroxyflavones. *Journal of Pharmaceutical and Biomedical Analysis*, *35*, 365-377.

Caltagirone, S., Ranelletti, F.O., Rinelli, A., Maggiano, N., Colasante, A., Musiani, P., Aiello, F.B., Piantelli, M. (1997). Interaction with type II estrogen binding sites and antiproliferative activity of tamoxifen and quercetin in human non-small-cell lung cancer. *American Journal of Respiratory Cell and Molecular Biology, 17*, 51–59.

Chaabi, M., Freund-Michel, V., Frossard, N., Randriantsoa, A., Andriantsitohaina, R., Lobstein, A. (2007). Anti-proliferative effect of Euphorbia stenoclada in human airway smooth muscle cells in culture. *Journal of Ethnopharmacology*, *109*, 134-139.

Chopra, M., Fitzsimons, P. E. E., Strain, J. J., Thurnham, D. I., Howard, A. N. (2000). Nonalcoholic red wine extract and quercetin inhibit LDL oxidation without affecting plasma antioxidant vitamin and carotenoid concentrations. *Clinical Chemistry, 46,* 1162-1170.

Comalada, M., Camuesco, D., Sierra, S., Ballester, I., Xaus, J., Gálvez, J., Zarzuelo, A. (2005). In vivo quercitrin anti-inflammatory effect involves release of quercetin, which inhibits inflammation through down-regulation of the NF-kappaB pathway. European Journal of Immunology, *35*, 584-592.

Cravotto, G., Binello, A., Baranelli, E., Carraro, P., & Trotta, F. (2006). Cyclodextrins as food additives and in food processing. *Current Nutrition & Food Science, 2*, 343-350.

Cushnie, T.P., Lamb, A.J. (2005). Antimicrobial activity of flavonoids. *International Journal of Antimicrobial Agents, 26*, 343–356.

Davis, J. M., Murphy, E. A., McClellan, J. L., Carmichael, M. D., Gangemi, J. D. (2008). Quercetin reduces susceptibility to influenza infection following stressful exercise. *American Journal of Physiology Regulatory, Integrative and Comparative Physiology, 295*, 505-509.

de Whalley, C.V., Rankin, S.M., Hoult, J.R., Jessup, W., Leake, D.S. (1990). Flavonoids inhibit the oxidative modification of low density lipoproteins by macrophages. *Biochemical Pharmacology, 39*, 1743–1750.

Desai, K. G. H., & Park, H. J. (2005). Recent developments in microencapsulation of food ingredients. *Drying Technology, 23*, 1361-1394.

Dias, A. S., Porawski, M., Alonso, M., Marroni, N., Collado, P. S., González-Gallego, J. (2005). Quercetin decreases oxidative stress, NF-kappaB activation, and iNOS overexpression in liver of streptozotocin-induced diabetic rats. *Journal of Nutrition, 135*, 2299-2304.

Ding, H., Chao, J., Zhang, G., Shuang, S., & Pan, J. (2003). Preparation and spectral investigation on inclusion complex of b-cyclodextrin with rutin. *Spectrochimica Acta Part A: Molecular and Biomolecular Spectroscopy, 59*, 3421-3429.

Erlund, I. (2004). Review of the flavonoids quercetin, hesperetin, and naringenin. Dietary sources, bioactivities, bioavailability, and epidemiology. *Nutrition Research. 24*, 851-874.

Frömming, K. H., & Szejtli, J. (1994). Cyclodextrins in pharmacy. Dordrecht: Kluwer Academic Publishers.

García-Río, L., Hervés, P., Leis, J. R., Mejuto, J. C., Pérez-Juste, J., & Rodríguez- Dafonte, P. (2006). Evidence for complexes of different stoichiometries between organic solvents and cyclodextrins. *Organic & Biomolecular Chemistry, 4*, 1038– 1048.

Gibbs, B.F., Kermasha, S., Alli, I. & Mulligan, C.N. (1999). Encapsulation in the food industry: A review. *International Journal of Food Sciences and Nutrition, 50*, 213-224.

Graf, B. A., Milbury, P. E., Blumberg, J. B. (2005). Flavonols, flavones, flavanones, and human health: epidemiological evidence. *Journal of Medicinal Food, 8*, 281-290.

Gulati, N., Laudet, B., Zohrabian, V.M., Murali, R., Jhanwar-Uniyal, M. (2006). The antiproliferative effect of quercetin in cancer cells is mediated via inhibition of the PI3K-Akt/PKB pathway. *Anticancer Research, 26*, 1177–1181.

Haenen, G.R.M.M., Bast, A. (1999). Nitric oxide radical scavenging of flavonoids. *Methods in Enzymology, 301*, 490–503.

Häkkinen, S.H., Kärenlampi, S.O., Heinonen, I.M., Mykkänen, H.M., Törrönen, A.R. (1999). Content of the flavonols quercetin, myricetin, and kaempferol in 25 edible berries. *Journal of Agricultural Food Chemistry, 47*, 2274-2279.

Hanasaki, Y., Ogawa, S., Fukui, S. (1994). The correlation between active oxygens scavenging and antioxidative effects of flavonoids. *Free Radical Biology & Medicine. 16*, 845–850.

Havsteen, B. H. (2002). The biochemistry and medical significance of the flavonoids. *Pharmacology & Therapeutics, 96*, 67-202.

Hayek, T., Fuhrman, B., Vaya, J., Rosenblat, M., Belinky, P., Coleman, R., Elis, A., Aviram, M. (1997). Reduced progression of atherosclerosis in apolipoprotein E-deficient mice after consumption of red wine, or its polyphenols quercetin or catechin, is associated with reduced susceptibility of LDL to oxidation and aggregation. *Arteriosclerosis, Thrombosis, and Vascular Biology, 17*, 2744-2752.

Hedges, R. A. (1998). Industrial applications of cyclodextrins. *Chemical Reviews, 98*, 2035–2044.

Heijnen, C.G., Haenen, G.R.M.M., van Acker, F.A., van der Vijgh, W.J., Bast, A. (2001). Flavonoids as peroxynitrite scavengers: the role of the hydroxyl groups. *Toxicology in Vitro, 15*, 3–6.

Heijnen, C.G., Haenen, G.R.M.M., Oostveen, R.M., Stalpers, E.M., Bast, A. (2002). Protection of flavonoids against lipid peroxidation: the structure activity relationship revisited. *Free Radical Research, 36*, 575–581.

Hertog, M.G., Kromhout, D., Aravanis, C., Blackburn, H., Buzina, R., Fidanza, F., et al. (1995). Flavonoid intake and longterm risk of coronary heart disease and cancer in the Seven Countries Study. *Archives of Internal Medicine, 155*, 381-386.

Higuchi, T., & Connors, K. A. (1965). Phase solubility techniques. *Advances in Analytical Chemistry and Instrumental, 4,* 56-63.

Hollman, P. C., Katan, M. B. (1997). Absorption, metabolism and health effects of dietary flavonoids in man. *Biomedicine & Pharmacotherapy, 51*, 305–310.

Hotamisligil, G. S. (2006). Inflammation and Metabolic Disorders. *Nature*, *444,* 860-867.

Jung, T. H., Ha, H. J., Ahn, J., & Kwak, H. S. (2008). Development of cholesterol reduced mayonnaise with crosslinked β-cyclodextrin and added phytosterol. Korean *Journal for Food Science of Animal Resources*, *28*, 211–217.

Justino, G.C., Santos, M.R., Canário, S., Borges, C., Florêncio, M.H., Mira, L. (2004). Plasma quercetin metabolites: structure–antioxidant activity relationships. *Archives of Biochemistry and Biophysics, 432*, 109–121.

Juzwiak, S., Wojcicki, J., Mokrzycki, K., Marchlewicz, M., Bialecka, M., Wenda-Rozewicka, L., Gawronska-Szklarz, B., Drozdzik, M. (2005). Effect of quercetin on experimental hyperlipidemia and atherosclerosis in rabbits. *Pharmacological Reports*, *57*, 604-609.

Kato, A., Minoshima, Y., Yamamoto, J., Adachi, I., Watson, A. A., Nash, R. J. (2008). Protective effects of dietary chamomile tea on diabetic complications *Journal of Agricultural Food Chemistry, 56*, 8206-8211.

Kim, S. H., Kim, H. Y., & Kwak, H. S. (2007). Cholesterol removal from lard with crosslinked b-cyclodextrin. Asian-Australasian Journal of Animal Sciences, 20, 1468–1472.

Knekt, P., Isotupa, S., Rissanen, H., Heliövaara, M., Järvinen, R., Häkkinen, S., Aromaa, A., Reunanen, A. (2000). Quercetin intake and the incidence of cerbrovascular disease. *European Journal of Clinical Nutrition*, *54*, 415-417.

Kühnau, J. (1976). The flavonoids. A class of semi-essential food components: their role in human nutrition. *World Review Of Nutrition And Dietetics, 24*, 117-191.

Kuo, S.M. (1996). Antiproliferative potency of structurally distinct dietary flavonoids on human colon cancer cells. *Cancer Letters, 110*, 41–48.

Kwak, H. S., Kim, S. H., Kim, J. H., Choi, H. J., & Kang, J. (2004). Immobilized □-cyclodextrin as a simple and recyclable method for cholesterol removal in milk. Archives of Pharmacology Research, 27, 873–877.

Lee, E.S., Lee, H.E., Shin, J.Y., Yoon, S., Moon, J.O. (2003). The flavonoid quercetin inhibits dimethylnitrosamine-induced liver damage in rats. *Journal of Pharmacy and Pharmacology, 55*, 1169–1174.

Liu, J., Mendoza, S., Román, R., Lynn, M., Xu, R., & Kaifer, A. (1999). Cyclodextrinmodified gold nanospheres. Host–guest interactions at work to control colloidal properties. *Journal of the American Chemical Society, 121*, 4304–4305.

Loftsson, T., Jarho, P., Másson, M. & Järvinen, T. (2005). Cyclodextrins in drug delivery. *Expert Opinion Drug Delivery*, 2, 335-351.

Loftsson, T., Másson, M., & Brewster, M. E. (2004). Self-Association of cyclodextrins and cyclodextrin complexes. *Journal of Pharmaceutical Science*, 93, 1091-1099.

Lubbers, S., Landy, P., & Voilley, A. (1998). Retention and release of aroma compounds in food containing proteins. *Journal of Food Technology*, 52, 68–74.

Lucas-Abellán, C., Fortea, M. I., Gabaldón, J. A., & Núñez-Delicado, E. (2008). Encapsulation of quercetin and myricetin in cyclodextrins at acidic pH. *Journal of Agricultural and Food Chemistry, 56,* 255-259.

Lucas-Abellán, C., Mercader-Ros, M.T., Zafrilla, M.P., Gabaldón J.A., & Núñez-Delicado, E. (2011). Comparative study of different methods to measure antioxidant activity of resveratrol in the presence of cyclodextrins. *Food and Chemical Toxicology, 49,* 1255-1260.

Manjeet, K. R., Ghosh, B. (1999). Quercetin inhibits LPS-induced nitric oxide and tumor necrosis factor-α production in murine macrophages. *International Journal of Immunopharmacology*, *21*, 435–443.

Martín del Valle, E. M. (2004). Cyclodextrins and their uses: a review. *Process Biochemistry, 39*, 1033–1046.

Mercader-Ros, M. T., Lucas-Abellán, C., Fortea, M. I., Gabaldón, J. A., & Núñez Delicado, E. (2010). Effect of HP-β-cyclodextrins complexation on the antioxidant activity of flavonols. *Food Chemistry*, 118, 769-773.

Min, Y. D., Choi, C. H., Bark, H., Son, H. Y., Park, H. H., Lee, S., Park, J. W., Park, E. K., Shin, H. I., Kim, S. H. (2007). Quercetin inhibits expression of inflammatory cytokines through attenuation of NF-κB and p38MAPK in HMC-1 human mast cell line. *Inflammation Research*, *56*, 210-215.

Moon, Y.J., Wang, X., Morris, M.E. (2006). Dietary flavonoids: effects on xenobiotic and carcinogen metabolism. *Toxicology in Vitro, 20*, 187–210.

Neznanov, N., Kondratova, A., Chumakov, K. M., Neznanova, L., Kondratov, R., Banerjee, A. K., Gudkov, A. V. (2008). Quercetinase pirin makes poliovirus replication resistant to flavonoid quercetin. *DNA and Cell Biology*, *27*, 191-198.

Núñez-Delicado, E., Serrano-Mejías, M., Pérez-López, A.J. & López-Nicolás, J.M. (2005). Polyphenol oxidase from Dominga table grape. *Journal of Agricultural and Food Chemistry*, *53*, 6087-6093.

Ono, K., Nakane, H., Fukushima, M., Chermann, J. C., Barré-Sinoussi, F. (1990). Differential inhibitory effects of various flavonoids on the activities of reverse transcriptase and cellular DNA and RNA polymerases. *European Journal of Biochemistry*, *190*, 469-476

Oršolić, N., Horvat, K. A., Šver, L., Terzić, S., Bašić, I. (2004). Immunomodulatory and antimetastatic action of propolis and related polyphenolic compounds. *Journal of Ethnopharmacolog, 94*, 307-315.

Pacifici, G.M. (2004). Inhibition of human liver and duodenum sulfotransferases by drugs and dietary chemicals: a review of the literatureInternational. *Journal of Clinical Pharmacology, Therapy, 42*, 488–495.

Peluso, M. R. (2006). Flavonoids Attenuate Cardiovascular Disease, Inhibit Phosphodiesterase, and Modulate Lipid Homeostasis in Adipose Tissue and Liver. *Experimental Biology and Medicine, 231*, 1287-1299.

Perez-Vizcaino, F., Bishop-Bailley, D., Lodi, F., Duarte, J., Cogolludo, A., Moreno, L., Bosca, L., Mitchell, J.A., Warner, T.D. (2006). The flavonoid quercetin induces apoptosis and inhibits JNK activation in intimal vascular smooth muscle cells. *Biochemical and Biophysical Research Communications, 346,* 919–925.

Piantelli, M., Maggiano, N., Ricci, R., Larocca, L.M., Capelli, A., Scambia, G., Isola, G., Natali, P.G., Ranelletti, F.O. (1995). Tamoxifen and quercetin interact with type II estrogen binding sites and inhibit the growth of human melanoma cells. *Journal of Investigative Dermatology, 105*, 248–253.

Pollard SE, Kuhnle GG, Vauzour D, Vafeiadou K, Tzounis X, Whiteman M, et al. (2006). The reaction of flavonoid metabolites with peroxynitrite. *Biochemical and Biophysical Research Communications, 350*, 960–968.

Procházková, D., Boušová, I., Wilhelmová, N. (2011). Antioxidant and prooxidant properties of flavonoids. *Fitoterapia, 82*, 513-523.

Rivera, L., Moron, R., Sanchez, M., Zarzuelo, A., Galisteo, M. (2008). Quercetin ameliorates metabolic syndrome and improves the inflammatory status in obese zucker rats. *Obesity, 16*, 2081-2087.

Rogerio, A. P., Kanashiro, A., Fontanari, C., da Silva, E. V. G., Lucisano-Valim, Y. M., Soares, E. G., Faccioli, L. H. (2007). Anti-inflammatory activity of quercetin and isoquercitrin in experimental murine allergic asthma. *Inflammation Research, 56*, 402-408.

Romero, M., Jiménez, R., Sánchez, M., López-Sepúlveda, R., Zarzuelo, M. J., O'Valle, F., Zarzuelo, A., Pérez-Vizcaíno, F., Duarte, J. (2009). Quercetin inhibits vascular superoxide production induced by endothelin-1: Role of NADPH oxidase, uncoupled eNOS and PKC. *Atherosclerosis, 202*, 58-67

Ross, J.A. and Kasum, C.M. (2002). Dietary flavonoids: bioavailability, metabolic effects, and safety. *Annual Reviews Nutrition, 22*, 19-34.

Sampson, L., Rimm, E., Hollman, P.C., de Vries, J.H., Katan, M.B. (2002). Flavonol and flavone intakes in US health professionals. *Journal of the American Dietetic Association, 102*, 1414- 1420.

Santos, M.R., Rodríguez-Goméz, M.J., Justino, G.C., Charro, N., Florencio, M.H., Miral, L. (2008). Influence of themetabolic profile on the in vivo antioxidant activity of quercetin under a low dosage oral regimen in rats. *British Journal of Pharmacology, 153*, 1750–1761.

Scalbert, A., Manach, C., Morand, C., Rémésy, C., & Jiménez, L. (2005). Dietary polyphenols and the prevention of diseases. *Critical Reviews in Food Science and Nutrition, 45*, 287-306.

Schlachterman, A., Valle, F., Wall, K. M., Azios, N. G., Castillo, L., Morell, L., Washington, A. V., Cubano, L. A., Dharmawardhane, S. F. (2008). Combined resveratrol, quercetin, and catechin treatment reduces breast tumor growth in a nude mouse model. *Translational Oncology, 1*, 19-27.

Schwarz, D., Kisselev, P., Roots, I. (2005). CYP1A1 genotype-selective inhibition of benzo [a]pyrene activation by quercetin. *European Journal of Cancer, 41*, 151–158.

Seyoum, A., Asres, K. & Kandeel El-Fiky, F. (2006). Structure-radical scavenging activity relationships of flavonoids. *Phytochemistry, 67*, 2058-2070.

Shahidi, F., & Han, X. Q. (1993). Encapsulation of food ingredients. *Critical Reviews in Food Science and Nutrition, 33*, 501-547.

Shim, S. Y., Ahn, J., & Kwak, H. S. (2003). Functional properties of cholesterol removed whipping cream treated by β-cyclodextrin. *Journal of Dairy Science, 86*, 2767–2772.

Shoskes, D. A. (1998). Effect of bioflavonoids quercetin and curcumin on ischemic renal injury: a new class of renoprotective agents. *Transplantation, 66*, 147-152.

Shutenko, Z., Henry, Y., Pinard, E., Seylaz, J., Potier, P., Berthet, F., Girard, P., Sercombe, R. (1999). Influence of the antioxidant quercetin in vivo on the level of nitric oxide determined by electron paramagnetic resonance in rat brain during global ischemia and reperfusion. *Biochemical Pharmacology, 57*, 199-208.

Singh, M., Arseneault, M., Sanderson, T., Murthy, V., Ramassamy, C. (2008). Challenges for research on polyphenols from foods in Alzheimer's disease: bioavailability, metabolism, and cellular and molecular mechanisms. *Journal of Agricultural and Food Chemistry', 56*, 4855–4873.

Singh, M., Sharma, R., & Banerjee, U. C. (2002). Biotechnological applications of cyclodextrins. *Biotechnology Advances*, 20, 341–359.

Szejtli, J. (1997). Utilization of cyclodextrins in industrial products and processes. *Journal of Materials Chemistry*, 7, 575–587.

Szente, L., Mikuni, K., Hasimoto, H., & Szejtli, J. (1998). Stabilization and solubilization of lipophilic natural colorants with cyclodextrins. *Journal of Inclusion Phenomena and Molecular Recognition in Chemistry,* 32, 81–89.

Terao J. (1999). Dietary flavonoids as antioxidants in vivo: conjugated metabolites of (−)-epicatechin and quercetin participate in antioxidative defence in blood plasma. *Journal of Investigative Medicine, 46*, 159–168.

Theoharides, T. C., Alexandrakis, M., Kempura, J. D., Lytinas, M. (2001). Anti-inflammatory actions of flavonoids and structural requirements for new design. *International Journal of Immunopharmacology, 14*, 119–127.

Tomás-Barberán, F. A., Espín, J. C. (2001). Phenolic compounds and related enzyme as determinants of quality in fruits and vegetables. *Journal of Agricultural and Food Chemistry, 81*, 853-876.

USDA http://www.ars.usda.gov/SP2UserFiles/Place/12354500/Data/Flav/Flav02-1.pdf.

van Acker, S.A., Tromp, M.N., Haenen, G.R.M.M., van der Vijgh, W.J., Bast, A. (1995). Flavonoids as scavengers of nitric oxide radical. *Biochemical and Biophysical Research Communications, 214*, 755–759.

van der Woude, H., Ter Veld, M. G., Jacobs, N., van der Saag, P. T., Murk, A. J., Rietjens, I. M. (2005). The stimulation of cell proliferation by quercetin is mediated by the estrogen receptor. *Molecular Nutrition & Food Research, 49*, 763-771.

Walle, T., Eaton, E.A., Walle, U.K., 1995. Quercetin, a potent and specific inhibitor of the human P-form phenosulfotransferase. *Biochemical Pharmacology, 50*, 731–734.

Williams, C.A., Harborne, J.B. (1994). The Flavonoids. Advances in research since 1986. In: Harborne, J.B., editor: Chapman & Hall. London. pp 337-385.

Wood, W. E. (2001). Improved aroma barrier properties in food packaging with cyclodextrins. TAPPI – Polymers, Laminations and Coatings Conference 367–377.

Yamashita, N., Kawanishi, S. (2000) Distinct mechanisms of DNA damage in apoptosis induced by quercetin and luteolin. *Free Radical Research*, *33*, 623-633.

Zang, M., Xu, S., Maitland-Toolan, K. A., Zuccollo, A., Hou, X., Jiang, B., Wierzbicki, M., Verbeuren, T. J., Cohen, R. A. (2006). Polyphenols stimulate AMP-activated protein Kinase, lower lipids, and inhibit accelerated atherogenesis in diabetic LDL receptor-deficient mice. *Diabetes*, *55*, 2180-2191.

Zeng, L. H., Wu, J., Fung, B., Tong, J. H., Mickle, D., Wu, T. W. (1997). Comparative protection *Biochemistry and Cell Biology*, *75*, 717-20.

In: Quercetin
Editors: Taiki Chikamatsu and Yuudai Hida
ISBN: 978-1 61942- 057-1

Chapter 8

QUERCETIN: DIETARY SOURCES, FUNCTIONS AND HEALTH BENEFITS

Qing-Yu Zhang and Ling-Dong Kong*
State Key Laboratory of Pharmaceutical Biotechnology, School of Life Sciences, Nanjing University, Nanjing, P. R. China

ABSTRACT

Quercetin (3, 3', 4', 5, 7-pentahydroxylflavone) is a typical flavonoid presented in various fruits and vegetables. More evidences have demonstrated that quercetin exhibits anti-oxidation, anti-cancer, anti-inflammation, anti-atherosclerosis, anti-bacteria, anti-virus, anti-diabetes, anti-aging, anti-hyperuricemia and so on. Quercetin is suggested to be a candidate for preventing various body disorders such as osteoporosis, certain forms of cancer, obesity-related disorder, pulmonary and cardiovascular diseases, neurodegenerative diseases, hyperuricemia and diabetes. Therefore, we reviewed the researching achievements of quercetin principally including its dietary sources, bioavailability and functions to health promotion and disease prevention as well as the related basic molecular mechanisms. Other aspects such as the metabolism of quercetin were covered briefly.

Keywords: Quercetin, dietary source, function, health benefit

ABBREVIATION

ROS: Reactive oxygen species;
RNS: reactive nitrogen species;
LDL: Low density lipoprotein;
LPS: Lipopolysaccharide;

* Address Correspondence to: Ling-Dong Kong, MD, State Key Laboratory of Pharmaceutical Biotechnology, Nanjing University, Nanjing, 210093, P. R. China. Tel/Fax: +86-25-8359-4691; E-mail address: kongld@nju.edu.cn.

XDH: xanthine dehydrogenase;
XOD: Xanthine oxidase;
TNF-α: Tumor necrosis factor alpha;
ERK: extracellular signal-regulated kinase;
MDR: multidrug resistance;
ER: estrogen receptor;
P-gp: P-glycoprotein.

INTRODUCTION

Quercetin (3, 3’, 4’, 5, 7-pentahydroxylflavone, Figure 1) belongs to an extensive class of polyphenolic flavonoid compounds almost ubiquitous in plant food sources [1]. Quercetin consists of three rings, 2 benzene rings (A and B) which are connected by an oxygen-containing pyrene ring (C). The three rings are planar and the molecule is relatively polarized. Three intermolecular hydrogen bonds are observed: two with the carbonyl group and the other between the hydroxyl groups in ring B. Thus, quercetin occurs mainly in leaves and the other parts of the plants as aglycones and glycosides, in which one or more sugar groups is bound to phenolic groups by β-glycosidic bond. Almost 180 different glycosides of quercetin have been described in nature, with rutin (quercetin-3-O-rutinoside) being one of the most common [2]. The water-solubility of quercetin increases with increasing number of sugar groups [3]. In addition, bioavailability of quercetin depends on its metabolic form. Quercetin exhibits a vary of bioactivities, such as anti-oxidation, anti-cancer, anti-inflammation, anti-atherosclerosis, anti-bacteria, anti-virus, anti-diabetes, anti-aging, anti-diarrhea, anti-hyperuricemia. Quercetin may have beneficial effects on many diseases, such as cancers, inflammation, cardiovascular diseases, hypertension, diabetes, gout, osteoporosis, neurodegenerative diseases. Therefore, we reviewed the researching achievements of quercetin principally including its dietary sources, bioavailability and functions to health promotion and disease prevention as well as the related basic molecular mechanisms. Other aspects such as the absorption of quercetin were covered briefly.

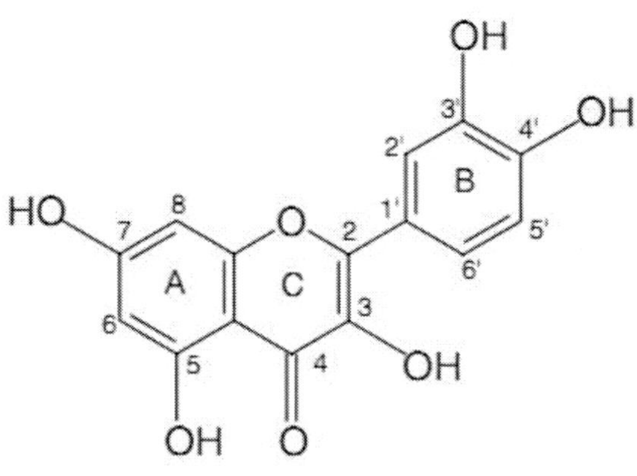

Figure 1. Chemical structure of quercetin.

Dietary Sources

Quercetin occur ubiquitously in human diet, with wide distribution in the edible portions of food plants, including oak tree, capers, red grapes, apples, onions, tea, citrus fruits, lovage, broccoli, other leafy green vegetables, cherries and many species of berries such as cranberries, blueberries etc [4]. Fruits and vegetables, particularly apples, cranberries, blueberries and onions, are the primary sources of naturally-occurring dietary quercetin [5]. Many food products, like black tea, red wine and various fruit juice, also are identified as rich dietary sources of quercetin [6-7].

Absorption of Quercetin

It is well known that diet is the primary source of quercetin for humans. Most quercetin present in food plants as hydrophilic glycosides are not easily absorbed directly because they are bound to sugars as glycosides[8]. Only free quercetin without a sugar molecule, the so-called aglycones, is considered to be able to pass through the gut wall [9]. The fate of dietary form of quercetin mainly quercetin glycosides in the major compartments of the gastro-intestinal tract is as follows. The β-glycosidic bond that link the aglycone and sugar groups together can be split up by the intestinal microflora[10]. Studies with human ileostomy volunteers show that quercetin aglycone is absorbed with different efficiencies, depending on quercetin source, *e.g.*, the absorption of quercetin aglycone is approximately 52 % from fried onions (containing mainly quercetin-4′-glucoside and quercetin-3, 4-diglucoside), 17% from rutin (quercetin-3-O-rhamnoglucoside) and 24% from quercetin aglycone [11]. The small intestine is the site of various mechanisms that allow the absorption of quercetin either as its aglycone or bound to a certain types of sugar groups. Some studies have confirmed that the absorption of quercetin is considerably enhanced by its conjugation with a sugar group [12-13]. The intestinal absorption of quercetin and its glycosides is believed to have two different mechanisms. First way is that lactase phlorizin hydrolase, which is bound to intestinal lumen for the hydrolysis of lactose, is capable of hydrolyzing quercetin glucosides effectively [14]. Second route of quercetin glycoside absorption appears to involve sodium dependent glucose transporter-1, which is responsible for the effective transport of quercetin glucosides from intestinal epithelial cells [15]. After uptake of quercetin glucosides into the enterocyte by interaction with glucose transporter-1, the glucoside is hydrolysed by intracellular cytosolic β-glucosidase activity. To date, lactase phlorizin hydrolase and glucose transporter-1 are generally recognized as important contributors to the absorption of quercetin glucosides. Most common routes of quercetin's metabolism in intestinal tract are oxidation, reduction and hydrolysis followed by conjugation. Furthermore, after absorbed by the intestinal epithelium, quercetin leaves the enterocytes as aglycone and undergoes metabolism once it enters the blood stream. In this compartment, quercetin is subject to O-methylation, glucuronidation, and/or sulfation and then bound to transport proteins [16-17].

On the other hand, quercetin glycosides that are not processed and absorbed by the small intestines are believed to be transported from the colon. The colonic microflora expresses considerable α, L-rhamnosidase and β, D-glucosidase activity, allowing efficient deglycosylation of quercetin glycosides [18]. In addition to deglycosylation reactions, the microflora present in the colon is also capable of other metabolic reactions including fission of A- and B-ring of quercetin, leading to the formation of lower molecular weight phenolics, such as phloroglucinol, 3, 4-dihydroxyphenylacetic acid and 3-methyl-4-hydroxybenzoic acid [19]. Presence of microflora with β, D-glucuronidase activity makes quercetin glucuronides excreted via the bile to get deglucuronidated, thereby liberating the aglycone and providing possibility for enterohepatic cycling. In the colon, both aglycone and degradation products of quercetin are either absorbed into the blood stream or excreted via feces. After absorption by the cells of the colon, quercetin and its degradation products may get glucuronidated, to a smaller extent, they are methylated by catechol-O-methyltransferase and uridine 5'-diphosphoglucuronosyltransferase activities present in the colonic mucosa.

FUNCTIONS

Anti-Oxidative Capacity

The best described property of quercetin is its ability to act as antioxidant. Quercetin seems to be the most powerful flavonoids for protecting the body against reactive oxygen species (ROS), including superoxide and reactive nitrogen species (RNS) such as nitric oxide is produced during the normal oxygen metabolism or induced by exogenous damage [20]. ROS generated *in vivo*, is powerful oxidizing agent, capable of damaging DNA, protein and other biomolecules to contribute to aging and several other degenerative processes such as cataracts, heart disease and cancer [21]. Human body comprises an elaborate antioxidant defense system to protect cellular compounds from damage induced by ROS, free radicals and other reactive species. Enzymatic antioxidants react with reactive species and are subsequently efficiently recycled. In fact, the enzyme functions as a catalyst. Consequently, only small amounts of these enzymes are needed to offer protection. Important antioxidant enzymes are superoxide dismutase (SOD), catalase (CAT) and glutathione peroxidase (GPx) [22]. Non-enzymatic antioxidants are represented by radical scavenging antioxidants such as vitamin C, vitamin A and plant phytochemicals including quercetin that inhibit the oxidation chain initiation and prevent chain propagation [23].

Quercetin acts as a free radical scavenger and prevents free radical-induced tissue injury directly or indirectly [24]. By scavenging free radicals, quercetin can inhibit low density lipoprotein (LDL) oxidation *in vitro*. This action can help protecting against atherosclerosis [25]. Quercetin also interferes with inducible nitric oxide synthase activity, resulting in a reduction in experimental ischemia–reperfusion injury and generation of damaging peroxynitrite from nitric oxide superoxide anions [26-27]. XOD is a main enzyme that is involved in the catalysis of oxidation of hypoxanthine to xanthine and finally xanthine to uric acid [28]. Quercetin interferes xanthine dehydrogenase/ xanthine oxidase (XDH/XOD) system to decrease oxidative injury occurring after ischemia or oxidative stress [28], indicating that quercetin may lower uric acid levels in hyperuricemia [29]. Moreover, quercetin substantially empower endogenous antioxidant shield due to its contribution to the total plasma antioxidant capacity which is 6.24 times higher than the reference antioxidant trolox [30]. The anti-oxidative capacity of quercetin is attributed to the presence of two antioxidant pharmacophores within its molecule that has the optimal configuration for free radical scavenging, e.g. the catechol group in B ring and OH group at position 3 of A and C ring [31].

Anti-Inflammatory Activity

Tumor necrosis factor alpha (TNF-α) is a typical pro-inflammatory cytokine involved in the pathogenesis of chronic inflammatory diseases [32]. It also enhances the transcription of other cytokines, chemokines, or inflammatory mediators. More evidence has demonstrated that quercetin suppress TNF-α production. Quercetin inhibits lipopolysaccharide-induced TNF-α production in macrophages [33]. Another explanation for its anti-inflammatory effects may be found in the interplay between oxidative stress and inflammation. ROS are not only important in the occurrence of oxidative stress, but also in the promotion of inflammatory processes via activation of transcription factors such as NF-κB and activator protein (AP)-1 which induce the production of cytokines like TNF-α [34]. Consequently, scavenging ROS would not only prevent the occurrence of oxidative stress but also help mitigate inflammation [35]. Indeed, study has been shown that quercetin can inhibit NF-κB activation, thereby directly reducing TNF-α production via this transcription factor [36]. Obesity is linked to chronic inflammation in white adipose tissue, which is exacerbated by infiltrating macrophages. Recent study demonstrates that grape powder extract, which is abundant in quercetin, reduces inflammation in human macrophages and prevents macrophage-mediated inflammation and insulin resistance in human adipocytes [37]. These observations indicate that quercetin has the ability to reduce chronic inflammation, and then relieve chronic inflammation-related diseases like diabetes and obesity.

Furthermore, in a Japanese study of mast cells from nasal mucosa of individuals with perennial allergic rhinitis, quercetin is confirmed to significantly inhibit antigen-stimulated histamine release [38]. Anti-inflammatory action of quercetin is also demonstrated on an experimental model of inflammation induced by histamine and serotonin [39], indicating that quercetin may help in preventing allergy and its related asthma attacks.

Anti-Cancer Effect

Carcinogenicity mainly relies on the cell's ability to proliferate abnormally, evade apoptosis, induce angiogenesis and metastasize to distant sites [40]. Quercetin has anti-proliferative effect on a variety of cancer cells, like breast adenocarcinoma, colon adenocarcinoma, chronic myelogenous leukemia and so on [41]. Several mechanisms for its anti-proliferative action have been proposed, such as the induction of DNA strand breakage, cell cycle arrest, and/or apoptosis [42]. For example, quercetin trigger DNA fragmentation, cleavage of poly polymerase, up-regulation of Bax and posttranslational modification of anti-apoptotic Bcl-2 in HL60 human leukemia cells [43]. Another study has proved that quercetin induces apoptotic cell death in HepG2 human hepatoma cells through the mitochondrial pathway and cell survival blockade sustained inhibition of the major survival signals, Akt and extracellular signal-regulated kinase (ERK) [44].

Tumor suppressor gene p53 plays an important role in regulating cellular response to exogenous and endogenous stress. Depending on the cell types and the nature of stress, p53 may cause cell cycle arrest or trigger apoptosis [45].

The inhibition of p53 expression by quercetin is found to arrest the cells in the G2-M phase of the cell cycle [46]. Furthermore, quercetin can prevent the accumulation of newly synthesized mutated forms of p53 protein in human breast cancer cell line MDA-MB468 [47]. The G1 checkpoint controlled by p53 gene is a major site for the control of cellular proliferation. Quercetin is demonstrated to arrest human leukemic T-cells in the late G1 phase of the cell cycle [48], possibly resulting in proliferation suppression.

Tyrosine kinase expression is involved in oncogenesis via an ability to override normal regulatory growth control [49]. In patients with the advanced cancers, intravenous administration of quercetin exhibits inhibition of lymphocyte tyrosine kinase activity in nine of eleven cases. Quercetin is the first natural compound with tyrosine kinase inhibitory activity tested in human phase I trial [50].

Estrogen receptor (ER) is a member of the super family of nuclear hormone receptors. The ratio ERα/ERβ is higher in breast tumors than in normal tissue. ERβ modulates ERα transcriptional activity, ERα may mediate the proliferative effects of estrogenic compounds, whereas, ERβ may have inhibitory action on this process [51-52]. The stimulation of cancer cell proliferation is dependent on ER, and appears to occur at the ER level that is physiologically relevant in humans [53]. Quercetin has been shown to induce ERβ expression in both type α estrogen receptor positive (ER+) and type α estrogen receptor negative (ER-) human breast cancer cells. The induction of ERβ allows for greater growth inhibition of ER- cells with quercetin treatment [54].

Quercetin can reverse multidrug resistance of the tumor cell. P-glycoprotein (P-gp), a glycoprotein encoded by human multidrug resistance 1 (MDR1) gene, is one of the best characterized multidrug efflux pumps. Earlier study demonstrates that quercetin interacts with the purified P-gp and efficiently inhibits its activity [55]. Quercetin is capable of decreasing P-gp expression in human cervical carcinoma KB-V1 cells [56]. Taken together, quercetin is an attractive natural compound for cancer prevention.

Antimicrobial Effect

Quercetin seems to exert antibacterial activity against almost all of bacteria strains known to cause respiratory, gastrointestinal, skin and urinary disorders [57]. Mechanism of quercetin's antiviral activity is related with its ability to bind with viral proteins whereby it interferes with the viral nucleic acid synthesis. For instance, methyl-quercetin is found to suppress polio virus replication by interfering with single strand RNA replicative intermediate in association with block of cellular protein synthesis both in infected cells and in cell-free systems [58].

Additionally, quercetin reduces susceptibility to influenza infection, in particular, following stressful exercise [59]. These health claims are supported by *in vitro* evidences associated with the ability of quercetin with strong antioxidant activity to modulate the activity of numerous enzymes involved in signal transduction, cell growth, and biotransformation [42].

Anti-Hypertension and Anti-Dyslipidemia Effect

Excessive production of ROS is a mark of hypertension. This is due, in large part, to excess production of oxidants, resulting in the decreased nitric oxide bioavailability and decreased antioxidant capacity in vasculature and kidney [60]. In fact, it has been suggested that oxidative stress is a pathogenetic factor in the development of essential hypertension [61]. More studies have demonstrated in animals and humans that antioxidants such as quercetin exhibit the anti-hypertension actions. For example, quercetin lowers blood pressure observed in the spontaneously hypertensive rat model [62]. It is well known that a major source for vascular and renal ROS is a family of nonphagocytic nicotinamide adenine dinucleotide phosphate (NADPH) oxidases [60]. Quercetin is proved to downregulate NADPH oxidase in spontaneously hypertensive rats [63]. Direct renal effects of quercetin may play some role in its anti-hypertension [62]. For instance, the downregulation of epithelial Na^+ channel in the kidney is suggested to contribute to blood pressure lowering effect in Dahl salt-sensitive hypertension[64].

Dyslipidemia, a strong predictor of cardiovascular disease, predict incident hypertension [65]. Quercetin has anti-dyslipidemia effect. The combined treatment with quercetin and α-tocopherol reduce the plasma levels of cholesterol, free fatty acids (FFA), very low density lipoprotein (VLDL) and LDL in cadmium-treated rats [66]. Chronic dietary intake of quercetin improves dyslipidemia in C56BL/6J mice with consumption of a Western-style diet [67] or in obese Zucker rats [68].

Leptin, the product of the ob gene, is a cytokine produced by adipose tissue and secreted into circulation. Leptin plays a critical role in body weight regulation by suppressing food intake and increasing energy expenditure [69]. The dysfunction of leptin can increase adiposity, dyslipidemia and insulin resistance [70]. More studies demonstrate that quecetin can regulate leptin secretion. For example, quercetin recovere fructose-induced alterations in serum TG, HDL and LDL in rats by improving hyperuricemia and hyperinsulinemia to normalize leptin secretion from adipose tissue [71].

Kidney Protection

Oxidative stress can promote the formation of a variety of vasoactive mediators that affect renal functions directly by causing renal vasoconstriction or decreasing the glomerular capillary ultrafiltration coefficient, and thus reducing the glomerular filtration rate [72]. Over burden of ROS can develop renal diseases. Because of anti-oxidative capacity of quercetin, it may play an important role in renal protection. Interstitial inflammation and tubular damage, is one of the earliest manifestations of nephropathy [73]. Pretreatment with quercetin preserves renal tubular damage and interstitial inflammation in ischemia-reperfusion rats [74]. In addition, quercetin reduces immune and nonimmune renal injury [75] and has protective effect against cadmium or glycerol-induced renal dysfunction [76] in rats.

Hyperuricemia may be a risk factor for renal dysfunction. In fact, kidney function depends on specific organic ion transporter molecule. The organic anion transporters OAT1 and OAT3 are responsible for the uptake of organic anions such as uric acid from the blood across the basolateral membrane into proximal tubule cells, which are recognized as the first step of renal organic anion secretion. The electrogenic urate transporter (UAT) is also involved in uric acid secretion across the luminal membrane in the kidney. The organic cation transporters OCT1 and OCT2 at the basolateral membrane of proximal renal tubules cooperate with each other in renal excretion of organic cations, mediating the first step during secretion of organic cations in proximal tubules. OAT1 and OAT3 take up anion toxic from the blood into the proximal tubular cells and significantly contribute to nephrotoxicity. Our previous studies showed that dysregulation of renal rOAT1, rUAT, rOCT1 and rOCT2 may be contributed to fructose-induced hyperuricemia and renal dysfunction in rats [77]. Moreover, the reduced endothelial NO levels possibly cause endothelial dysfunction, and then renal dysfunction. Quercetin can restore dysregulation of these organic ion transporters and make NO elevation in the kidney of fructose-fed rats, resulting in reduction of hyperuricemia and alleviation of renal dysfunction [77]. In addition, quercetin reduces serum creatinine and blood urea nitrogen concentrations in ischemia-reperfusion-induced renal injury of rats and decreased plasma creatinine levels in cadmium-induced nephrotoxicity, thus relieving renal injury [77]. These observations further demonstrate nephroprotection of quercetin[78].

Health Benefits

Various Cancers

Results of some, but not all, *in vivo* and *in vitro* laboratory studies, clinical trials and human epidemiological investigations suggest that quercetin may protect against various cancers. Quercetin inhibits the growth of MCF-7 human breast adenocarcinoma, HT-29 human colon adenocarcinoma and K562 human chronic myelogenous leukemia cell lines [79]. It has also been shown to inhibit carcinogen-induced mammary, colonic, oral and lung neoplasia in rodents and DNA adducts in human hepatoma cells [80]. Quercetin seems to be a strong anti-proliferative agent against colorectal, ovarian, lymphoid and breast cancer.

Although the etiology of cancer may be multifactorial (*e.g.* diet, genetic, environment), there is wide recognition that ROS/RNS play an important role in the pathophysiological process. ROS/RNS have been shown to be carcinogenic and may exert their deleterious effects by causing DNA damage, altering cell signaling pathways and gene expression. Quercetin with anti-oxidant property prevents DNA damage-induced ROS, leading to mutational changes. Furthermore, quercetin inhibits angiogenesis [81]. Angiogenesis is normally a strictly controlled process in human body. Pathological, unregulated angiogenesis occurs in cancers [82]. Among the angiogenesis inhibitors, quercetin appears to be important compound. However, the mechanism behind its anti-angiogenic effect is unclear. A possible mechanism could be the inhibition of protein kinase. Quercetin is confirmed to be effective in inhibiting radiation-induced protein kinase C (PKC) activity. Activation of PKC is one of the means of conferring radioresistance on tumor cells. Suppression of PKC activity by quercetin may prevent the development of radioresistance following radiotherapy.

A number of phase I clinical trials have been performed with quercetin pharmacokinetics and evidence for tyrosine kinase inhibition [50] and adenoma regression [83]. A combination of quercetin and curcumin is found to regress the adenomas in patients with familialadenomatous polyposis, an autosomal-dominant disorder characterized by the development of colorectal adenomas and eventual colorectal cancer [83].

Inflammatory Diseases

For quercetin shows anti-inflammatory action with inhibition of the production and release of histamine and other allergic/inflammatory substances, it is suggested to be useful in the treatment of some allergies and inflammation-related diseases. Results from clinical trials show that quercetin acts rapidly within a few days to ease swelling of the inflamed joints and banish pain. In addition, patients with rheumatoid arthritis experience an improvement in their symptoms, when they switch from a typical western diet to a vegan diet with lots of uncooked berries, fruits and vegetables containing amongst antioxidants, quercetin [84]. Other clinical study demonstrates that supplement of a high dose of quercetin (4×500 mg orally within 24 h) over a 24 h-period can reduce biomarkers of oxidative stress and inflammation in sarcoidosis [85]. These observations suggest that quercetin has enormous benefit to those suffering from arthritis and sarcoidosis.

Cardiovascular Diseases and Hypertension

Oxidative damage is a common underlying mechanism in the progression of a large number of disorders such as coronary heart disease, stroke and atherosclerosis [86]. Epidemiological data have demonstrated an association between quercetin rich diet and significant reduction of mortality risk for coronary heart disease and stroke [87-88]. Oxidative modification of LDL is believed to be an initial step for foam cell formation leading to cardiovascular diseases and atherosclerosis [89]. Moreover, proliferation of vascular smooth muscles is a characteristic feature of atherosclerosis and ROS can cause growth of vascular smooth muscle cells. Therefore, the excellent scavenger of ROS, antioxidant quercetin, is strongly considered to act as an effective anti-atherosclerotic agent. Platelet aggregation contributes to both the development of atherosclerosis and acute platelet thrombus formation. The activated platelets adhering to vascular endothelium generate lipid peroxides and oxygen free radicals, which suppress endothelial formation of prostacyclin and nitrous oxide. Interestingly, quercetin directly scavenges free radicals, thereby maintaining proper concentrations of endothelial prostacyclin and nitric oxide [90].

On the other hand, high blood pressure is known to cause abnormal growth and remodeling of the heart, a cardiac hypertrophy. Clinical study demonstrates that daily supplementation with 730 mg quercetin for 28 d can reduce systolic, diastolic and mean arterial pressure in patients with stage 1 hypertension [91].

Diabetes

Diabetes is one of the most common endocrine metabolic disorders. Specific microvascular disease in diabetes is a leading cause of blindness, renal failure and nerve damage. Diabetes-accelerated atherosclerosis causes the elevated risk of myocardial infarction, stroke and limb amputation. Normal secretion of insulin by pancreatic β cells can control serum glucose level, reduce the risk of diabetes. Quercetin promotes glucose- and glibenclamide-induced insulin secretion and protects pancreatic β cells against oxidative damage through ERK1/2 pathway in rats [92]. It also enhances glucose metabolism through activation of both silent mating type information regulation 2 homolog 1 (SIRT1) and AMPK in HepG2 cells [93]. On the other hand, diabetes is usually associated with inflammation. Chronic subclinical inflammation may aggravate insulin resistance, a situation of increased risk for developing diabetes [94]. Quercetin has anti-inflammatory effects, which further suggest that quercetin has benefit to diabetes.

Anti-Aging

Compounds with strong antioxidative activity are considered as anti-aging agents. Quercetin has already been shown to exert protective effects on ageing of specific tissues and functions in cellular and animal models. For example, upon supplementation with quercetin, the enhancement of exploratory behavior, spatial learning and memory has been revealed in aged mice [95].

Proteasome is the major cellular non-lysosomal threonine protease, implicating in the removal of normal as well as abnormal, denatured or otherwise damaged proteins [96]. More studies have reported loss of proteasome function upon ageing of several human tissues and senescent primary cultures. Quercetin is confirmed to be a potent proteasome activator with anti-oxidant property that consequently influences cellular lifespan, survival and viability [97]. The rejuvenating effect of quercetin on middle-aged and terminally senescent primary fibroblasts is also demonstrated [97]. These observations suggest that quercetin may have anti-aging effect. Therefore, proteasome may be related to the function of anti-oxidant quercetin upon senescence [98].

Hyperuricemia

Hyperuricemia is the most important risk factor for the development of gout and has been linked to renal dysfunction, cardiovascular diseases, hypertension, hyperlipidemia, cancer and diabetes. Hyperuricemia occurs as a result of increased uric acid production, impair renal uric acid excretion, or combination of both mechanisms [99]. Controlling of hyperuricemia is mainly achieved by reducing uric acid production with an inhibitor of XOD, main enzyme that is involved in the catalysis of oxidation of hypoxanthine to xanthine and finally xanthine to uric acid during uric acid synthesis [100]. Quercetin has a C_2–C_3 double bond with hydroxyl groups at position 3, 5, and 7 possess hypouricemic activity as a result of their ability to reduce serum urate levels by inhibiting XOD [101]. Furthermore, our previous studies showed that quercetin can reduce serum urate level through regulation of renal urate transport-related proteins [102]. This indicate that querctin have benefit effect on hyperuricemia and its related disorders.

Neurodegenerative Diseases

Neurodegenerative diseases such as Alzheimer's (AD) and Parkinson's (PD) diseases are defined by a progressive neuronal dysfunction and an ensuing behavioral dysfunction.

Although protein aggregation (*i.e.* β-amyloid and α-synuclein) plays a pivotal role in both AD and PD, there is increasing evidence that excessive accumulation of ROS that occurs during normal and pathological brain aging contributes to neuronal losses and dysfunction [103-104]. Quercetin has been attributed with many physiological benefits including the prevention of neurodegenerative diseases due to its antioxidant and free radical scavenging properties in subjects [103-104].

Osteoporosis

Quercetin has the stimulatory effect on alkaline phosphatase activity and rapidly activates ERKs in osteoblasts by the ER-dependent pathway [105]. This indicates that quercetin can stimulate osteoblastic activity, show anti-osteoporosis effect.

The elder women, who drank tea containing quercetin have higher bone mineral density than those who did not drink tea [106]. Therefore, quercetin in the tea may be responsible for the prevention of osteoporosis.

Toxicity and Incompatibility

A single oral dose of up to 4 g of quercetin is not associated with side-effects in human. Single intravenous bolus doses of 100 mg are apparently well tolerated as well [107]. It has been well described that oxidation products like semiquinone radicals and quinones display various toxic effects due to their abilities of arylating protein thiols [108-109], thus, quercetin with anti-oxidative activity, becomes oxidized into various oxidation products.

Quercetin has also been reported to display genotoxic effects *in vitro*. However, these mutagenic effects are predominantly shown in bacteria and suggested to require quinine formation as mediators as well [110-111]. Quercetin is consistently tested positive for mutagenic activity in most standard strains of *Salmonella typhimurium* [112-113] and reverse mutations, and DNA single strand breaks in *Escherichia coli* [114]. Additionally, quercetin induces chromosomal aberrations, DNA single strand breaks and micronucleus formation in hamster and mouse cells and human lymphocytes [115]. Mutagenic activity of quercetin is dependent on the presence of an ortho-3′, 4′-dihydroxygroup in B-ring allowing the formation of quinone-type metabolites. When this catechol group is present in the parent molecule, the compound is mutagenic even without metabolic activation [116]. In contrast to mammalian cells, the presence of C_7-OH group is not a prerequisite for genotoxic effects of quercetin in bacterial test systems [117]. Of note, quercetin displays genotoxic effects in bacteria [118]. However, the significance of this finding for humans is not clear. The results of quercetin-related mutagenicity observed *in vitro* have not been confirmed by *in vivo* experiments. Taken together, it is suggested that quercetin should be avoided by pregnant women and nursing mothers. More research is required to explain the discrepancy observed between the *in vitro* and *in vivo* quercetin genotoxicity studies in order to further elucidate the possible genotoxic effects of quercetin for man.

Therapeutic Dosages

To quercetin, therapeutic dosages can range from 250 to 500 mg three times per day. Quercetin is available in the form of capsules (250, 300 and 500 mg) and tablets (50, 250 and 500 mg). The recommended adult dosages of quercetin vary depending on the health condition being treated. For allergic condition, 250-600 mg quercetin per day in the divided doses or for chronic hives, 200-400 mg quercetin thrice daily is recommended, respectively [119]. Study with ^{14}C-labeled quercetin aglycone administered orally to normal, healthy volunteers confirm that oral absorption is high, ranging from 36 to 53 %, and biological half-life is as long as 20–72 h [120]. In addition, quercetin is found to interact with various drugs. For example, quercetin significantly affects the pharmacokinetics of cyclosporine in healthy volunteers, particularly resulting in bioavailability elevation of cyclosporine [118].

Conclusion

The flavonoid quercetin has been proved to have excellent bioactivities, such as anti-oxidation, anti-inflammation, anti-cancer and other capacities. As occurrence of quercetin is directly associated with human daily dietary intake of antioxidants, it is important to evaluate quercetin sources in food. Fruits and vegetables are the main dietary sources of quercetin for humans, along with tea and wine. More evidence shows that quercetin has the potent effects on reduction of clinical symptoms in humans, especially the diseases such as cancer, diabetes, hypertension and renal injury that are associated with ROS, inflammation and hyperuricemia. Most of the studies have been conducted *in vitro* studies; therefore, it is difficult to draw definite conclusion about the usefulness of quercetin in the diet. As expected, quercetin exerts some toxicity as well. It is suggested that quercetin should be avoided by pregnant women and nursing mothers. The toxicity of quercetin is only proved *in vitro*. All in all, the intake of fruits, vegetables and beverages (e.g., tea and moderate amounts of red wine) containing quercetin is recommended.

Acknowledgments

The work was co-financed by grants from NSFC (Nos. 81025025 and J1103512), PCSIRT (IRT1020) and JSNSF (BK2010365).

References

[1] Lamson, D. W. and Brignall, M. S. (2000). Antioxidants and cancer, part 3: quercetin. *Alternative Medecine Review*, 5, 196-208.

[2] Hollman, P. C. H. and Arts, I. C. W. (2000). Flavonols, flavones and flavanols - nature, occurrence and dietary burden. *Journal of the Science of Food and Agriculture,* 80, 1081-1093.

[3] Mendoza-Wilson, A. M. and Glossman-Mitnik, D. (2004). CHIH-DFT determination of the molecular structure, infrared and ultraviolet spectra of the flavonoid quercetin. *Journal of Molecular Structure-Theochem*, 681, 71-76.

[4] Brown, J. P. (1980). A Review of the Genetic-Effects of Naturally-Occurring Flavonoids, *Anthraquinones and Related-Compounds. Mutation Research,* 75, 243-277.

[5] Day, A. J. and Williamson, G. (2000). Human metabolism of dietary quercetin glycosides. *Plant Polyphenols 2: Chemistry, Biology, Pharmacology, Ecology*, 66, 415-434.

[6] Hertog, M. G. L.; Hollman, P. C. H. and Vandeputte, B. (1993). Content of Potentially Anticarcinogenic Flavonoids of Tea Infusions, Wines, and Fruit Juices. *Journal of Agricultural and Food Chemistry*, 41, 1242-1246.

[7] Sampson, L.; Rimm, E.; Hollman, P. C. H.; de Vries, J. H. M. and Katan, M. B. (2002). Flavonol and flavone intakes in US health professionals. *Journal of the American Dietetic Association*, 102, 1414-1420.

[8] Bischoff, S. C. (2008). Quercetin: potentials in the prevention and therapy of disease. *Curr. Opinion in Clinical Nutrition and Metabolic Care*, 11, 733-740.

[9] Kuhnau, J. (1976). The flavonoids. A class of semi-essential food components: their role in human nutrition. *World Review of Nutrition and Dietetics,* 24, 117-191.

[10] Manach, C.; Scalbert, A.; Morand, C.; Remesy, C. and Jimenez, L. (2004). Polyphenols: food sources and bioavailability. *The American Journal of Clinical Nutrition,* 79, 727-747.

[11] Hollman, P. C.; de Vries, J. H.; van Leeuwen, S. D.; Mengelers, M. J. and Katan, M. B. (1995). Absorption of dietary quercetin glycosides and quercetin in healthy ileostomy volunteers. *The American Journal of Clinical Nutrition,* 62, 1276-1282.

[12] Hollman, P. C. and Katan, M. B. (1997). Absorption, metabolism and health effects of dietary flavonoids in man. *Biomed Pharmacother*, 51, 305-310.

[13] Erlund, I.; Kosonen, T.; Alfthan, G.; Maenpaa, J.; Perttunen, K.; Kenraali, J.; Parantainen, J. and Aro, A. (2000). Pharmacokinetics of quercetin from quercetin aglycone and rutin in healthy volunteers. *European Journal of Clinical Pharmacology*, 56, 545-553.

[14] Kuhnle, G.; Spencer, J. P.; Schroeter, H.; Shenoy, B.; Debnam, E. S.; Srai, S. K.; Rice-Evans, C. and Hahn, U. (2000). Epicatechin and catechin are O-methylated and glucuronidated in the small intestine. *Biochemical and Biophysical Research Communications*, 277, 507-512.

[15] Hollman, P. C.; de Vries, J. H.; van Leeuwen, S. D.; Mengelers, M. J. and Katan, M. B. (1995). Absorption of dietary quercetin glycosides and quercetin in healthy ileostomy volunteers. *The American Journal of Clinical Nutrition,* 62, 1276-1282.

[16] Conquer, J. A.; Maiani, G.; Azzini, E.; Raguzzini, A. and Holub, B. J. (1998). Supplementation with quercetin markedly increases plasma quercetin concentration without effect on selected risk factors for heart disease in healthy subjects. *Journal of Nutrition*, 128, 593-597.

[17] Hollman, P. C.; vd Gaag, M.; Mengelers, M. J.; van Trijp, J. M.; de Vries, J. H. and Katan, M. B. (1996). Absorption and disposition kinetics of the dietary antioxidant quercetin in man. *Free Radical Biology and Medicine,* 21, 703-707.

[18] Day, A. J.; DuPont, M. S.; Ridley, S.; Rhodes, M.; Rhodes, M. J.; Morgan, M. R. and Williamson, G. (1998). Deglycosylation of flavonoid and isoflavonoid glycosides by human small intestine and liver beta-glucosidase activity. *FEBS Letters*, 436, 71-75.

[19] Hackett, A. M. (1986). The metabolism of flavonoid compounds in mammals. Progress in clinical and biological research, 213, 177-194.

[20] de Groot, H. (1994). Reactive oxygen species in tissue injury. *Hepatogastroenterology*, 41, 328-332.

[21] Scalbert, A.; Manach, C.; Morand, C.; Remesy, C. and Jimenez, L. (2005). Dietary polyphenols and the prevention of diseases. *Critical Reviews in Food Science and Nutrition,* 45, 287-306.

[22] Diplock, A. T.; Charleux, J. L.; Crozier-Willi, G.; Kok, F. J.; Rice-Evans, C.; Roberfroid, M.; Stahl, W. and Vina-Ribes, J. (1998). Functional food science and defence against reactive oxidative species. *British Journal of Nutrition*, 80, S77-S112.

[23] Lakhanpa, P. and Rai, D. K. (2007). Quercetin: *A Versatile Flavonoid. Internet Journal of Medical Update*, 2, 22-37.

[24] Santos, A. C.; Uyemura, S. A.; Lopes, J. L. C.; Bazon, J. N.; Mingatto, F. E. and Curti, C. (1998). Effect of naturally occurring flavonoids on lipid peroxidation and membrane permeability transition in mitochondria. *Free Radical Biology and Medicine*, 24, 1455-1461.

[25] Croft, K. D.; Loke, W. M.; Proudfoot, J. M.; Mckinley, A. J.; Needs, P. W.; Kroon, P. A. and Hodgson, J. M. (2008). Quercetin and its in vivo metabolites inhibit neutrophil-mediated low-density lipoprotein oxidation. *Journal of Agricultural and Food Chemistry*, 56, 3609-3615.

[26] Shutenko, Z.; Henry, Y.; Pinard, E.; Seylaz, J.; Potier, P.; Berthet, F.; Girard, P. and Sercombe, R. (1999). Influence of the antioxidant quercetin in vivo on the level of nitric oxide determined by electron paramagnetic resonance in rat brain during global ischemia and reperfusion. *Biochemical Pharmacology*, 57, 199-208.

[27] Huk, I.; Brovkovych, V.; Vili, J. N.; Weigel, G.; Neumayer, C.; Partyka, L.; Patton, S. and Malinski, T. (1998). Bioflavonoid quercetin scavenges superoxide and increases nitric oxide concentration in ischaemia-reperfusion injury: an experimental study. *British Journal of Surgery*, 85, 1080-1085.

[28] Chang, W. S.; Lee, Y. J.; Lu, F. J. and Chiang, H. C. (1993). Inhibitory Effects of Flavonoids on Xanthine-Oxidase. *Anticancer Research*, 13, 2165-2170.

[29] Zhu, J. X.; Wang, Y.; Kong, L. D.; Yang, C. and Zhang, X. (2004). Effects of Biota orientalis extract and its flavonoid constituents, quercetin and rutin on serum uric acid levels in oxonate-induced mice and xanthine dehydrogenase and xanthine oxidase activities in mouse liver. *Journal of Ethnopharmacology*, 93, 133-140.

[30] Arts, M. J. T. J.; Dallinga, J. S.; Voss, H. P.; Haenen, G. R. M. M. and Bast, A. (2004). A new approach to assess the total antioxidant capacity using the TEAC assay. Food Chemistry, 88, 567-570.

[31] Heijnen, C. G.; Haenen, G. R.; Oostveen, R. M.; Stalpers, E. M. and Bast, A. (2002). Protection of flavonoids against lipid peroxidation: the structure activity relationship revisited. *Free Radical Research*, 36, 575-581.

[32] Taylor, P. C.; Williams, R. O. and Feldmann, M. (2004). Tumour necrosis factor alpha as a therapeutic target for immune-mediated inflammatory diseases. Current opinion in biotechnology, 15, 557-563.

[33] Manjeet K, R. and Ghosh, B. (1999). Quercetin inhibits LPS-induced nitric oxide and tumor necrosis factor-alpha production in murine macrophages. International *Journal of Immunopharmacology*, 21, 435-443.

[34] Boots, A. W.; Haenen, G. R. M. M. and Bast, A. (2008). Health effects of quercetin: from antioxidant to nutraceutical. *European Journal of Pharmacology,* 585, 325-337.

[35] Boots, A. W.; Haenen, G. R. and Bast, A. (2008). Health effects of quercetin: from antioxidant to nutraceutical. *European Journal of Pharmacology,* 585, 325-337.

[36] Nair, M. P.; Mahajan, S.; Reynolds, J. L.; Aalinkeel, R.; Nair, H.; Schwartz, S. A. and Kandaswami, C. (2006). The flavonoid quercetin inhibits proinflammatory cytokine (tumor necrosis factor alpha) gene expression in normal peripheral blood mononuclear cells via modulation of the NF-kappa beta system. *Clinical and Vaccine Immunology*, 13, 319-328.

[37] Overman, A.; Chuang, C. C. and McIntosh, M. (2011). Quercetin attenuates inflammation in human macrophages and adipocytes exposed to macrophage-conditioned media. *International Journal of Obesity* (Lond),

[38] Thornhill, S. M. and Kelly, A. M. (2000). Natural treatment of perennial allergic rhinitis. Alternative medicine review : *a journal of clinical therapeutic,* 5, 448-454.

[39] Borissova, P.; Valcheva, S. and Belcheva, A. (1994). Antiinflammatory effect of flavonoids in the natural juice from Aronia melanocarpa, rutin and rutin-magnesium complex on an experimental model of inflammation induced by histamine and serotonin. *Acta Physiologica et Pharmacologica Bulgaric*a, 20, 25-30.

[40] Manson, M. M.; Farmer, P. B.; Gescher, A. and Steward, W. P. (2005). Innovative agents in cancer prevention. *Recent Results in Cancer Research,* 166, 257-275.

[41] Neto, C. C. (2007). Cranberry and its phytochemicals: a review of in vitro anticancer studies. *The Journal of Nutrition*, 137, 186S-193S.

[42] JAN, A. T.; KAMLI, M. R.; MURTAZA, I.; SINGH, J. B.; ALI, A. and HAQ, Q. M. R. (2010). Dietary Flavonoid Quercetin and Associated Health Benefits—An Overview. *Food Reviews International*, 26, 302-317.

[43] Duraj, J.; Zazrivcova, K.; Bodo, J.; Sulikova, M. and Sedlak, J. (2005). Flavonoid quercetin, but not apigenin or luteolin, induced apoptosis in human myeloid leukemia cells and their resistant variants. *Neoplasma*, 52, 273-279.

[44] Granado-Serrano, A. B.; Martin, M. A.; Bravo, L.; Goya, L. and Ramos, S. (2006). Quercetin induces apoptosis via caspase activation, regulation of Bcl-2, and inhibition of PI-3-kinase/Akt and ERK pathways in a human hepatoma cell line (HepG2). *The Journal of Nutrition*, 136, 2715-2721.

[45] Mu, C.; Jia, P.; Yan, Z.; Liu, X.; Li, X. and Liu, H. (2007). Quercetin induces cell cycle G(1) arrest through elevating Cdk inhibitors p21 and p27 in human hepatoma cell line (HepG2). *Methods and Findings in Experimental and Clinical Pharmacology*, 29, 179-183.

[46] Lamson, D. W. and Brignall, M. S. (2000). Antioxidants and cancer, part 3: quercetin. Alternative medicine review : *a journal of clinical therapeutic,* 5, 196-208.

[47] Avila, M. A.; Velasco, J. A.; Cansado, J. and Notario, V. (1994). Quercetin mediates the down-regulation of mutant p53 in the human breast cancer cell line MDA-MB468. *Cancer Research*, 54, 2424-2428.

[48] Yoshida, M.; Yamamoto, M. and Nikaido, T. (1992). Quercetin arrests human leukemic T-cells in late G1 phase of the cell cycle. *Cancer Research*, 52, 6676-6681.

[49] Boutin, J. A. (1994). Tyrosine Protein-Kinase Inhibition and Cancer. *International Journal of Biochemistry*, 26, 1203-1226.

[50] Ferry, D. R.; Smith, A.; Malkhandi, J.; Fyfe, D. W.; deTakats, P. G.; Anderson, D.; Baker, J. and Kerr, D. J. (1996). Phase I clinical trial of the flavonoid quercetin: Pharmacokinetics and evidence for in vivo tyrosine kinase inhibition. *Clinical Cancer Research*, 2, 659-668.

[51] Benassayag, C.; Perrot-Applanat, M. and Ferre, F. (2002). Phytoestrogens as modulators of steroid action in target cells. Journal of chromatography B, *Analytical technologies in the biomedical and life sciences,* 777, 233-248.

[52] McDonnell, D. P. and Hall, J. M. (1999). The estrogen receptor beta-isoform (ER beta) of the human estrogen receptor modulates ER alpha transcriptional activity and is a key regulator of the cellular response to estrogens and antiestrogens. *Endocrinology*, 140, 5566-5578.

[53] van der Woude, H.; Gliszczynska-Swiglo, A.; Struijs, K.; Smeets, A.; Alink, G. M. and Rietjens, I. M. C. M. (2003). Biphasic modulation of cell proliferation by quercetin at concentrations physiologically relevant in humans. *Cancer Letters*, 200, 41-47.

[54] Scambia, G.; Ranelletti, F. O.; Panici, P. B.; Piantelli, M.; Devincenzo, R.; Ferrandina, G.; Bonanno, G.; Capelli, A. and Mancuso, S. (1993). Quercetin Induces Type-Ii Estrogen-Binding Sites in Estrogen-Receptor-Negative (Mda-Mb231) and Estrogen-Receptor-Positive (Mcf-7) Human Breast-Cancer Cell-Lines. *International Journal of Cancer*, 54, 462-466.

[55] Chen, C.; Zhou, J. and Ji, C. (2010). Quercetin: a potential drug to reverse multidrug resistance. *Life Sciences*, 87, 333-338.

[56] Limtrakul, P.; Khantamat, O. and Pintha, K. (2005). Inhibition of P-glycoprotein function and expression by kaempferol and quercetin. *Journal of Chemotheraphy*, 17, 86-95.

[57] Rigano, D.; Formisano, C.; Basile, A.; Lavitola, A.; Senatore, F.; Rosselli, S. and Bruno, M. (2007). Antibacterial activity of flavonoids and phenylpropanoids from Marrubium globosum ssp. libanoticum. *Phytotherapy Research*, 21, 395-397.

[58] Castrillo, J. L. and Carrasco, L. (1987). Action of 3-methylquercetin on poliovirus RNA replication. *Journal of virology*, 61, 3319-3321.

[59] Neznanov, N.; Kondratova, A.; Chumakov, K. M.; Neznanova, L.; Kondratov, R.; Banerjee, A. K. and Gudkov, A. V. (2008). Quercetinase pirin makes poliovirus replication resistant to flavonoid quercetin. *DNA and Cell Biology,* 27, 191-198.

[60] Datla, S. R. and Griendling, K. K. (2010). Reactive Oxygen Species, NADPH Oxidases, and Hypertension. *Hypertension* (Baltimore), 56, 325-330.

[61] Harrison, D. and Kojda, G. (1999). Interactions between NO and reactive oxygen species: pathophysiological importance in atherosclerosis, hypertension, diabetes and heart failure. *Cardiovascular Research,* 43, 562-571.

[62] Mackraj, I.; Govender, T. and Ramesar, S. (2008). The antihypertensive effects of quercetin in a salt-sensitive model of hypertension. *Journal of Cardiovascular Pharmacolo*gy, 51, 239-245.

[63] Sanchez, M.; Galisteo, M.; Vera, R.; Villar, I. C.; Zarzuelo, A.; Tamargo, J.; Perez-Vizcaino, F. and Duarte, J. (2006). Quercetin downregulates NADPH oxidase, increases eNOS activity and prevents endothelial dysfunction in spontaneously hypertensive rats. *Journal of hypertensio*n, 24, 75-84.

[64] Aoi, W.; Niisato, N.; Miyazaki, H. and Marunaka, Y. (2004). Flavonoid-induced reduction of ENaC expression in the kidney of Dahl salt-sensitive hypertensive rat. *Biochemical Biophysical Research Communicat*ions, 315, 892-896.

[65] Halperin, R. O.; Sesso, H. D.; Ma, J.; Buring, J. E.; Stampfer, M. J. and Gaziano, J. M. (2006). Dyslipidemia and the risk of incident hypertension in men. *Hypertension* (Baltimore), 47, 45-50.

[66] Prabu, S. M.; Shagirtha, K. and Renugadevi, J. (2010). Amelioration of Cadmium-Induced Oxidative Stress, Impairment in Lipids and Plasma Lipoproteins by the Combined Treatment with Quercetin and alpha-Tocopherol in Rats. *Journal of Food Science*, 75, T132-T140.

[67] Kobori, M.; Masumoto, S.; Akimoto, Y. and Takahashi, Y. (2009). Dietary quercetin alleviates diabetic symptoms and reduces streptozotocin-induced disturbance of hepatic gene expression in mice. *Molecular Nutrition and Food Research*, 53, 859-868.

[68] Rivera, L.; Moron, R.; Sanchez, M.; Zarzuelo, A. and Galisteo, M. (2008). Quercetin ameliorates metabolic syndrome and improves the inflammatory status in obese Zucker rats. *Obesity* (Silver Spring, Md), 16, 2081-2087.

[69] Halaas, J. L.; Gajiwala, K. S.; Maffei, M.; Cohen, S. L.; Chait, B. T.; Rabinowitz, D.; Lallone, R. L.; Burley, S. K. and Friedman, J. M. (1995). Weight-reducing effects of the plasma protein encoded by the obese gene. *Science* (New York, N Y), 269, 543-546.

[70] Huan, J.-N.; Li, J.; Han, Y.; Chen, K.; Wu, N. and Zhao, A. Z. (2003). Adipocyte-selective reduction of the leptin receptors induced by antisense RNA leads to increased adiposity, dyslipidemia, and insulin resistance. *Journal of Biological Chemistry*, 278, 45638-45650.

[71] Li, J.-M.; Wang, C.; Hu, Q.-H. and Kong, L.-D. (2008). Fructose Induced Leptin Dysfunction and Improvement by Quercetin and Rutin in Rats. *Chinese Journal of Natural Medicines*, 6, 466-472.

[72] Salvi, A.; Carrupt, P.; Tillement, J. and Testa, B. (2001). Structural damage to proteins caused by free radicals: asessment, protection by antioxidants, and influence of protein binding. *Biochemical Pharmacolo*gy, 61, 1237-1242.

[73] Thomson, S. C.; Deng, A.; Bao, D. J.; Satriano, J.; Blantz, R. C. and Vallon, V. (2001). Ornithine decarboxylase, kidney size, and the tubular hypothesis of glomerular hyperfiltration in experimental diabetes. *Journal of Clinical Investigation*, 107, 217-224.

[74] Singh, D.; Chander, V. and Chopra, K. (2004). Quercetin, a bioflavonoid, attenuates ferric nitrilotriacetate-induced oxidative renal injury in rats. *Drug and Chemical Toxicology*, 27, 145-156.

[75] Shoskes, D. A. (1998). Effect of bioflavonoids quercetin and curcumin on ischemic renal injury: a new class of renoprotective agents. *Transplantation*, 66, 147-152.

[76] Prabu, S. M. and Renugadevi, J. (2010). Quercetin protects against oxidative stress-related renal dysfunction by cadmium in rats. *Experimental and Toxicologic Pathology*, 62, 471-481.

[77] Kong, L. D.; Hu, Q. H.; Wang, C. A.; Li, J. M. and Zhang, D. M. (2009). Allopurinol, rutin, and quercetin attenuate hyperuricemia and renal dysfunction in rats induced by fructose intake: renal organic ion transporter involvement. *American Journal of Physiology-Renal Physiology*, 297, F1080-F1091.

[78] Moore, P. K.; Griffiths, R. J. and Lofts, F. J. (1983). The effect of some flavone drugs on the conversion of prostacyclin to 6-oxoprostaglandin E1. *Biochemical Pharmacology*, 32, 2813-2817.

[79] Neto, C. C. (2007). Cranberry and its phytochemicals: a review of in vitro anticancer studies. *The Journal of Nutrition*, 137, 186S-193S.

[80] Hirvonen, T.; Virtamo, J.; Korhonen, P.; Albanes, D. and Pietinen, P. (2001). Flavonol and flavone intake and the risk of cancer in male smokers (Finland). *Cancer Causes and Control* : CCC, 12, 789-796.

[81] Fotsis, T.; Pepper, M. S.; Aktas, E.; Breit, S.; Rasku, S.; Adlercreutz, H.; Wahala, K.; Montesano, R. and Schweigerer, L. (1997). Flavonoids, dietary-derived inhibitors of cell proliferation and in vitro angiogenesis. *Cancer Research*, 57, 2916-2921.

[82] Fan, T. P.; Jaggar, R. and Bicknell, R. (1995). Controlling the vasculature: angiogenesis, anti-angiogenesis and vascular targeting of gene therapy. *Trends in Pharmacological Sciences*, 16, 57-66.

[83] Cruz-Correa, M.; Shoskes, D. A.; Sanchez, P.; Zhao, R.; Hylind, L. M.; Wexner, S. D. and Giardiello, F. M. (2006). Combination treatment with curcumin and quercetin of adenomas in familial adenomatous polyposis. *Clinical Gastroenterology and Hepatology*, 4, 1035-1038.

[84] Hanninen; Kaartinen, K.; Rauma, A. L.; Nenonen, M.; Torronen, R.; Hakkinen, A. S.; Adlercreutz, H. and Laakso, J. (2000). Antioxidants in vegan diet and rheumatic disorders. *Toxicology*, 155, 45-53.

[85] Boots, A. W.; Drent, M.; de Boer, V. C. J.; Bast, A. and Haenen, G. R. M. M. (2011). Quercetin reduces markers of oxidative stress and inflammation in sarcoidosis. *Clinical Nutrition* (Edinburgh, Scotland), 30, 506-512.

[86] Walgren, R. A.; Karnaky, K. J., Jr.; Lindenmayer, G. E. and Walle, T. (2000). Efflux of dietary flavonoid quercetin 4'-beta-glucoside across human intestinal Caco-2 cell monolayers by apical multidrug resistance-associated protein-2. Th*e Journal of Pharmacology and Experimental Therapeutics*, 294, 830-836.

[87] Manach, C.; Mazur, A. and Scalbert, A. (2005). Polyphenols and prevention of cardiovascular diseases. *Current Opinion in Lipidology*, 16, 77-84.

[88] Knekt, P.; Jarvinen, R.; Reunanen, A. and Maatela, J. (1996). Flavonoid intake and coronary mortality in Finland: a cohort study. *British Medical Journal* (Clinical research ed), 312, 478-481.

[89] Terao, J.; Kawai, Y. and Murcita, K. (2008). Vegetable flavonoids and cardiovascular disease. *Asia Pacific Journal of Clinical Nutrition*, 17, 291-293.

[90] Gryglewski, R. J.; Korbut, R.; Robak, J. and Swies, J. (1987). On the mechanism of antithrombotic action of flavonoids. *Biochemical Pharmacology*, 36, 317-322.

[91] Edwards, R. L.; Lyon, T.; Litwin, S. E.; Rabovsky, A.; Symons, J. D. and Jalili, T. (2007). Quercetin reduces blood pressure in hypertensive subjects. *The Journal of nutrition*, 137, 2405-2411.

[92] Oiry, C.; Youl, E.; Bardy, G.; Magous, R.; Cros, G.; Sejalon, F.; Virsolvy, A.; Richard, S.; Quignard, J. F.; Gross, R.; Petit, P. and Bataille, D. (2010). Quercetin potentiates insulin secretion and protects INS-1 pancreatic beta-cells against oxidative damage via the ERK1/2 pathway. *British Journal of Pharmacology*, 161, 799-814.

[93] Suchankova, G.; Nelson, L. E.; Gerhart-Hines, Z.; Kelly, M.; Gauthier, M. S.; Saha, A. K.; Ido, Y.; Puigserver, P. and Ruderman, N. B. (2009). Concurrent regulation of AMP-activated protein kinase and SIRT1 in mammalian cells. *Biochemical and Biophysical Research Communications*, 378, 836-841.

[94] Du, L. and Xie, W. (2011). Diabetes is an inflammatory disease: evidence from traditional *Chinese medicines. Diabetes Obesity and Metabolism,* 13, 289-301.

[95] Liu, J.; Yu, H. and Ning, X. (2006). Effect of quercetin on chronic enhancement of spatial learning and memory of mice. Science China Series C: *Life Sciences*, 49, 583-590.

[96] Navon, A. and Ciechanover, A. (2009). The 26 S proteasome: from basic mechanisms to drug targeting. *The Journal of Biological Chemistry*, 284, 33713-33718.

[97] Chondrogianni, N.; Kapeta, S.; Chinou, I.; Vassilatou, K.; Papassideri, I. and Gonos, E. S. (2010). Anti-ageing and rejuvenating effects of quercetin. *Experimental gerontology*, 45, 763-771.

[98] Gonos, E. S. and Chondrogianni, N. (2005). Proteasome dysfunction in mammalian aging: Steps and factors involved. *Experimental gerontology*, 40, 931-938.

[99] Saag, K. G. and Choi, H. (2006). Epidemiology, risk factors, and lifestyle modifications for gout. *Arthritis Research and Therapy*, 8 Suppl 1, S2.

[100] Nuki, G. and Simkin, P. A. (2006). A concise history of gout and hyperuricemia and their treatment. *Arthritis Research and Therapy*, 8,

[101] Kong, L. D.; Mo, S. F.; Zhou, F.; Lv, Y. Z.; Hu, Q. H. and Zang, D. M. (2007). Hypouricemic action of selected flavonoids in mice: Structure-activity relationships. *Biological and Pharmaceutical Bulletin*, 30, 1551-1556.

[102] Hu, Q.-H.; Wang, C.; Li, J.-M.; Zhang, D.-M. and Kong, L.-D. (2009). Allopurinol, rutin, and quercetin attenuate hyperuricemia and renal dysfunction in rats induced by fructose intake: renal organic ion transporter involvement. *American Journal of Physiology* - Renal Physiology, 297, F1080-F1091.

[103] Floyd, R. A. (1999). Antioxidants, oxidative stress, and degenerative neurological disorders. *Experimental Biology and Medicine*, 222, 236-245.

[104] Heo, H. J. and Lee, C. Y. (2004). Protective effects of quercetin and vitamin C against oxidative stress-induced neurodegeneration. *Journal of Agricultural and Food Chemistry,* 52, 7514-7517.

[105] Prouillet, C.; Maziere, J.-C.; Maziere, C.; Wattel, A.; Brazier, M. and Kamel, S. (2004). Stimulatory effect of naturally occurring flavonols quercetin and kaempferol on alkaline phosphatase activity in MG-63 human osteoblasts through ERK and estrogen receptor pathway. *Biochemical Pharmacology*, 67, 1307-1313.

[106] Hegarty, V. M.; May, H. M. and Khaw, K. T. (2000). Tea drinking and bone mineral density in older women. *The American Journal of Clinical Nutrition,* 71, 1003-1007.

[107] Gugler, R.; Leschik, M. and Dengler, H. J. (1975). Disposition of Quercetin in Man after Single Oral and Intravenous Doses. *European Journal of Clinical Pharmacology*, 9, 229-234.

[108] Jorgensen, L. V.; Cornett, C.; Justesen, U.; Skibsted, L. H. and Dragsted, L. O. (1998). Two-electron electrochemical oxidation of quercetin and kaempferol changes only the flavonoid C-ring. *Free Radical Research*, 29, 339-350.

[109] Awad, H. M.; Boersma, M. G.; Boeren, S.; van Bladeren, P. J.; Vervoort, J. and Rietjens, I. M. (2002). The regioselectivity of glutathione adduct formation with flavonoid quinone/quinone methides is pH-dependent. *Chemical Research in Toxicology*, 15, 343-351.

[110] Vrijsen, R.; Michotte, Y. and Boeye, A. (1990). Metabolic activation of quercetin mutagenicity. *Mutation Research*, 232, 243-248.

[111] Jurado, J.; Alejandre-Duran, E.; Alonso-Moraga, A. and Pueyo, C. (1991). Study on the mutagenic activity of 13 bioflavonoids with the Salmonella Ara test. *Mutagenesis*, 6, 289-295.

[112] Cross, H. J.; Tilby, M.; Chipman, J. K.; Ferry, D. R. and Gescher, A. (1996). Effect of quercetin on the genotoxic potential of cisplatin. *International Journal of Cancer*, 66, 404-408.

[113] Czeczot, H. (1994). Mutagenic activity of quercetin in derivatives of Escherichia coli WP2 uvrA with increased permeability. *Acta Biochimica Polonica,* 41, 144-147.

[114] Czeczot, H. and Kusztelak, J. (1993). A study of the genotoxic potential of flavonoids using short-term bacterial assays. *Acta biochimica Polonica,* 40, 549-554.

[115] Caria, H.; Chaveca, T.; Laires, A. and Rueff, J. (1995). Genotoxicity of quercetin in the micronucleus assay in mouse bone marrow erythrocytes, human lymphocytes, V79 cell line and identification of kinetochore-containing (CREST staining) micronuclei in human lymphocytes. *Mutation Research*, 343, 85-94.

[116] Silva, I. D.; Gaspar, J.; da Costa, G. G.; Rodrigues, A. S.; Laires, A. and Rueff, J. (2000). Chemical features of flavonols affecting their genotoxicity. Potential implications in their use as therapeutical agents. *Chemico-Biological Interactions*, 124, 29-51.

[117] Vanderhoeven, J. C. M.; Bruggeman, I. M. and Debets, F. M. H. (1984). Genotoxicity of Quercetin in Cultured Mammalian-Cells. *Mutation Research,* 136, 9-21.

[118] Choi, K. E.; Choi, J. S. and Choi, B. C. (2004). Effect of quercetin on the pharmacokinetics of oral cyclosporine. *American Journal of Health-System Pharmacy*, 61, 2406-2409.

[119] Joseph, L. W. (1993). Nutritional Influences on Mental-Illness - a Sourcebook of Clinical Research - Werbach, Mr. *Canadian Journal of Psychiatry*-Revue Canadienne De Psychiatrie, 38, 235-235.

[120] Walle, T.; Otake, Y.; Walle, U. K. and Wilson, F. A. (2000). Quercetin glucosides are completely hydrolyzed in ileostomy patients before absorption. *The Journal of nutrition*, 130, 2658-2661.

In: Quercetin
Editors: Taiki Chikamatsu and Yuudai Hida

ISBN: 978-1 61942- 057-1

Chapter 9

FORMULATIONS FOR PHARMACEUTICAL ADMINISTRATION OF QUERCETIN

Paola Scarfato*

University of Salerno, Department of Industrial Engineering,
Via Ponte don Melillo, Fisciano (SA), Italy

ABSTRACT

Quercetin is a polyphenolic compound synthesized by many food plants and is an abundant micronutrient in human diet. It is attracting a large interest by virtue of its numerous beneficial biological effects: in fact, it has demonstrated anti-oxidative, free-radical scavenging and anticancer activities, protective effects towards cardiovascular disease, antiviral action, etc. Nevertheless, its bioavailability and bioefficacy is generally low due to its very poor aqueous solubility and scant stability in some environments and biological fluids. Several research efforts have been recently devoted to overcome these limitations by designing and testing appropriate formulations able to improve the quercetin bioavailability, to modulate the release kinetic and to target the release to specific tissue. This review presents the most interesting quercetin delivery systems till now developed.

INTRODUCTION

Quercetin (Q, 3,5,7,3',4'-pentahydroxyflavone) is a common dietary component occurring in various edible plant and herbal medicines [1-2]. This flavonoid has been shown to have a variety of biological activities and pharmacological actions in numerous mammalian cell systems, in vitro as well as in vivo: such as dilating coronary arteries, decreasing blood lipid, anti-platelet aggregation, anti-cancer, antioxidation, anti-anemia, anti-inflammation, and

* Email: pscarfato@unisa.it.

anti-anaphylaxis effects [3-8]. Moreover, it might contribute to reduce toxicant-induced cellular damage and to diminish UV radiation-mediated oxidative damage to the skin [9-10].

Although the variety of its biological effects, clinical studies investigating different programs of quercetin administration have been limited by its poor water solubility and its instability in some physiological media. In fact, essential for quercetin to exert its action in vivo is the extent of its absorption after ingestion and its ability to be distributed in various body tissues. However, quercetin has minimal absorption in gastrointestinal tract, and its oral bioavailability is less than 17% in rats, even 1% in men [11-12]. As a result, the clinical application of the drug is greatly restricted. Therefore, a safe, stable and efficient method for quercetin delivering is highly desired.

This review will mainly focus on the several strategies investigated to improve quercetin bioavailability and efficacy, including the use of solubilizers or cosolvents, the micro- and nanoencapsulation, the emulsification and the nanosuspension technology, the complexation with cyclodextrin and liposomes.

1. Microparticles

Some of the first systems intended for quercetin delivering have been developed by Lauro et al. [13]. The authors formulated sustained release dosage forms for oral administration of flavonoids included quercetin, succeeding at the same time in enhancing the dissolution rate of this low soluble drug and in modulating its delivery. The reported drug/carrier systems consist of fast- and slow-release tablets. The first ones were formulated using cross-linked sodium carboxymethylcellulose (CMC-XL), sodium carboxymethylstarch (E) or cross-linked polyvinylpirrolidone (P) as hydration enhancer; the latter were formulated using hydroxypropylmethylcellulose (HPMC) of different viscosity grades as hydrophilic swellable retarding polymer. The drug/carrier systems, containing 20 wt% of quercetin and, if the case, sodium lauryl sulphate, sodium starch glycolate, magnesium stearate, colloidal silicon dioxide and microcrystalline cellulose as excipients, were prepared either by mixing or co-milling techniques. The obtained tablets were submitted to in vitro dissolution/release tests at 37°C in distilled water and in simulated intestinal fluid (SIF, pH 7.5), according to the USP 24 drug release test – method A. Comparing the results of the dissolution studies performed on the fast-release Q tablets, based on the different polymeric carriers and prepared with or without excipients either by mixing and co-milling techniques, the authors demonstrate the following points: (1) the co-milled tablets show dissolution rates faster than the respective mixed ones; (2) the CMC-XL and E polymers are more efficient than P one in enhancing the drug dissolution rate: in fact, in the absence of excipients the first systems release in distilled water about 35-42% of drug in 15 min, the latter only the 6% in the same time; (3) the addition of the excipients into the tablets formulation improves the release rate of the drug, leading to about 53% of released Q from the systems based on CMC-XL and E polymers and to about 20% of released Q from those based on P after 15 min in distilled water; (4) similar efficiency differences among the three polymeric carriers were also obtained in SIF, even if the amounts of released Q in the same time were higher in this case, as expected considering that the Q solubility increases with pH, being Q weakly acid; (5) no more than 55% of Q in water and 85% of Q in IF was released from these formulations at long times (60 min). The slow-release formulations, on the other hand, were demonstrated able to deliver all the Q content at long times; however, only the use of HPMC matrices with high viscosities (> 4000 cP) seems able to effectively slow the dissolution rate of the drug.

In order to better comply with the necessity to protect the quercetin in the gastric medium after an oral administration, in a following paper Lauro et al. [14] produced microparticulated gastro-resistant dosage forms obtained by spray-drying. In particular, the authors prepared spray-dryed quercetin microparticles using cellulose acetate trimellitate and cellulose acetate phthalate as gastro-resistant polymer matrices. They tested several formulations with different drug/polymer ratios (1:1, 1:3 and 1:5) and different conditions of the spray-drying process, evaluating the effectiveness of the preparation procedure, the morphology and the release properties of the obtained systems. Even if the production yield of the process and the encapsulation efficiency resulted to be acceptable in some cases, the morphology of the systems was far from the expected. SEM observation, in fact, demonstrated the presence of cluster of microparticles and needle crystals of not encapsulated Q. Moreover, the in vitro release tests, carried out according to the pH change method according to USP 25 (USP 25 Drug Release Test, method A for Enteric Coated Articles), demonstrated that both the enteric polymers in gastric conditions (pH 1.0) slow the dissolution rate of the microencapsulated Q compared to that of Q alone, but they protect only partially the flavonoids. Moreover, they are not able to promote the complete release of Q in the intestinal medium (pH 6.8).

Improved gastro-resistant quercetin microspheres were firstly developed by our group in a research program focused on the development of microparticulated formulations for controlled release of active molecules. [15]. In our study we prepared several formulations by water-in-oil (W/O) emulsion solvent evaporation using cellulose derivatives as matrix materials. In particular, two different cellulose derivatives were tested: an enteric polymer (cellulose acetate phthalate, CAP), insoluble at low pH and soluble at slightly acidic pH values, and a rather impermeable polymer (cellulose acetate propionate, CAPr). Their mixtures in 3:1, 1:1, and 1:3 ratios were also investigated in the attempt to modulate the drug release rate from the microspheres. Table 1 reports the nomenclature adopted for the Q-loaded microspheres having different matrix composition and the encapsulation efficiency of the drug. The data demonstrated that the W/O emulsion solvent evaporation technique allows to microencapsulate the quercetin with high efficiency and high production yields.

Table 1. Nomenclature adopted for the Q-loaded microspheres

Microspheres nomenclature	Matrix composition		Polymer/drug ratio	Production yields (%)	Encapsulation efficiency of Q (%)
	CAP (%)	CAPr (%)			
M1-Q	100	0	4:1	97.8	96.5
M2-Q	75	25	4:1	99.3	100
M3-Q	50	50	4:1	97.2	99.0
M4-Q	25	75	4:1	95.4	92.5
M5-Q	0	100	4:1	84.5	89.5

Source: ref. [15] – reprinted with permission.

In terms of morphology, SEM micrographs (Figure 1) show that the obtained microspheres exhibit regular geometry with a well defined spherical shape. The surfaces are quite smooth and nonporous and no coalescence phenomena are evident. Only the M1-Q sample evidences the presence of small drug particles on the surface.

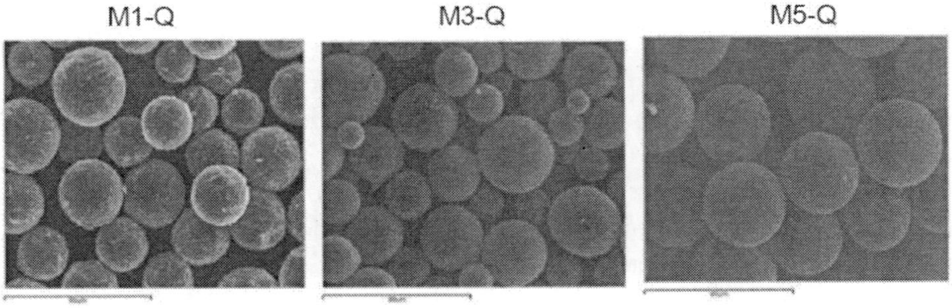

Source: ref. [15] – reprinted with permission.

Figure 1. Scanning electron micrographs of Q-loaded microspheres M1-Q, M3-Q and M5-Q.

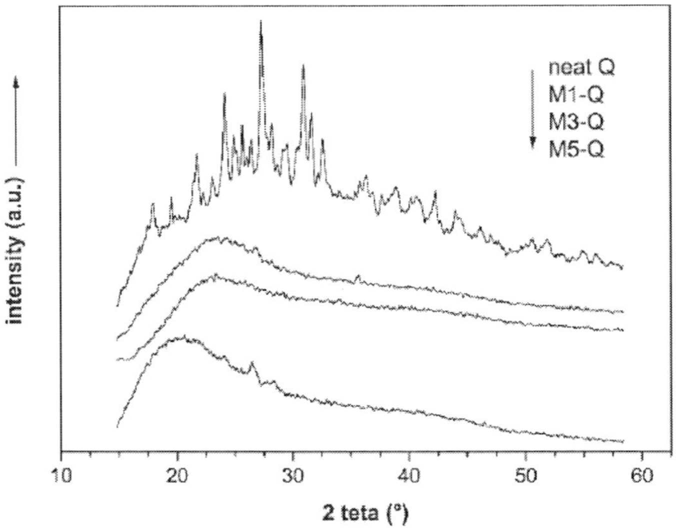

Source: ref. [15] – reprinted with permission.

Figure 2. Comparison between the X-ray patterns of crystalline neat Q and Q-loaded microspheres (M1-Q, M3-Q, and M5-Q).

Moreover, X-ray diffraction (XRD) tests demonstrates that the drug was molecularly dispersed in all the Q-loaded microsphere samples, like a solid solution (Figure 2). The diffractograms reveal that Q incorporation into the CAP and/or CAPr matrices, in our experimental conditions, reduces the crystallinity of Q to practical insignificance, giving amorphous drug/polymer blends. The obtainment of such solid solutions is a very important result since it has been proved to be an effective strategy for enhancing drug solubility and bioavailability for other crystalline and poorly soluble drugs [16].

In vitro release studies for Q loaded microspheres were carried out using a pH change method according the USP 28 procedure to investigate the release behavior both in simulated gastric fluid (SGF) and simulated intestinal fluid (SIF) medium. The dissolution profiles are plotted in Figure 3 together with that of neat Q, reported for comparison. As expected, Q is poorly soluble both in SGF and in SIF even if, being a weak acid, its solubility increases with pH, according to the dissolution profile shown in the graph. All microsphere samples exhibit a pH-dependent biphasic drug release, typical of gastro-resistant dosage forms. In the SGF medium, after an initial Q release (about 20% for M1-Q and 15% for M3-Q and M5-Q samples in 30 min), which can be related to the solubilization of the small drug particles adhering on the microspheres surface, only a very slow and incomplete release of the encapsulated drug occurs. So, a satisfactory gastric protection was gained in all cases.

After the pH change, strong differences among the drug release behaviors of the three samples are present. In fact, the M1-Q microspheres release more than 90% of Q within 30 min after the pH change, since the CAP matrix is fairly soluble in SIF medium; on the other hand, the M5-Q ones release only 25% of Q at the same time and the M2-Q, M3-Q, and M4-Q ones have an intermediate behavior, since the CAPr polymer is only slightly swelled at intestinal pH but remains insoluble. As a consequence, the drug must diffuse through the matrix to be released and only the drug near the surface undergoes to dissolution. So, the pH-dependent solubility of the two cellulose derivatives used as matrices, together with the amorphous state of the microencapsulated quercetin, as evidenced from X-ray measurements, has a key role in determining the release behavior of the final microspheres. On the whole, from a comparison of all the release profiles reported in Figure 3, the M1-Q formulation, based on the cellulose acetate phthalate polymer, appears as a very efficient system for controlled delivery of quercetin to the intestinal tract, by enhancing the solubility and thus the bioavailability of this drug.

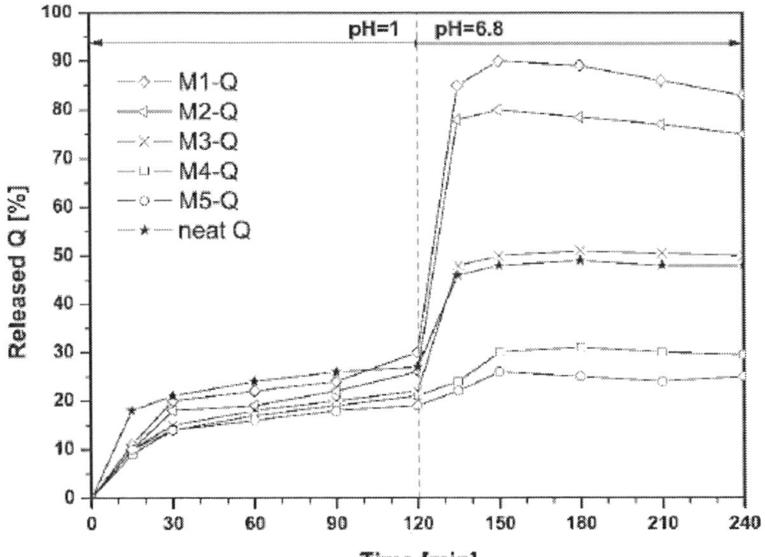

Source: ref. [15] – reprinted with permission.

Figure 3. Dissolution profiles of Q-loaded microspheres, in comparison with the dissolution profile of the neat Q.

Recently, Sansone et al. [17] have been able to obtain by spray-drying quercetin microparticles that, thanks to the use of opportune enhancers, assure in the same time a satisfactory protection in SGF and an almost complete release in SIF.

In particular, they prepared several microparticles formulations loaded with about 17-22 wt% of quercetin, using cellulose acetate phthalate (CAP) as enteric polymer matrix and three different enhancers: cross-linked sodium carboxymethylcellulose (CMC), sodium dodecylbenzensulfonate (SDBS), and polyoxyethylene sorbitan trioleate (Tween 85). For comparison, they prepared also a formulation of Q-loaded CAP microparticles without enhancers. All the produced systems were submitted to dissolution/release study (according to USP 31, 2008) and the results are shown in Figure 4, compared with the neat quercetin.

The release profiles evidence that the amounts of Q released from the microparticles in SGF are always significantly lower compared to the neat Q, demonstrating the gastro-resistance of the CAP/Q/enhancers microparticles. The best gastro-protection was provided by the enhancers-free system (CAP/Q, batch #2d) that release only the 7.5% of Q after 2 h in SGF. Nevertheless, its release remains low also in SIF, where the amount of dissolved Q (50.9%) is similar to that of the neat Q (43.1%).

On the other hand, all the enhancer-containing microparticles show a large improvement of the drug dissolution rate. In particular, the CAP/Q/CMC (batch #2a) and CAP/Q/Tween (batch # 2c) systems give a practically complete release in 45 min after the pH change. The authors related these good results to the enhancers ability to increase the quercetin solubility.

The authors have also verified that their systems maintain the functional stability during the storage. In this aim, they measured during 12 months of storage the free-radical scavenging activity of the produced systems using the stable 1,1-diphenyl-2-picrylhydrazyl radical (DPPH test) and the strong antioxidant α-tocopherol as positive control of the assay [18]. The mean effective scavenging concentrations (E_{50}), reported in Table 2, evidences that the microencapsulated Q keeps its antioxidant activity quite unaltered up to 12 months of storage, while the unencapsulated Q about doubles its effective scavenging concentration during the same period.

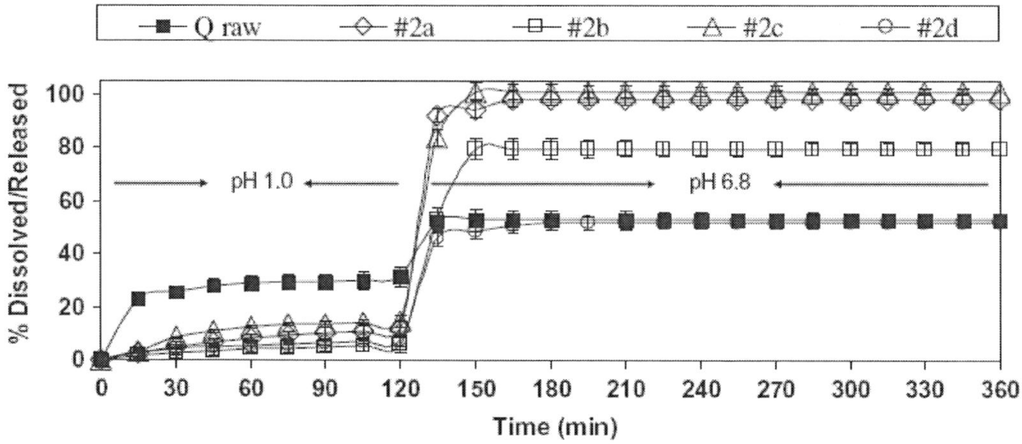

Source: ref. [17] – reprinted with permission.

Figure 4. Release profile of CAP/Q/enhancers microparticles (CAP/Q/CMC #2a, CAP/Q/SDBS #2b, CAP/Q/Tween #2c) compared to Q as raw material, and CAP/Q (batch #2d) microparticles.

Similar results about the improvement of the quercetin stability through its microencapsulation were also reported by Scalia et al. [19]. The authors incorporated quercetin in lipid microparticles (LMs) in order to enhance the photo- and chemical-stability of this flavonoid in topical formulations. The Q-loaded lipid microparticles were prepared through a hot emulsion technique that does not require organic solvents, using only physiologically compatible substances. Tristearin was selected as lipidic material and hydrogenated phosphatidylcholine as surfactant. The technique allowed to obtain isolated microparticles with irregular shapes and uneven surfaces, having particle size in the range 15-35 micron, suitable for topical applications [20-21].

Photodecomposition experiments were performed irradiating for 2 h, with a solar simulator test, creams preparations consisting of oil-in-water emulsions and containing microencapsulated quercetin (0.5%, w/w) or an equivalent amount of the unencapsulated flavonoids, for comparison purpose. The data, listed in Table 3, show that the quercetin loss measured after irradiation of microencapsulated flavonoid samples is about half of that measured for formulations containing free Q. Moreover, the photostabilization effect of the Q-loaded LMs in the cream preparation was retained after 3-month storage.

Table 2. Free-radical scavenging activity of encapsulated and unencapsulated Quercetin during 12 months of storage

Materials	Months			
	0	3	6	12
DPPH test EC_{50} µg/mL[a]				
Q	2.3 ± 0.4[a]	2.5 ± 0.2	4.5 ± 0.5	5.1 ± 0.4
CAP/Q/CMC	2.8 ± 0.3	3.0 ± 0.3	3.0 ± 0.4	3.2 ± 0.3
CAP/Q/SDBS	2.7 ± 0.2	2.8 ± 0.3	2.8 ± 0.3	3.1 ± 0.2
CAP/Q/Tween	2.5 ± 0.3	2.6 ± 0.3	2.6 ± 0.2	2.8 ± 0.3
α-Tocopherol[b]	10.1 ± 1.3	10.2 ± 1.3	10.1 ± 1.6	10.3 ± 1.3

[a] Mean ± standard deviation.

[b] Positive control of the assay.

Source: ref. [18] – reprinted with permission.

Table 3. Photodegradation values for free and microparticle-entrapped quercetin in cream formulations, immediately after preparation and after 3-month storage

Sample	% quercetin loss[a]		P^b
	$t = 0$	$t = 90$ days	
Free quercetin	23.1 ± 3.6	20.9 ± 5.2	
Quercetin-loaded LMs	11.9 ± 2.5	11.3 ± 2.4	< 0.01

[a] Each value is the mean ± S.D. of eight determinations.

[b] *P* values (unpaired *t*-test) vs. free quercetin.

Source: ref. [19] – reprinted with permission.

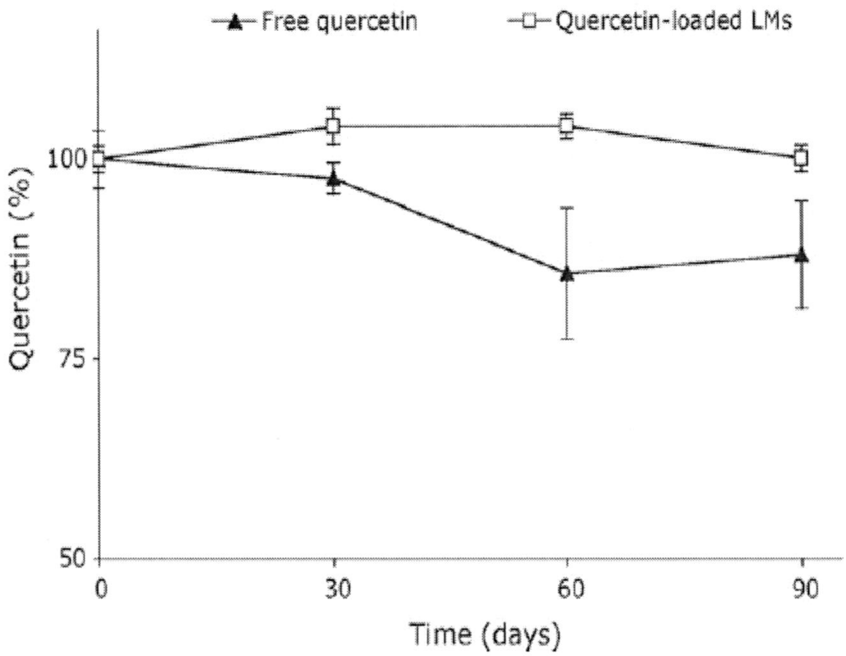

Source: ref. [19] – reprinted with permission.

Figure 5. Quercetin content in its formulations at different storing times. Operating conditions as described in Section 2. Values are means±S.D. (n = 5).

The incorporation of Q in lipid microparticles affect positively also its chemical stability, evaluated by aging the cream formulations over 3 months at room temperature and in the dark. The results, reported in Figure 5, evidence that in the unencapsulated formulations the Q level falls below 86% of the initial concentration within 3 months, whereas it remains unchanged in the formulations containing the Q-loaded LMs.

2. Nanoparticles and Liposomes

The development of nanoparticles for delivery of quercetin has recently attracted the interest of many researchers looking for formulations capable of widening the applications of this flavonoid in pharmaceutical field. Several matrices (chitosan, poly-D,L-lactide, poly(lactide-co-glycolide), Eudragit E, polyvinyl alcohol, lipid mixtures) and preparation techniques were experimented to prepare these nanosized drug carrier systems [20-28].

Zhang et al. [22] prepared quercetin-loaded chitosan nanoparticles by ionic gelation of chitosan with tripolyphosphate and characterized the obtained samples in terms of morphology, internal structure and antioxidant activity. They verified that the used technique allows to produce uniform ellipsoidal nanoparticles having average size of about 76 nm and containing the drug in the amorphous state.

They also demonstrated that the quercetin incorporated into the nanoparticles maintained its antioxidant activity, as shown in Figure 6 that compares the scavenging potential of the blank and quercetin-loaded chitosan nanoparticles on 1,1-diphenyl-2-picrylhydrazyl radical as a function of the concentration of nanoparticles.

Wu et al. [23] used Eudragit E (EE) and polyvinyl alcohol (PVA) as carriers and a nanoprecipitation technology [24] to produce the quercetin-loaded nanoparticles (QUEN). They formulated several systems having different ratios of Q:EE:PVA (1:1:1, 1:5:5, and 1:10:10 w/w/w). Also these nanoparticles have good morphology, with spherical shape and uniform size distribution, and entrap the quercetin in the amorphous state.

The dissolution behavior in the simulated gastric fluid, evaluated according to USP 24 method, is compared in Figure 7 with that of the neat Q and its physical mixtures with the polymer carrier.

The dissolution profiles demonstrate that Q was released faster from the nanoparticles than from the corresponding physical mixtures. In particular, the QUEN 1:10:10 formulation releases more than 95% of Q within 20 min.

The QUEN 1:10:10 system, tested for its antioxidant power in comparison with pure Q dissolved in DMSO or distilled water, showed also excellent activity in vitro. Figure 8 reports the results of the antioxidant activities assay (DPPH free radical-scavenging activity, anti-superoxide anion formation activity, superoxide anion-scavenging activity and anti-lipid peroxidation activity).

It clearly emerges that the nanoencapsulation of Q, improving the dissolution behavior of the drug, markedly enhances its antioxidant power, too. This suggest that the QUEN may be positively applied in clinical setting.

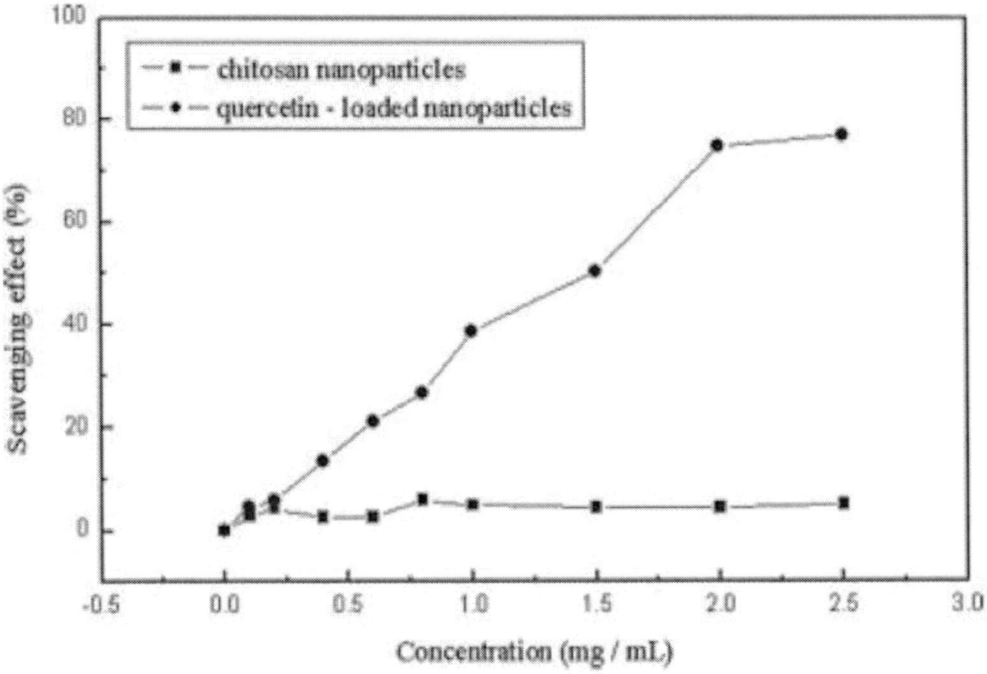

Source: ref. [22] – reprinted with permission.

Figure 6. Scavenging effect of chitosan nanoparticles and quercetin-loaded nanoparticles on 1,1-diphenyl-2-picrylhydrazyl radical. Each value is expressed as mean ± SD (n = 3).

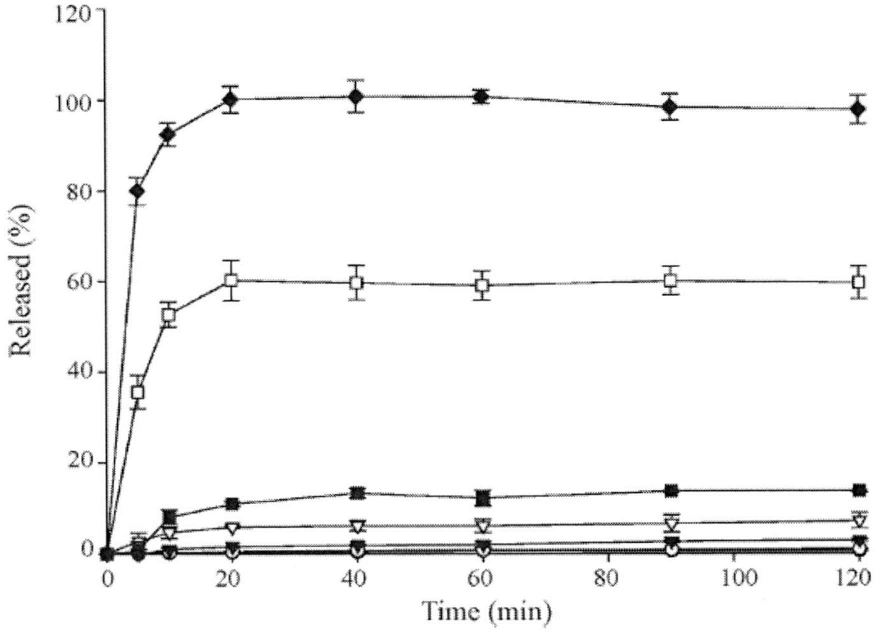

Source: ref. [23] – reprinted with permission.

Figure 7. Dissolution profiles of Q, the physical mixtures (PM), and the quercetin-loaded nanoparticles (QUEN) with various weight ratios of Q:EE:PVA. Quercetin (●), PM 1:1:1 (o), PM 1:5:5 (▼), PM 1:10:10 (∇), QUEN 1:1:1 (■), QUEN 1:5:5 (□), and QUEN 1:10:10 (♦). Values were expressed as mean±S.D., n=6.

Kumari et al. [25] developed biodegradable nanoparticles based on poly-L,D-lactide (PLA) using the emulsion solvent evaporation technique.

They successfully loaded quercetin in the PLA nanoparticles with a very high encapsulation efficiency (96.7%) and an actual drug loading of 19.4wt%. In terms of morphology and particle size and distribution, AFM analyses evidenced that the quercetin loaded PLA nanoparticles are smooth and spherical with uniform size distribution and average particle sizes of 130±30 nm (Figure 9).

In terms of quercetin bioavailability, in vitro tests, performed evaluating the antioxidant activity of the nanoencapsulated Q by 1,1-diphenyl-2-picrylhydrazyl (DPPH) assay and the Q cumulative release by HPLC assay, evidenced that incorporated drug, after an initial burst effect, shows a sustained release behavior (Figure 10).

The release occurring in the burst step (40-45% of Q released within 0.5 h) was due to the rapid dissolution in the surrounding medium of the drug adsorbed close to the nanoparticles surface. The subsequent sustained release (87.6% of released Q after 96 h) was due to the drug incorporated into the core of the nanoparticles, which must diffuse through the polymer matrix to be solubilized.

Li et al. [26] designed and characterized quercetin-loaded solid lipid nanoparticles (QT-SLNs) demonstrating through in vivo tests that their systems are valuable as an oral delivery carrier to enhance the absorption of this poorly water soluble drug. The authors, after having characterized the physicochemical properties of their systems, measured the release of the quercetin in vitro by dynamic dialysis using aqueous ethanol (35% v/v) as receptor medium.

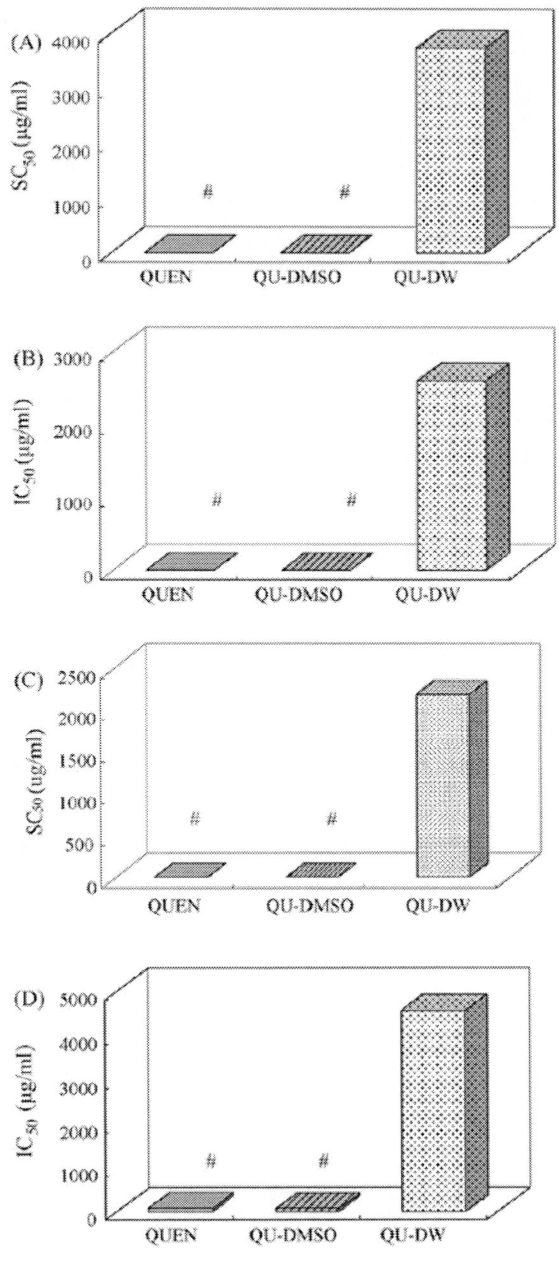

Source: ref. [23] – reprinted with permission.

Figure 8. The antioxidant activities of QUEN, Q–DMSO, and Q–DW in different studies: (A) DPPH radical-scavenging activity; (B) anti-superoxide anion formation; (C) superoxide anion-scavenging effect; (D) anti-lipid peroxidation. All determinations were performed in triplicate and values were expressed as mean±S.D., n=5. $^{\#}$Significantly different from the QU–DW ($P < 0.001$). SC_{50} is the scavenging concentration of each sample at 50%. IC_{50} is the inhibition concentration of each sample at 50%.

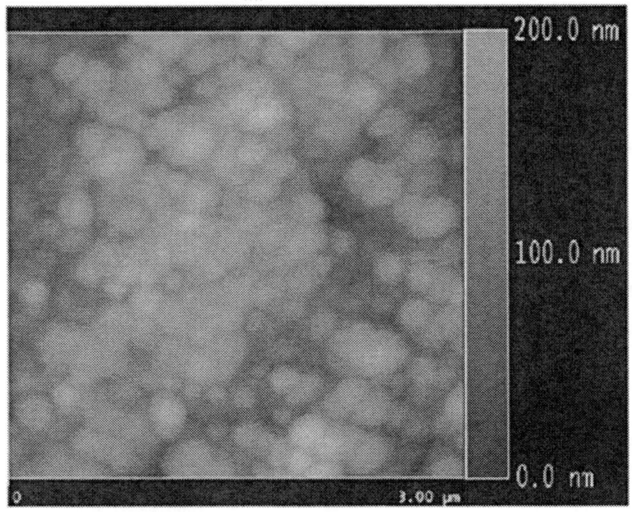

Source: ref. [25] – reprinted with permission.

Figure 9. AFM image of quercetin loaded PLA nanoparticles. The nanoparticles have been characterized using tapping mode.

Similarly to the PLA systems above discussed, also these QT-SLNs samples show a biphasic release profile of Q: in the first phase there is a fast release of the drug, which accumulated percentage is 50% within 6 h; in the second extended release phase the drug is released in a more sustained way giving an accumulated percentage of 87.5% at 48 h. When the QT-SLNs suspension was administrated by oral route in rats (at quercetin dose of 50 mg/kg), the amount of quercetin absorbed in the rat's stomach after 2 h was only 6.20±1.46 %, which indicated that the stomach was not a good absorption segment for the drug in this formulation. On the other hand, the intestine was able to absorb the QT-SLNs suspension in all segments with the following absorption percentages: duodenum 13.00±2.41%, jejunum 17.57±1.84%, ileum 30.44±2.21% and colon 22.03±1.77%.

Tabile 4. Pharmacokinetic parameters of quercetin and QT-SLNs in rat plasma (n=5, x±s)

Parameter	Quercetin	QT-SLNs
A (µg/mL)	8.95±1.12	14.22±2.15
Ke (1/h)	0.12±0.03	0.04±0.01
Ka (1/h)	0.50±0.12	0.32±0.11
Lag time (h)	0.04±0.02	0.02±0.01
$t_{1/2Ka}$ (h)	1.39±0.41	2.16±0.38
$t_{1/2Ke}$ (h)	5.79±1.22	17.96±2.22
Tmax (h)	5.00±1.18	8.00±1.38
Cmax (µg/mL)	5.90±1.24	12.22±2.15
$AUC_{(0\rightarrow 48h)}$[(µg/mL) h]	56.73±9.23	324.18±41.35
CLs (L/h)	0.23±0.03	0.04±0.01
Vc (L)	1.91±0.32	1.04±0.02
MRT (h)	12.46±2.11	27.48±3.42

Source: ref. [26] – reprinted with permission.

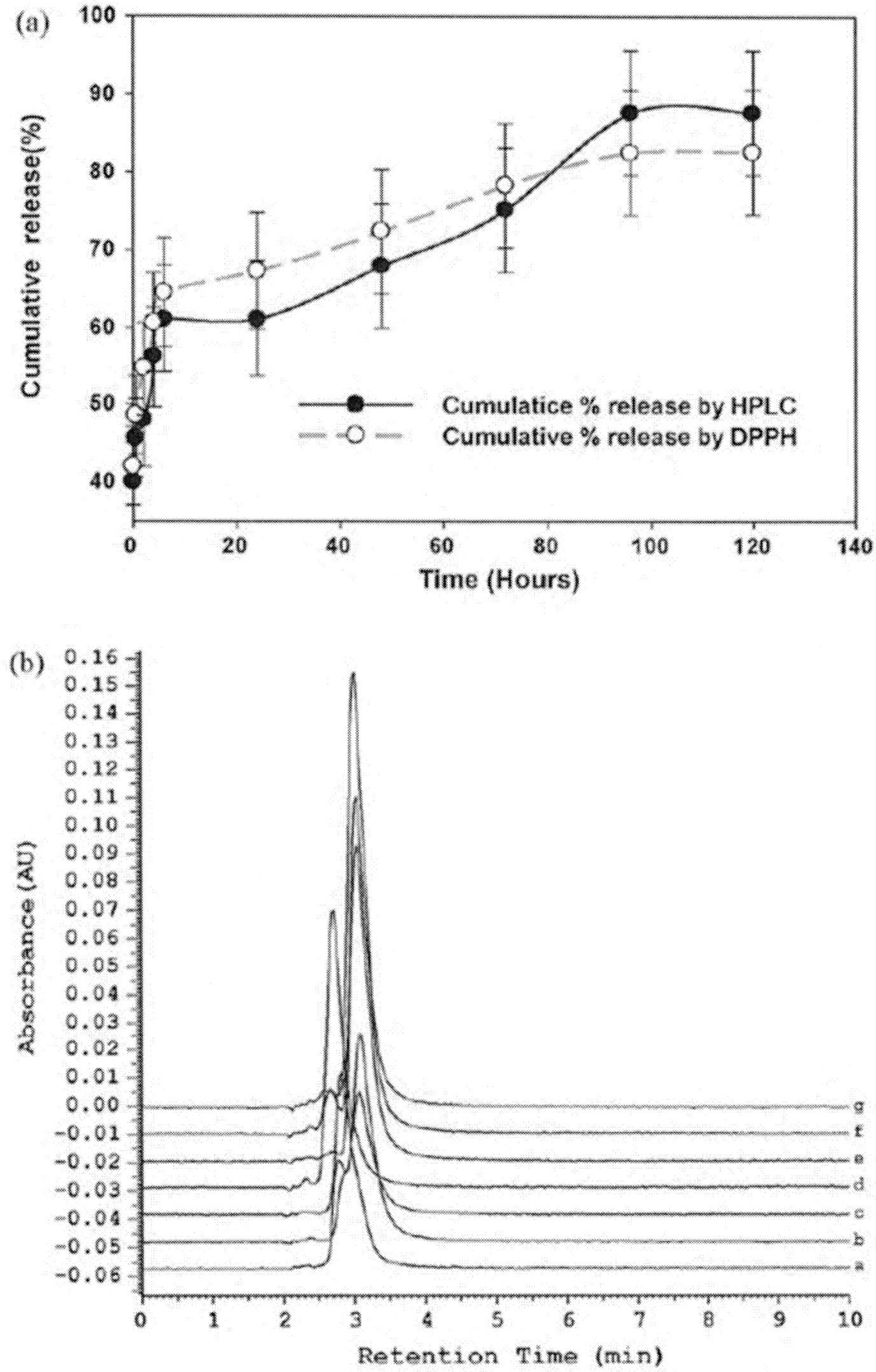

Source: ref. [25] – reprinted with permission.

Figure 10. (a) Release profile of quercetin from quercetin loaded PLA nanoparticles by HPLC and DPPH method. Release curve was obtained by plotting % of quercetin released vs. time. (b)HPLC chromatograms of release solutions after regular intervals recorded on HPLC.

The pharmacokinetic parameters of quercetin and QT-SLNs in rat plasma (Table 4) and the mean plasma concentration-time curve of quercetin in rat after a single oral dose (50 mg/kg) of quercetin suspension and QT-SLNs (Figure 11) demonstrated that the time of peak concentration (T_{max}) and mean residence time (MRT) were both prolonged, and the relative bioavailability of QT-SLNs to quercetin suspension (calculated as the ratio between the area under the curves of Figure 11) was 571.4%, with an improvement of more than 5 fold.

Another research group [9, 27] nanoencapsulated quercetin in poly(lactide-co-glycolide) (PLGA) using an emulsion-diffusion-evaporation method and investigated the therapeutic potential of their formulation in an oral route against arsenite-induced hepatic and neuronal cell damage in a rats model.

In this aim, the authors analyzed the liver and brain tissues of three experimental groups of rats exposed to an injection of sodium arsenite (13 mg/kg) and sacrificed 24 h after the treatment schedule. 90 min prior the arsenite injection the rats were fed with free quercetin (8.98 μmol/kg), nanoencapsulated quercetin (8.98 μmol/kg) or an empty nanocapsule suspension (control).

The effects of the free quercetin (QC) or nanoencapsulated quercetin (NPQC) on the changes in various components of the antioxidant defense system in hepatic and neuronal cells of rats by the induction of sodium arsenite were listed in Table 5.

The data demonstrate that the nanoencapsulated quercetin is very effective in prevent the liver and brain oxidative injury of arsenite-treated rats, whereas the free quercetin does not. The authors attributed the better performances of the nanoencapsulated formulation to the enhanced intracellular accumulation of quercetin by selective tissue-targeted delivery of nanocapsules.

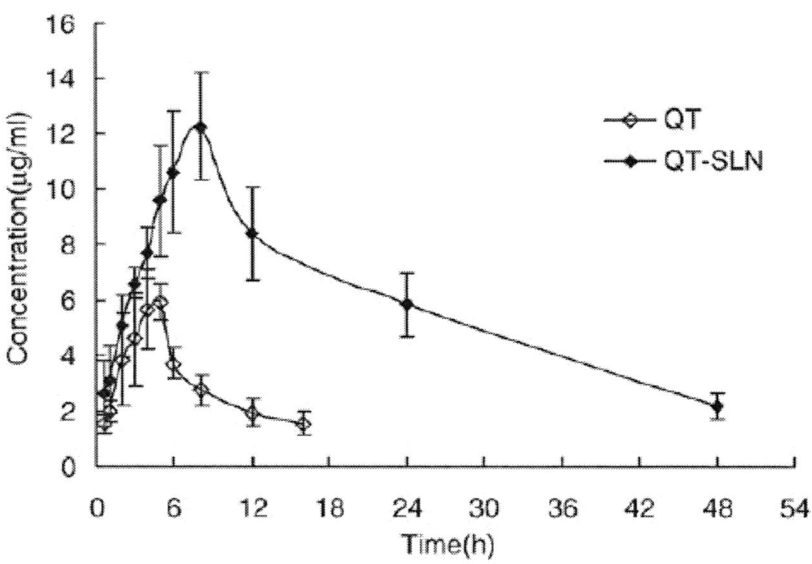

Source: ref. [26] – reprinted with permission.

Figure 11. The mean plasma concentration-time curve of quercetin in rat after a single oral dose (50 mg/kg) of quercetin suspension and QT-SLNs. Each data represents the mean±standard deviation of 5 rats.

In other studies the same authors [27-28] investigated for their hepatoprotective activity against arsenite quercetin-loaded liposomes. Comparing the results with those of a nanoencapsulated formulation, the researchers demonstrated that the quercetin has higher biological effectiveness in nanocapsule delivery systems than in liposomes in combating the acute arsenite induced hepatocellular oxidative damage.

In this regard, they prepared the multilamellar liposomes using phosphatidyl ethanolamine, cholesterol, dicetyl phosphate (DCP) and quercetin (QC) in molar ratio 7:1:1:1 and the nanocapsules using PLA as polymer matrix and QC in weigh ratio 4:1. The incorporation efficiency of quercetin was 89.9% for the liposomes and 45.5% for the nanocapsules.

The formulations were applied in the in vivo tests in order to evaluate the protective effects of quercetin in different delivery systems (free, liposomal and nanoencapsulated form) against the damage induced by arsenite in liver tissue of rats. The results of the tests are compared in Figure 12 and Table 6. The authors explained the higher activity of the nanoencapsulated quercetin compared to the liposomal formulation presuming that nanocapsules are more efficient in targeting the drug to hepatic cells giving a better accumulation of quercetin in liver.

Yuan et al. [8] found that liposomal quercetin efficiently suppresses growth of solid tumors in murine models.

The liposomes were chosen as quercetin vehicle for their ability to extravasate through the defects in the capillary endothelium of tumor tissues, where they are accumulated.

The authors investigated the pharmacokinetic properties and biodistribution in tumor-bearing and tested the anticancer efficacy of liposomal quercetin in vivo and in vitro. The study was performed using pegylated liposomal quercetin (Q-PEGL) and empty pegylated liposomes (PEGL), which sizes were in the range of 130±20nm and 100±20nm, respectively.

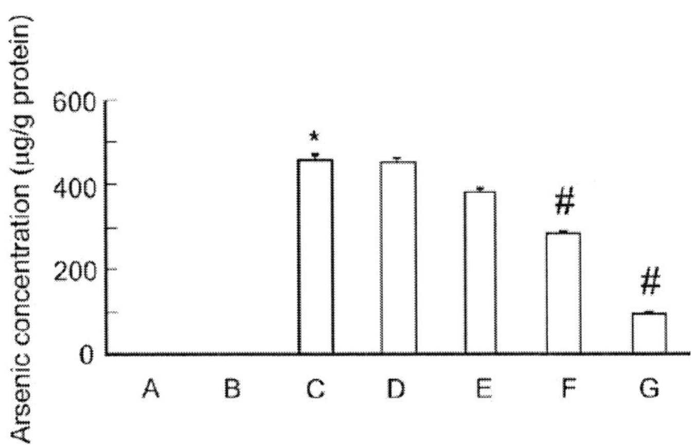

Source: ref. [27] – reprinted with permission.

Figure 12. Values of arsenic levels in liver tissue from normal, sodium arsenite and nanocapsulated QC treated rats. The groups are Normal (A), Normal + Nanoencapsulated QC treated (B), Arsenite treated (C), C + Empty nanocapsule treated (D), C + Free QC treated (E), C + Liposomal QC treated (F) and C + Nanoencapsulated QC treated (G). Values are mean±S.E. of five rats. *P < 0.001 significantly different from normal. #P < 0.001 significantly different from sodium arsenite treated rats.

Table 5. Effects of free quercetin (QC) or nanoencapsulated quercetin (NPQC) on the changes in various components of the antioxidant defense system in hepatic and neuronal cells of rats by the induction of sodium arsenite

	GP_x		G6PDH		Glutathione reductase		Catalase		Glutathione S transferase	
	Liver	Brain	Liver	Brain	Liver	Brain	Liver	Brain	Liver	Brain
	μmol NADPH oxidation/min/mg protein		nmol NADPH reduced/min/mg protein		μmol NADPH oxidation/min/mg protein		μmol H_2O_2 reduced/min/mg protein		nmol product/min/mg	
Normal	8.75±0.45	5.23±0.27	10.33±0.51	6.32±0.48	28.52±2.13	18.72±1.77	8.32±0.52	7.31±0.83	128.2±21.21	108.76±13.21
Sodium arsenite-treated (A)	3.92±0.18	2.17±0.09	6.17±0.48	3.61±0.29	13.79±1.67	9.92±0.87	4.69±0.31	2.79±0.54	73.91±11.76	69.26±9.88
(A)+Free QC-treated	4.22±0.21	2.81±0.13	6.82±0.39	3.97±0.18	11.82±0.96	10.11±1.33	5.17±0.62	3.17±0.82	98.72±17.32	72.66±5.98
(A)+empty nanocapsule-treated	3.87±0.19	2.23±0.17	6.72±0.51	3.58±0.27	14.82±2.32	10.73±2.11	4.87±0.39	2.92±0.61	78.72±12.11	62.18±10.26
(A)+QC Entrapped nanocapsule-treated	8.56±0.39	4.98±0.31	9.89±0.72	6.07±0.39	27.91±3.01	17.92±2.33	7.96±0.81	6.87±0.72	116.86±19.26	97.86±7.22

Results are expressed as mean±SD. The sodium arsenite-treated group was compared with the normal group, and the value was significantly different with $P<0.001$. The nanocapsulated QC-treated group was also compared with the sodium arsenite-treated group, and the value was also significantly different with $P<0.001$.

Source: ref. [9] – reprinted with permission.

Table 6. Effect of QC in free, liposomal and nanoencapsulated forms on the changes in the generation of reactive oxygen species (ROS) and lipid peroxidation levels in rat liver by the induction of sodium arsenite

Groups	DCF-fluorescence (% of normal)	Lipohydroperoxide (μmol/mg protein)
Normal (A)	100 ± 6.32	1.45 ± 0.01
(A) + Nanoencapsulated QC treated	103 ± 2.73	1.36 ± 0.06
$NaAsO_2$-treated (B)	300 ± 15.30*	2.75 ± 0.04*
(B) + Empty nanocapsule treated	290 ± 14.72*	2.63 ± 0.02*
(B) + Free QC treated	270 ± 13.55*	2.60 ± 0.03*
(B) + Liposomal QC treated	200 ± 10.02#	2.20 ± 0.04#
(B) + Nanoencapsulated QC treated	110 ± 7.11#	1.50 ± 0.01#

Spectrofluorimetric determination of DCF fluorescence as a measure of ROS generation in normal and experimental liver tissues. Results are expressed as % of normal cells, $n = 5$; mean ± S.E. *$P < 0.001$ represent significant differences from normal values (A). #$P < 0.001$ represent significant differences from sodium arsenite treated (B) values.

For Lipohydroperoxide levels, results are expressed as mean ± S.E. of five rats. *$P < 0.001$ significantly different from normal. #$P < 0.001$ significantly different from sodium arsenite treated (B).

Source: ref. [27] – reprinted with permission.

The authors found that the Q-PEGL prolonged blood circulation times of quercetin up to 2 h in plasma, whereas the lifetime of free quercetin was only 5 min.

They also verified that the encapsulation with PEGL induced highly accumulation of Q at the tumor sites, whereas free Q was widely distributed also in normal organs. Consequently, even if the antiproliferative activity in vitro of Q-PEGL was similar to that of free quercetin, in vivo the Q-PEGL treatment demonstrated higher efficacy.

Anyway, it should be pointed out that the treatment of mice with Q-PEGL did not result in the complete eradication of the tumor cells with the dose and schedules used in the study.

3. Cyclodextrin Inclusion Complexes

Vijaia et al. [29] investigated the possibility to improve the aqueous solubility and the dissolution properties of quercetin, preparing and characterizing cyclodextrin (CD) inclusion complexes of this flavonoid. CD inclusion complexes have been already demonstrated to be able to effectively improve the stability, solubility, dissolution rate and bioavailability of other drugs [30-33]. Morover, CD complexes with quercetin have been also prepared, but only their physicochemical and structural characterization has been reported [34-35].

In their study Vijaia et al. examined quercetin inclusion complexes with β-cyclodextrin (β-CD) and hydroxyl propyl-β-cyclodextrin (HP-β-CD), prepared by kneading and coevaporation methods.

The authors demonstrated that in the inclusion complexes Q reduces its crystallinity but it does not become completely amorphous. The dissolution studies evidences that the complexation with both CDs increases the solubility and the dissolution rate of the quercetin.

The amount of the effect depends on both system formulation and preparation method. Highest solubility and dissolution rate values were obtained in the case of HP-β-CD complexes prepared by the kneading method. The better effectiveness of HP-β-CD may be explained as a consequence of its greater water solubility and higher wetting and complexation ability.

4. NANOSUSPENSIONS

Gao et al. [36] obtained chemical- and photo-stable quercetin formulations through the nanosuspension technology.

Nanosuspensions are colloidal drug delivery systems stabilized by surfactants and containing pure drug particles with a nanometric particle sizes, typically ranging between 10 and 1000nm [37-38]. In their study Gao and co-workers prepared Q nanosuspensions using two different nanosuspension methods, the evaporative precipitation into aqueous solution (EPAS) and the high pressure homogenization (HPH), and characterized the obtained formulations in terms of chemical- and photo-stability. A control water solution containing about 0.8 mg/100mL of quercetin was tested in parallel. The results were reported in Figure 13 and 14.

The histograms show that both EPAS and HPH nanosuspensions stored at the same conditions do not undergo significant alterations in drug content over the monitoring period. Similar results were observed in the photostability studies (Figure 14). Only the control water solutions exhibit a reduction in drug content of 28.3% after 1-month conservation at 25°C (no light) and of 19.9% after 10 days of exposition to a fluorescent lamp.

To explain their findings the authors hypothesized that the nanosized drug particles may be protected by: (1) a layer of suspension stabilizer that cover their surface; and (2) a degraded outer monolayer of drug that shields the inner part of the nanoparticle from further degradation.

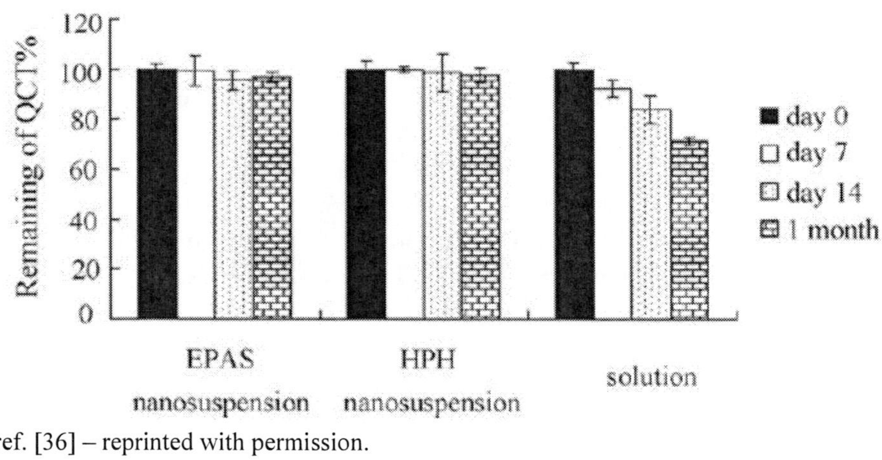

Source: ref. [36] – reprinted with permission.

Figure 13. Degradation of quercetin (QCT) in different formulations stored at 25°C in the light-shielding condition.

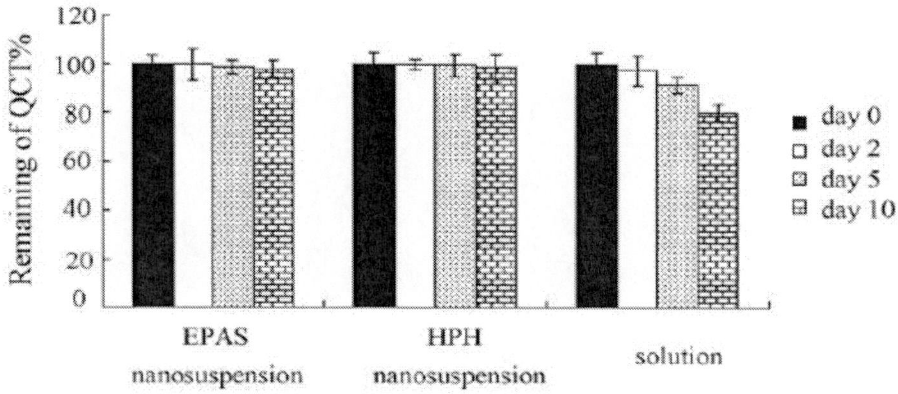

Source: ref. [36] – reprinted with permission.

Figure 14. Degradation of quercetin (QCT) in different formulations exposed to a continuous illuminance (2500 Lx supplied by a fluorescent lamps) for 10 days.

The authors also verified that both EPAS and HPH nanosuspensions give a quite complete release of Q after 40 min in phosphate buffer solution (PBS, pH 6.8), demonstrating that their method can be an effective route for improving the quercetin stability and bioavailability in skin delivery formulations.

5. MICROEMULSIONS

Several other researchers investigated the possibility to improve the efficiency of the intradermal delivery of the quercetin. Among them, Kitagawa et al. [39] experimented the usefulness of microemulsions evaluating the skin incorporation of Q through an in vitro study and measuring the anti-peroxidative activity of Q retained in the skin. After an initial screening of either water-in-oil (w/o) and oil-in-water (o/w) microemulsions targeted to formulate a system able to assure high quercetin solubility, the researchers choose as Q vehicle a w/o microemulsion, referred as microemulsion D, having the following composition: isopropyl myristate (33 wt%), NaCl solution 150 mM (7 wt%), Tween 80 (30 wt%) and ethanol (30 wt%). Then, this microemulsion was saturated with Q (Q solubility in the system is 78.6 ± 8.9 mM) and tested. Figure 15 shows the results of the in vitro experiments of skin accumulation of quercetin in Yucatan micropig skin.

The graph demonstrates that microemulsion D at saturated concentration of Q gives a very marked improvement of quercetin incorporation into the skin compared with that obtained when Q is applied as a suspension in NaCl solution or in isopropyl myristate. Moreover, the concentration–depth profile of quercetin in guinea-pig skin, shown in Figure 16, evidences that Q penetrates in deep skin layers, even if its concentration is higher near the surface. The Q retained in the skin was also resulted able to significantly inhibit the lipid peroxidation in a dose dependent manner (Figure 17).

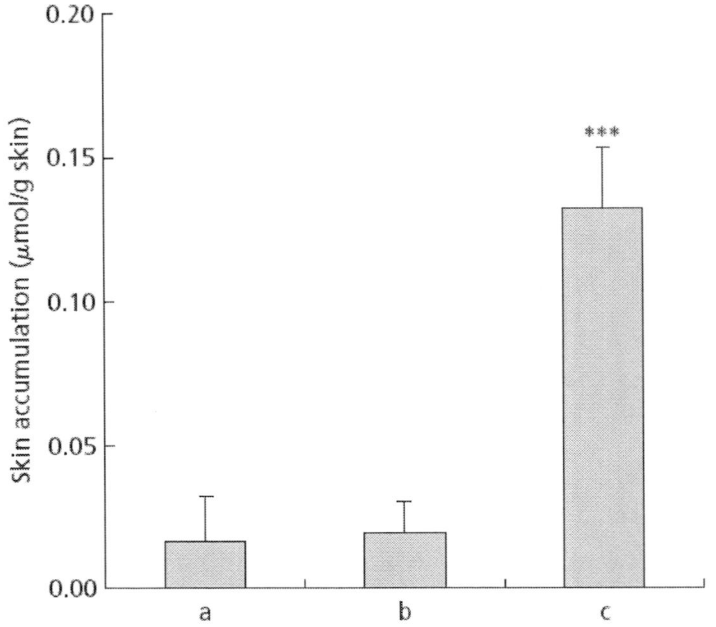

Source: ref. [39] – reprinted with permission.

Figure 15. Skin accumulation of quercetin in Yucatan micropig skin. Microemulsions were applied as a suspension in either 150 mM NaCl solution (a) or isopropyl myristate (b), as microemulsion D at saturated concentration (78.6 mM) (c). Data are the means ± SD of four experiments. ***$P < 0.001$, significantly different compared with the values in NaCl and isopropyl myristate.

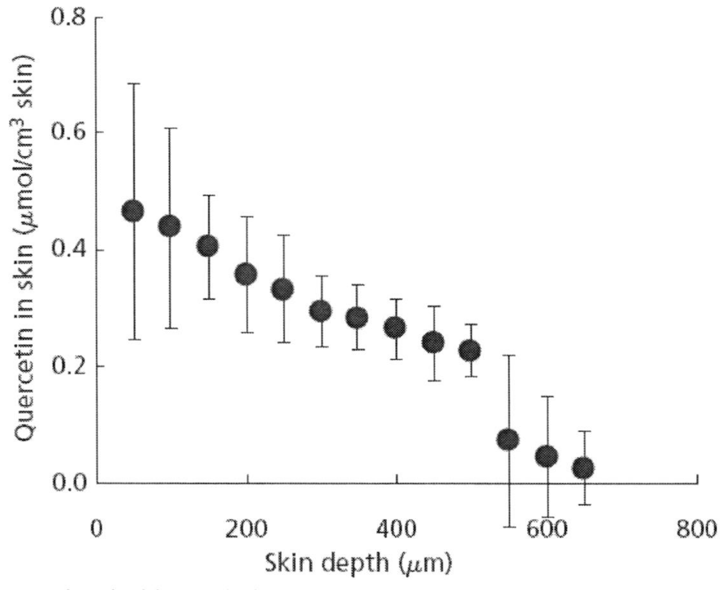

Source: ref. [39] – reprinted with permission.

Figure 16. Concentration–depth profile of quercetin in guinea-pig skin. Quercetin was applied with microemulsion D at saturated concentration (78.6 mM of Q). Data are the means ± SD of four experiments.

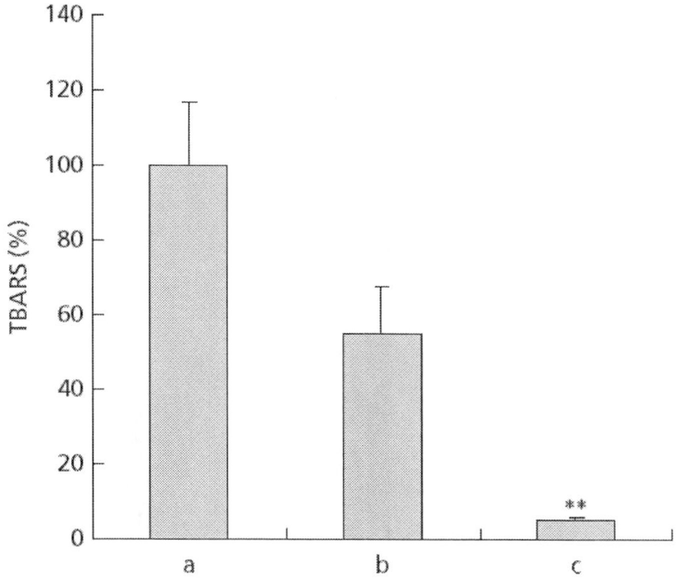

Source: ref. [39] – reprinted with permission.

Figure 17. Effect of quercetin on lipid peroxidation. The effect of quercetin was tested by using ammonium iron(II) sulfate and sodium citrate when applied with microemulsion D in guinea-pig skin at 0 mM (a), 20 mM (b) or saturated concentration (78.6 mM) (c). Data are the means ± SD of four experiments. TBARS, thiobarbituric acid reactive substances. **$P < 0.01$, significantly different compared with the value in the absence of quercetin.

Vicentini et al. [40] investigated the potential of another w/o microemulsion measuring in vitro and in vivo skin penetration of Q and evaluating in vivo the efficacy of their formulation against skin damages induced by UVB irradiation.

The microemulsion that they tested has the following composition: mixture of polypropylene glycol and water 3:1 (15 wt%); mixture of Span 80 and Tween 80 3:1 (46.75 wt%); canola oil (38.25 wt%). Quercetin was incorporated to the w/o microemulsion by dissolving it in the oil phase at saturation level (0.3 wt%).

Using this formulation Vicentini and co-workers measured quercetin skin penetration by in vitro and in vivo tests, obtaining results similar to those reported by Tanaka and above described. In particular, Figure 18 shows the in vivo skin penetration of quercetin at 6 h following its topical application on hairless mice using the w/o microemulsion or a control formulation (i.e. a solution of quercetin in polypropylene glycol at 0.3 wt%).

The histogram evidences that the w/o microemulsion increases the quercetin level both in the stratum corneum and in the epidermis + dermis of 1.5 and 2 times, respectively.

The authors verified also the good tolerability of the developed formulation by evaluating three established endpoints of skin irritation: erythema formation, epidermis thickening and infiltration of inflammatory cells.

After 2 days of daily application of the w/o microemulsion no erythema formation or histopathological alteration were induced.

The w/o microemulsion resulted also effective against skin damage induced by UVB irradiation. In fact, it was able to significantly inhibit the UVB irradiation-induced depletion of the glutathione (GSH) skin content compared to the control groups (untreated-unexposed), as shown in Figure 19. The results are in agreement with those reported by Skaper et al. [41] and Casagrande et al. [42] about the protective effectiveness of Q against the GSH depletion induced by several stress factors.

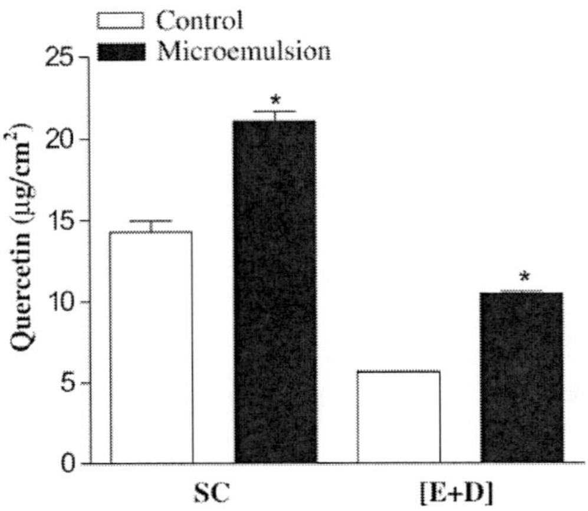

Source: ref. [40] – reprinted with permission.

Figure 18. In vivo skin penetration of quercetin at 6 h following its topical application using the w/o microemulsion or control formulation. SC, stratum corneum, [E + D]: epidermis (without SC) plus dermis. Results are represented by means ± S.D. (n = 5). Statistical analysis was performed by one-way ANOVA followed by Bonferroni's test of multiple comparisons. *Significant statistical difference compared to control (propylene glycol formulation) ($p < 0.05$).

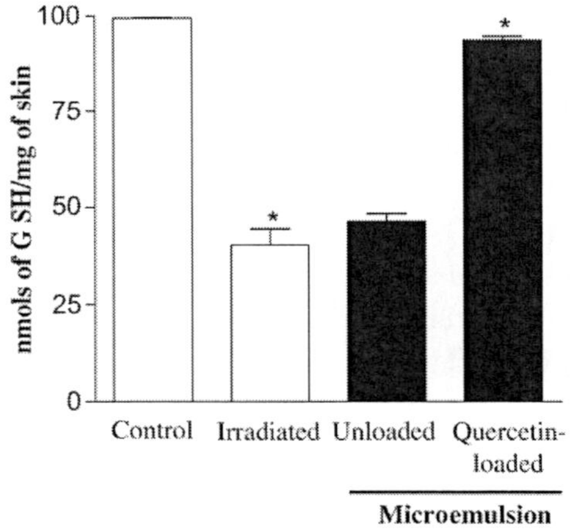

Source: ref. [40] – reprinted with permission.

Figure 19. Effect of w/o microemulsion containing quercetin on the decrease of the endogenous antioxidant GSH system induced by UVB irradiation. Bars represent means ± S.E.M. of three separated experiments, 3–5 animals per group. Statistical analysis was performed by one-way ANOVA followed by Bonferroni's test of multiple comparisons. *$p < 0.05$ compared to the respective control (untreated–unexposed or irradiated treated with unloaded microemulsion groups).

All the findings about the effectiveness of the above reported microemulsions in promoting the skin quercetin delivery can be explained considering that: (1) the flavonoid is introduced into the formulations at saturation level, which ensures the highest thermodynamic activity and consequently the higher permeation rate of the drug; (2) due to low interfacial tension and low droplet size of microemulsions, the contact surface between the skin and the drug carrier system is particularly high and hence the drug absorption is improved [43]; (3) several constituents of the microemulsion (surfactants and oil molecules) act as enhancers either by disrupting the lipid structure of the stratum corneum, increasing the drug diffusivity through this barrier layer, or by increasing the solubility of the drug in the skin.

6. Transdermal Systems

Dias et al. [44] used supercritical carbon dioxide to develop natural-based wound dressings impregnated with quercetin for transdermal delivery applications.

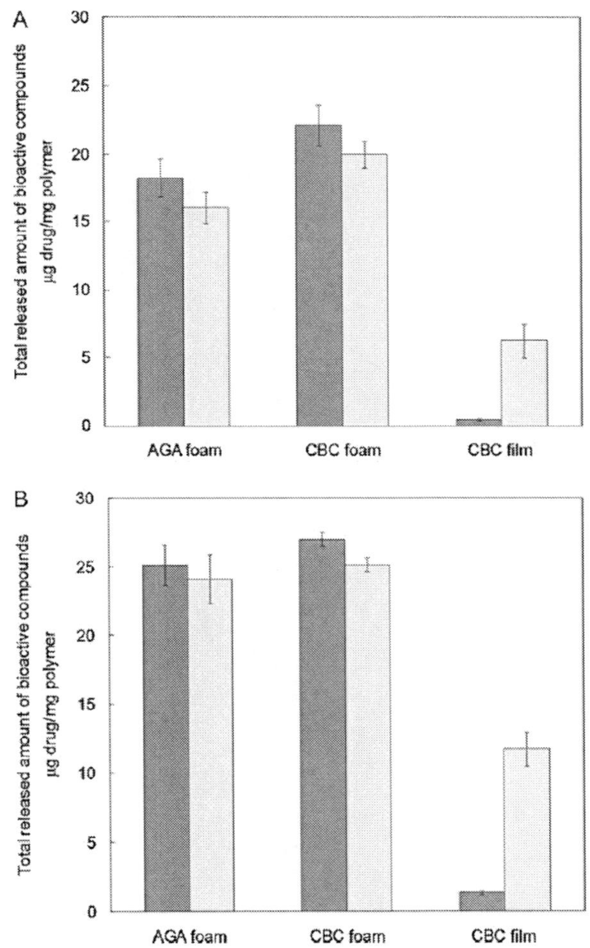

Source: ref. [44] – reprinted with permission.

Figure 20. Quercetin and thymol total/cumulative released amounts from AGA (foams) and from CBC (films and foams) after a 9 h release period. Experiments performed at different SSI experimental conditions: (A) 10MPa and 303 K; (B) 20MPa and 313 K. Results for quercetin (•) and for thymol (▲) loaded separately.

Film- and foam-like structures of N-carboxybutylchitosan (CBC) and of agarose (AGA) were prepared, loaded with quercetin or a mixture of quercetin and thymol by supercritical solvent impregnation (SSI) method using different operative conditions, then submitted to in vitro release tests.

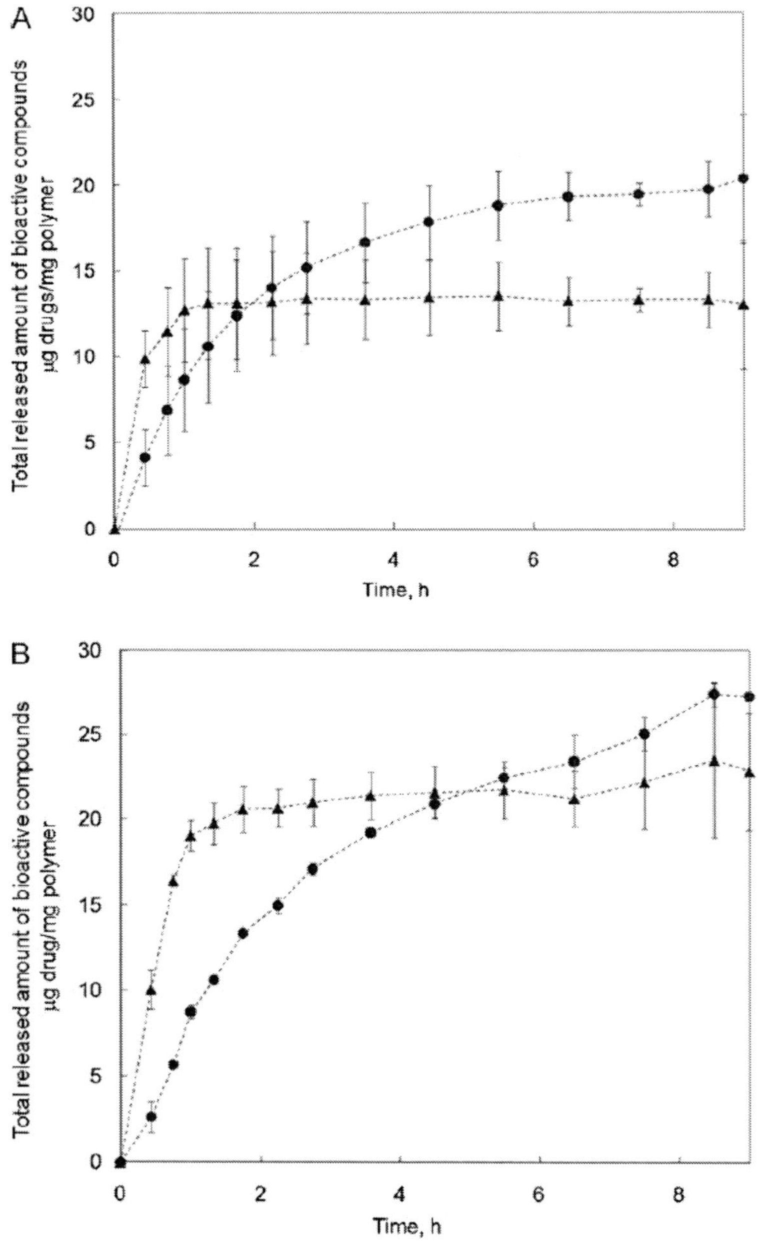

Source: ref. [44] – reprinted with permission.

Figure 21. Quercetin and thymol total/cumulative released amounts from CBC foams for a 9 h release period. Experiments performed with the simultaneous loading of quercetin (●) and thymol (▲), at different SSI experimental conditions: (A) 10MPa and 303 K; (B) 20MPa and 313 K. Lines serve only as guides for the eye.

Figure 20 compares the quercetin and thymol total/cumulative released amounts from AGA (foams) and from CBC (films and foams) after a 9 h release period (the results are for quercetin and for thymol loaded separately).

The histogram shows that: (1) the loaded amounts of quercetin are always slightly higher than the loaded amounts of thymol at both experimental pressure–temperature conditions; (2) the foam structures give the highest cumulative release amounts of both quercetin and thymol at each operative condition of the SSI process, as a consequence of their high porosity that allowed higher loadings of the drugs compared to the film substrate. On the basis of these findings, the authors focused the dissolution studies on the CBC foams.

Figure 21 shows the dissolution profiles of CBC foams simultaneously loaded with quercetin and thymol. The graphs evidence that the total released amount of the drugs at the end of the test depends on the operative conditions of the SSI process, being higher at higher pressure/temperature conditions.

Moreover, quercetin has a more sustained release than thymol. This can be justified considering its lower solubility in water, its higher molecular volume (which slows its diffusion through the polymeric network) and some specific favorable interactions between quercetin and CBC. Based on these results, the authors demonstrated that the SSI loading can be a feasible and advantageous process for loading of bioactive substances, even as a mixture, into previously prepared polymeric matrixes and that the loaded amounts of these substances can be tuned by opportunely changing the operational pressure-temperature conditions. Therefore, several pharmaceutical and tissue engineering applications can be envisaged for the SSI technique.

CONCLUSION

The development of drug carrier systems for delivering of quercetin and other very poor soluble drugs is a challenge issue. The need to have appropriate formulations able not only to improve the quercetin solubility, bioavailability and stability, but also to target the flavonoid to a particular destination in the body has attracted the interest of many researchers. A lot of quercetin delivery systems differing for the preparation technique, the physical nature, the constituents and the intended administration route were investigated in order to evaluate their effectiveness. Although the high variety of the considered systems makes difficult to organically systematize the reported results, some general remarks can be made. The incorporation of quercetin in particulated and vesicular systems (i.e. microparticles, nanoparticles, nanoemulsions, liposomes) is an effective tool to increase the bioavailability of the flavonoid and its chemical- and photo-stability when exposed to degradative environments. The largest improvements in terms of quercetin solubility and release behavior were obtained in formulations containing the drug in the amorphous state. The correct choice of the co-formulating agents (polymeric vehicles, surfactants, enhancers, etc.) can allow to modulate the release kinetic and to target the release to specific tissue, as demonstrated by in vitro and in vivo assays. Therefore, the application of devices with different quercetin release capacities may be useful as therapeutic approach for the treatment of several diseases.

REFERENCES

[1] Kuhnau, *J. World Rev. Nutr. Diet* 1976, 24, 117-191.
[2] Olthof, M. R.; Hollman, P. C.; Vree, T. B.; Katan, M. B. *J. Nutr.,* 2000, 130, 1200-1203.
[3] Lamson, D. W.; Brignall, M. S. *Altern. Med. Rev.,* 2000, 5, 196-208.
[4] Morand, C.; Crespy, V.; Manach, C.; Besson, C.; Demigne, C.; Remesy, *C. Am. J. Physiol. Regul. Integr. Comp. Physiol.* 1998, 44, R212-r219.
[5] Memorial Sloan-Kettering Cancer Center. About herbs: Quercetin. 2005. Available at: http://www. mskcc.org/mskcc /html/ 69346.cfm# ClinicalFindings. Accessed April 2 2007.
[6] Pe´rez-Mateos, M.; Bravo, L.; Goya, L.; Go´mez-Guille´n, C.; Montero, P. *J. Sci. Food Agric.,* 2005, 85, 1651-1659.
[7] Wadworth, A. N.; Faulds, D. Drugs 1992, 44, 1013-1032.
[8] Yuan, Z.P., Chen, L.J., Fan, L.Y., Tang, M.H., Yang, G.L., Yang, H.S., Du, X.B., Wang, G.Q., Yao, W.X., Zhao, Q.M., Ye, B., Wang, R., Diao, P., Zhang, W., Wu, H.B., Zhao, X., Wei, Y.Q., *Clin. Cancer. Res*., 2006, 12, 3193–3199.
[9] Ghosh, A.; Mandal, A.K.; Sarkar, S.; Panda, S.; Das, N. *Life Sci*., 2009, 84, 75–80.
[10] Vicentini, F.; Simi, T.; Del Ciampo, J.; Wolga, N.; Pitol, D.; Iyomasa, M.; Bentley, M.V.; Fonseca, M.J.V.; Eur. *J. Pharm. Biopharm*. 2008, 69, 948-957.
[11] Bhattaram, V.A.; Graefe, U.; Kohlert, C.; Veit, M.; Derendorf, H.; *Phytomedicine.* 2002, 9, 1–33.
[12] Ader, P.; Wessmann, A.; Wolffram, S.; *Free Radic. Biol. Med*., 2000, 28, 1056-1067.
[13] Lauro, M.R.; Torre, M.L.; Maggi, L.; De Simone, F.; Conte, U.; Aquino, R.P. *Drug Dev Ind Pharm.,* 2002, 28(4), 372-379.
[14] Lauro, M.R.; Maggi, L.; Conte, U.; De Simone, F.; Aquino, R.P. *J. Drug Del. Sci. Tech.,* 2005, 15(5), 363-369.
[15] Scarfato, P.; Avallone, E.; Iannelli, P.; Aquino, R. P.; Lauro, M. R.; Rossi, A.; Acierno, D. *J. Appl. Polym. Sci*., 2008, 109, 2994–3001.
[16] Edgar, K. *J. Cellulose.,* 2007, 14, 49-64.
[17] Sansone, F.; Picerno, P.; Mencherini, T.; Villecco, F.; D'Ursi, A.M.; Aquino, R.P.; Lauro, M.R. *J. Food Eng.,* 2011, 103, 188–196.
[18] Mencherini, T., Picerno, P., Scesa, C., Aquino, R.P. *J. Nat., Prod* 2007, 70(12), 1889–1894.
[19] Scalia, S.; Mezzena, M. *J. Pharmaceut. Biomed. Anal.,* 2009, 49, 90–94.
[20] Wiechers, *J.W. Cosmet. Toil*., 2000, 115, 39–46.
[21] Song, X.; Zhao, Y.; Hou, S.; Xu, F.; Zhao, R.; He, J.; Cai, Z.; Li, Y.; Chen, Q. *Eur. J. Pharm. Biopharm.,* 2008, 69, 445–453.
[22] Zhang, Y.; Yang, Y.; Tang, K.; Hu, X.; Zou, G. *J. Appl. Polym. Sci*., 2008, 107, 891–897.
[23] Wu, T.-H.; Yen, F.-L.; Lin, L.-T.; Tsai, T.-R.; Lin, C.-C.; Cham, T.-M. *Int. J. Pharm*., 2008, 346, 160–168.
[24] Bilati, U., Allemann, E., Doelker, E. Eur. *J. Pharm. Sci*., 2005, 24, 67–75.
[25] Kumari, A.; Yadav, S. K.; Pakade, Y.B.; Singh, B.; Yadav, *S.C. Colloids Surf. B Biointerfaces*., 2010, 80, 184–192.

[26] Li, H.; Zhao, X.; Ma, Y.; Zhai, G.; Li, L.; Lou, H. *J. Control. Rel.,* 2009, 133, 238–244.
[27] Ghosh, D.; Ghosh, S.; Sarkar, S.; Ghosh, A.; Dasa, N.; Das Saha, K.; Mandal, A.K. *Chem. Biol. Interact.,* 2010, 186, 61–71.
[28] Mandal, A.K.; Das, S.; Basu, M. K.; Chakrabarti, R. N.; Das, N. *J. Pharmacol. Exp. Ther.*, 2007, 320(3), 994-1001.
[29] Vijaya Sri, K.; Kondaiah, A.; Vijaya Ratna, J.; Annapurna, A. *Drug. Dev. Ind. Pharm.*, 2007, 33, 245–253.
[30] Stella, V.J.; Rajewski, R. A. *Pharm. Res*., 1997, 14, 556–567.
[31] Rajewski, R. A.; Stella, V.J. *J. Pharm. Sci*., 1996, 85(11), 1142–1168.
[32] Loftsson, T.; Brewster, M. E. *J. Pharm. Sci*., 1996, 85(10), 1017–1025.
[33] Arun, R.; Ashok, K.C.K.; Sravanthi, V.V.N.S.S. *Sci Pharm*., 2008, 76, 567–598.
[34] Zheng, Y.; Haworth, I. S.; Zuo, Z.; Chow, M. S. S.; Chow, A. H. L. *J. Pharm. Sci*., 2005, 94(5), 1079–1086.
[35] Pralhad, T.; Rajendrakumar, K. *J. Pharm. Biomed Anal*., 2004, 34, 333–339.
[36] Gao, L.; Liu, G.; Wang, X.; Liu, F.; Xu, Y.; Ma, *J. Int J Pharm.,* 2011, 404, 231–237.
[37] Keck, C.M.; Müller, R.H. *Eur. Pharm. Biopharm*., 2006, 62, 3–16.
[38] Gao, L., Zhang, D., Chen, M. *J. Nanopart., Res*. 2008, 10, 845–862.
[39] Kitagawa, S.; Tanaka, Y.; Tanaka, M.; Endo, K.; Yoshii, A. *J Pharm Pharmacol.,* 2009; 61, 855–860.
[40] Vicentini, F.T.M.C.; Simi, T.R.M.; Del Ciampo, J.O.; Wolga, N.O.; Pitol, D.L.; Iyomasa, M.M.; Bentley, M.V.L.B.; Fonseca, M.J.V. *Eur. J. Pharm. Biopharm*., 2008, 69, 948–957.
[41] Skaper, S.D.; Fabris, M.; Ferrari, V.; Carbonare, M.D.; Leon, A. *Free Radic. Biol. Med*., 1997, 22, 669–678.
[42] Casagrande, R.; Georgetti, S.R.; Verri W.A. Jr.; Dorta, D.J.; dos Santos, A.C.; Fonseca, M.J.V. *J. Photochem. Photobiol. B: Biol*., 2006, 84, 21–27.
[43] Kreilgaard, M. Adv. Drug Deliv. Rev. 2002, 54, S77–S98.
[44] Dias, A.M.A.; Braga, M.E.M.; Seabra, I.J.; Ferreira, P.; Gil, M.H.; de Sousa, H.C. *Int. J. Pharm*., 2011, 408, 9–19.

In: Quercetin
Editors: Taiki Chikamatsu and Yuudai Hida
ISBN: 978-1 61942- 057-1

Chapter 10

THE ACTION OF QUERCETIN ON OXYGEN UPTAKE BY UNCOUPLED MITOCHONDRIA OXIDIZING VARIOUS SUBSTRATES

Jorgete Constantin, Nair Seiko Yamamoto,* Gisele Dias Buss, Rodrigo Polimeni Constantin, Emy Luiza Ishii-Iwamoto and Adelar Bracht
Laboratory of Liver Metabolism, University of Maringá, Maringá, Brazil

ABSTRACT

The action of quercetin on oxygen uptake by uncoupled rat liver mitochondria was measured. Quercetin clearly inhibited oxygen uptake with several substrates. With 300 μM quercetin the inhibition degrees with the following substrates were: citrate, 73%; β-hydroxybutyrate, 68%; α-ketoglutarate, 67%; isocitrate, 41%, α-glycerophosphate, 38%. With fumarate, oxaloacetate and succinate no significant inhibition was found. Quercetin also inhibited oxygen uptake during the oxidation of various activated fatty acids with well-defined concentration dependencies.

The degrees of inhibition with 300 μM quercetin were: octanoyl-carnitine, 83%; octanoyl-CoA, 82%; palmitoyl-CoA, 74%; oleoyl-CoA, 74%; palmitoyl-carnitine, 70%; and stearoyl-CoA, 67%. An action of quercetin on the fatty acyl-carnitine transferases is unlikely because octanoyl-CoA permeates the inner mitochondrial membrane as easily as octanoyl-carnitine or long-chain fatty acyl-carnitines and oxygen uptake with octanoyl-CoA was equally inhibited.

Although direct action on dehydrogenases cannot be ruled out, the inhibition of NADH-oxidase activity suggests inhibitory effects on electron flow probably by acting on the respiratory chain complex I. This assumption was corroborated by experiments with disrupted mitochondria in which the effects of quercetin on membrane-bound enzymatic activities were measured. Quercetin did not affect succinate-oxidase activity, but inhibited NADH-oxidase activity in a dose dependent manner. There is also the possibility of generation of prooxidant metabolites in the respiratory chain by quercetin

* E-mail: nsyamamoto@uem.br, Fax: 55-44-3011-4896.

which could lead to a competition for NADH between the respiratory chain and the quercetin metabolites, anticipating NADH oxidation.

Keywords: Flavonoids, quercetin, liver metabolism, mitochondrial metabolism, NADH oxidation, prooxidant mechanisms

INTRODUCTION

Flavonoids are members of a class of natural compounds that has recently been the subject of considerable scientific and therapeutic interest. The flavonoids are usually classified as secondary plant metabolites and are a class of variable polyphenolic compounds (Constantin and Bracht, 2008). In general, the flavonoids are compounds of low molecular weight and its basic structure is formed by three rings, as illustrated in Figure 1. The first ring, A, is aromatic and is conjugated to the second ring, C, which is heterocyclic with an oxygen atom. These two rings are linked by means of a C-C bond to a third ring, B, which is also aromatic (Peterson and Dwyer, 1998; Strack, 1997). According to the chemical structures around the heterocyclic ring C, the flavonoids can be divided into six main classes: flavonols, flavones, flavanones, catechins, anthocyanidins and isoflavonoids, as illustrated in Figure 1. Substitutions in the aromatic rings A and B, such as hydroxylations, glycosylations, methylations, sulfations and glucuronidations, are equally possible (Hollman and Katan, 1997). Over 4000 structurally unique flavonoids have been identified in plant sources (Harborne, 1986; Harbone, 1988a,b). Primarily recognized as the pigments responsible for the autumnal burst of hues and the many shades of yellow, orange, and red in flowers and food (Timberlake and Henry, 1986; Brouillard and Cheminant, 1988), the flavonoids are widely distributed in foods and beverages of plant origin, such as fruits, vegetables, tea, cocoa, and wine. Actually, a large body of literature exists regarding their content in various foods, but they are prominent components of citrus fruits (Kefford and Chandler, 1970) and other particular food sources (Herrmann, 1976) and are regular constituents of the normal human diet. Within the class of flavonols, the flavonoid quercetin (3,5,7,3',4'-pentahydroxyflavone, Figure 1) is the most frequently occurring compound in foods. Also common are kaempferol, myricetin, and the flavones apigenin and luteolin. Tea and onions are the main dietary sources of flavonols and flavones. Quercetin is the most abundant flavonol present in apples and onions, whereas tea contains notable amounts of both quercetin and kaempferol (Ross and Kasum, 2002).

The dietary flavonoids are more frequently found with a sugar moiety linked in the position 3 of ring C (Day *et al.*, 1998) or in positions 5 and 7 of ring A. Flavonoids with sugar moieties linked to the B ring, though uncommon, have also been described. Glucose, galactose, rhamnose, xylose and arabinose are the sugars most frequently found in association with the flavonoids, linked most frequently by O and C glycosylation. When not linked to sugars, the flavonoids are termed aglycones and they appear in several structural classes according to the oxidation state of the central pyrene ring (Strack, 1997).

As previously mentioned, the flavonoids are commonly part of the human diet, but there is no general agreement about the quantities that are ingested daily. For example, the average daily intake in the Netherlands is estimated to be 23 mg/day (Hertog *et al.*, 1993). However, flavonoid intakes seem to vary greatly between countries, the lowest intakes (≈2.6 mg/day) are in Finland and the highest intakes (68.2 mg/day) are in Japan (Hertog *et al.*, 1995; Friesenecker *et al.*, 1995; Haenen and Bast, 1999).

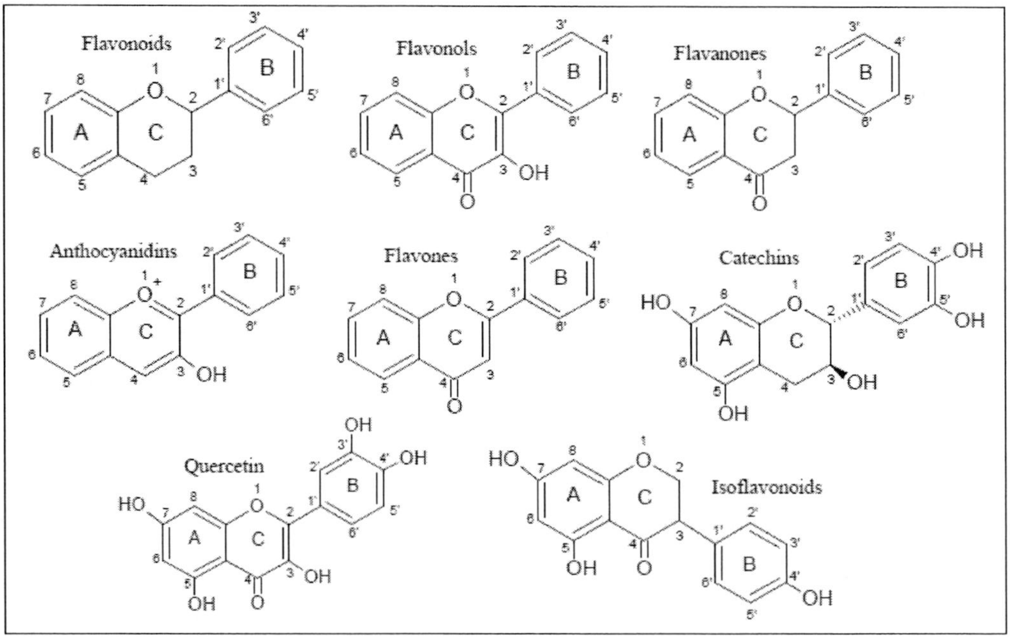

Figure 1. The basic structure of the flavonoids and its main classes with numbering scheme and ring labels. The structure of quercetin, the most abundant flavonoid, with numbering scheme and ring labels.

Intakes of flavonoids exceed those of vitamin E and β-carotene, whereas the average intake of vitamin C is three times higher than the intake of flavonoids. Quercetin is the most important contributor to the estimated intake of flavonoids, mainly from the consumption of tea, apples and onions (Knekt *et al.*, 1997). A major problem in studies on flavonoid intakes is that only a limited number of flavonoids can be measured in biological samples, and more importantly, only a relatively small number of fruits and vegetables are used to make an accurate estimation (Nijveldt *et al.*, 2001). It is assumed for sure that the amounts of flavonoids that are ingested in a normal diet are unable to induce mutations or cytotoxicity. However, the supplementary ingestion of flavonoids, particularly as antioxidants, has been currently recommended in terms of grams and not milligrams, a practice that could well result in toxic levels of exposition (Constantin and Bracht, 2008). For some manufactured formulas containing quercetin, for example, doses of 500 and 1000 mg per day are being indicated. This corresponds to 10 or 20 times of what would be ingested daily in a typical vegetarian diet. This suggests that commercialized formulations containing flavonoids, which are recommended for their real or imaginary beneficial effects, could be equally provoking reactions that are adverse to human health (Skibola and Smith, 2000). This is particularly true for quercetin, the compound of this class that possibly exerts the greatest variety of biological effects in mammalian cells (Constantin and Bracht, 2008). Biological activities ascribed to quercetin include its antiviral (Boers *et al.*, 1998; ElAttar and Virji, 1999), anti-inflammatory (Kim *et al.*, 1998), antiproliferative (Ferry *et al.*, 1996; Kawaii *et al.*, 1999), and antimicrobial properties (Aziz *et al.*, 1998). Due to absorption differences in conjugated forms, the bioavailability of quercetin varies greatly in foods. Researchers found that the absorption of quercetin-β-glycosides was far greater than the absorption of quercetin without its sugar moiety (Hollman *et al.*, 1999). Additionally, the quercetin glycosides in onions are more readily absorbed than those found in tea (de Vries *et al.*, 1997). The substantial daily exposure of the human body to the flavonoids, mainly to quercetin, in the normal diet or in commercial formulations containing flavonoids, is a good reason for scientists from several areas (for example, biochemistry, toxicology and nutrition) to develop studies involving flavonoids (Skibola and Smith, 2000). Work in our laboratory has demonstrated that quercetin affects liver metabolism in many ways. It increases glycogenolysis and glycolysis from endogenous sources (Gasparin *et al.,* 2003a), decreases gluconeogenesis from lactate and pyruvate and decreases glycolysis from exogenous glucose (Gasparin *et al.*, 2003b). It also decreases the cytosolic as well as the mitochondrial NADH to NAD^+ ratios, shifting the cellular environment to a more oxidized state (Gasparin *et al.*, 2003b; Buss *et al.*, 2005). This action seems to result from the ability of quercetin in promoting the oxidation of NADH in a reaction which depends on endogenous hydrogen peroxide (H_2O_2) and on the generation of *o*-hemiquinones by liver peroxidases or similar enzymatic systems (Chan *et al.*, 1999; Buss *et al.*, 2005). The action of quercetin on oxygen uptake, on the other hand, is quite complex: stimulation tends to occur at lower concentrations and inhibition at higher ones. The turning point from stimulation to inhibition depends on the metabolic state of the liver and on the perfusion conditions (Gasparin *et al.*, 2003a,b; Buss *et al.*, 2005). In isolated rat liver mitochondria, inhibition of oxygen consumption by quercetin was found only during the phosphorylation of exogenously added ADP (state III respiration). This inhibition can be partly caused by an inhibition of the ATP-synthase/ATPase; a phenomenon which was indeed detected experimentally (Gasparin *et al.*, 2003a). On the other hand, mitochondria phosphorylating exogenous ADP are in a condition where respiration is accelerated to levels which can be relatively close to the maximal capacities of the enzymatic systems catalyzing the oxidation-reduction reactions (electron transport chain and soluble dehydrogenases). In this respect, the possibility exists that inhibition of the enzymes catalyzing the oxidation-reduction reactions coupled to the ATP-synthase occurs in such a way that oxygen uptake is affected only when the former are the rate-limiting components. From the available experimental data (Gasparin *et al.*, 2003a; Buss *et al.*, 2005) it is difficult or even impossible to deduce the relative contribution of both the oxidation-reduction reactions and the ATP-synthase reaction to the whole process of oxygen uptake inhibition by quercetin. There is another experimental condition, however, where oxygen uptake by isolated mitochondria depends solely on the capacities of the enzymatic systems involved in electron transfer (a specific dehydrogenase + respiratory chain), without any limitation by the ATP-synthase. Such a condition can be induced by uncoupling oxidative phosphorylation from the electron transport chain using uncouplers such as 2,4-dinitrophenol, for example. In order to gain more information about the action of quercetin on the mitochondrial metabolism, several experiments were done in which oxygen uptake by uncoupled rat liver mitochondria was measured at various quercetin concentrations and using various substrates as sources of reducing equivalents. These substrates were several Krebs cycle intermediates, β-hydroxybutyrate, α-glycerophosphate and several forms of activated fatty acids. A second series of experiments was done in which oxygen consumption by freeze-thawing disrupted rat liver mitochondria was measured at various quercetin concentrations using NADH and succinate as sources of reducing equivalents. These mitochondrial preparations allow a direct assessment of quercetin actions on NADH- and succinate-oxidases activities. Furthermore additional sets of experiments were done to evaluate if quercetin causes catalytic oxidation of NADH by alternative mechanisms in disrupted rat liver mitochondria. The results presented in this chapter, amongst others from previous works, should provide a better understanding about the actions of quercetin on mitochondrial and liver metabolism. This additional information could increase our knowledge about the physiological and toxicological effects of the flavonoid quercetin.

MATERIALS AND METHODS

Materials

Enzymes and coenzymes used in the assay procedures and quercetin were purchased from Sigma Chemical Co. (St. Louis, USA). All other chemicals were from the best available grade.

Isolation of Rat Liver Mitochondria

Fasted rats (Wistar strain), weighing between 200 and 280 g, were decapitated and their livers removed immediately and cut into small pieces. These tissue fragments were suspended in a medium containing 0.2 M mannitol, 75 mM sucrose, 1.0 mM Tris-HCl (pH 7.4), 1 mM ethylene glycol-bis-(b-aminoethylether) tetraacetic acid (EGTA) and 50 mg% fatty acid-free bovine serum albumin. Homogenization was carried out in the same medium by means of a van Potter–Elvehjem homogenizer. After homogenization, the mitochondria were isolated by differential centrifugation (Voss *et al.*, 1961; Bracht *et al.*, 2003) and suspended in the same medium, which was kept at 0–4°C. Protein content of the mitochondrial suspensions was measured by means of the method described by Lowry *et al.* (1951), using the Folin-phenol reagent and bovine-serum albumin as a standard.

Oxygen Uptake of Uncoupled Mitochondria Oxidizing Fatty Acids

Oxygen in the incubation medium was measured polarographically using a teflon-shielded platinum electrode (Clark, 1956; Voss *et al.,* 1961). The incubation medium was composed of 2 mM potassium phosphate, 10 mM 4-(2-hydroxyethyl)-1-piperazine-ethanesulfonic acid (HEPES pH 7.2), 0.1 mM ethylene glycol-bis(β-aminoethyl ether)-N,N′,N′,N′-tetraacetic acid (EGTA), 130 mM potassium chloride, 2.5 mM magnesium chloride, 0.1 mM 2,4-dinitrophenol (DNP), 2.5 mM L-malate, 200 mg% fatty acid-free bovine-serum albumin (Garland *et al.*, 1969), several activated forms of fatty acids and various quercetin concentrations. The fatty acids were: (a) 20 μM palmitoyl-L-carnitine; (b) 20 μM palmitoyl-CoA + 2.0 mM L-carnitine; (c) 20 μM octanoyl-L-carnitine; (d) 20 μM octanoyl-CoA + 2.0 mM L-carnitine; (e) 20 μM stearoyl-CoA + 2.0 mM L-carnitine; (f) 20 μM oleoyl-CoA + 2.0 mM L-carnitine. The mitochondria were added to the incubation for a final protein concentration around 2 mg/ml. Quercetin was added to the incubation medium as a dimethylformamide solution for final concentrations between 50 and 300 μM.

Oxygen Uptake of Isolated Mitochondria Oxidizing Krebs Cycle Intermediates and Other Substrates

Oxygen in the incubation medium was measured polarographically using a teflon-shielded platinum electrode (Clark, 1956; Voss *et al.*, 1961). The incubation medium contained 2 mM potassium phosphate monobasic, 10 mM 4-(2-hydroxyethyl)-1-piperazine-ethanesulfonic acid (HEPES pH 7.2), 0.1 mM ethylene glycol-bis(β-aminoethyl ether)-N,N,N′,N′-tetraacetic acid (EGTA), 130 mM potassium chloride, 2.5 mM magnesium chloride, 0.1 mM 2,4-dinitrophenol (DNP), 2 mg/ml fatty acid-free bovine-serum albumin and substrates (Garland *et al.*, 1969). The substrates were 10 Mm α-ketoglutarate, 10 mM citrate, 10 mM fumarate, 5 mM isocitrate, 5 mM oxaloacetate, 10 mM succinate, 10 mM β-hydroxybutyrate and 30 mM α-glycerophosphate. Mitochondria were added to the incubation for a final protein concentration around 2 mg/ml. Quercetin was added to the incubation medium as a dimethylformamide solution for final concentrations between 50 and 300 μM.

Oxygen Uptake of Isolated Disrupted Mitochondria Oxidizing NADH and Succinate (NADH-Oxidase and Succinate-Oxidase Activities)

Oxygen in the incubation medium was measured polarographically using a teflon-shielded platinum electrode (Clark, 1956; Voss *et al.,* 1961). Freeze–thawing disrupted mitochondria were used as an enzyme source for assaying the succinate- and NADH-oxidase activities (Singer, 1974). Mitochondria were frozen in liquid nitrogen and rapidly thawed at 37°C. This procedure was repeated three times. The disrupted mitochondria were incubated in the closed chamber of an oxygraph (1 mg protein/ml) in a medium containing 20 mM Tris–HC1 (pH 7.4) and 1 mM NADH or 10 mM succinate. Quercetin was added to the incubation medium as a dimethylformamide solution for final concentrations between 50 and 300 μM. Another series of experiments were done in order to obtain a better understanding about the mechanisms of quercetin actions on NADH-oxidase activity. In such experiments, disrupted rat liver mitochondria were incubated in the same conditions as related above; however, in this case, the protein amount was 2 mg/ml and the NADH concentration was equal to 130 μM. Instead of evaluating only the initial rates of NADH oxidation in the presence or absence of quercetin, the reaction was accompanied until total NADH oxidation. This allowed us to verify if quercetin affects the NADH oxidation by any alternative mechanism.

Data Analysis

Data were shown as means±standard errors of the mean (SEM). Statistical significance of the differences between parameters was evaluated by means of the Student-Newman-Keuls test after variance analysis; $p \leq 0.05$ was adopted as a criterion of significance.

Results

Figure 2 shows the results of a series of experiments in which the actions of quercetin on oxygen uptake by uncoupled mitochondria oxidizing substrates dependent on NADH-NAD$^+$ dehydrogenases were investigated. Uncoupling was achieved by the addition of 100 μM 2,4-

dinitrophenol. Oxygen uptake rates were evaluated from the slopes of the polarographic recordings. Figure 2 reveals that quercetin clearly inhibited oxygen uptake when the substrates were citrate, isocitrate, β-hydroxybutyrate and α-ketoglutarate. With 300 μM quercetin the inhibition degrees were: citrate, 73%; β-hydroxybutyrate, 68%; α-ketoglutarate, 67%; isocitrate, 41%. With fumarate and oxaloacetate a tendency toward inhibition was apparent, but statistical significance was lacking.

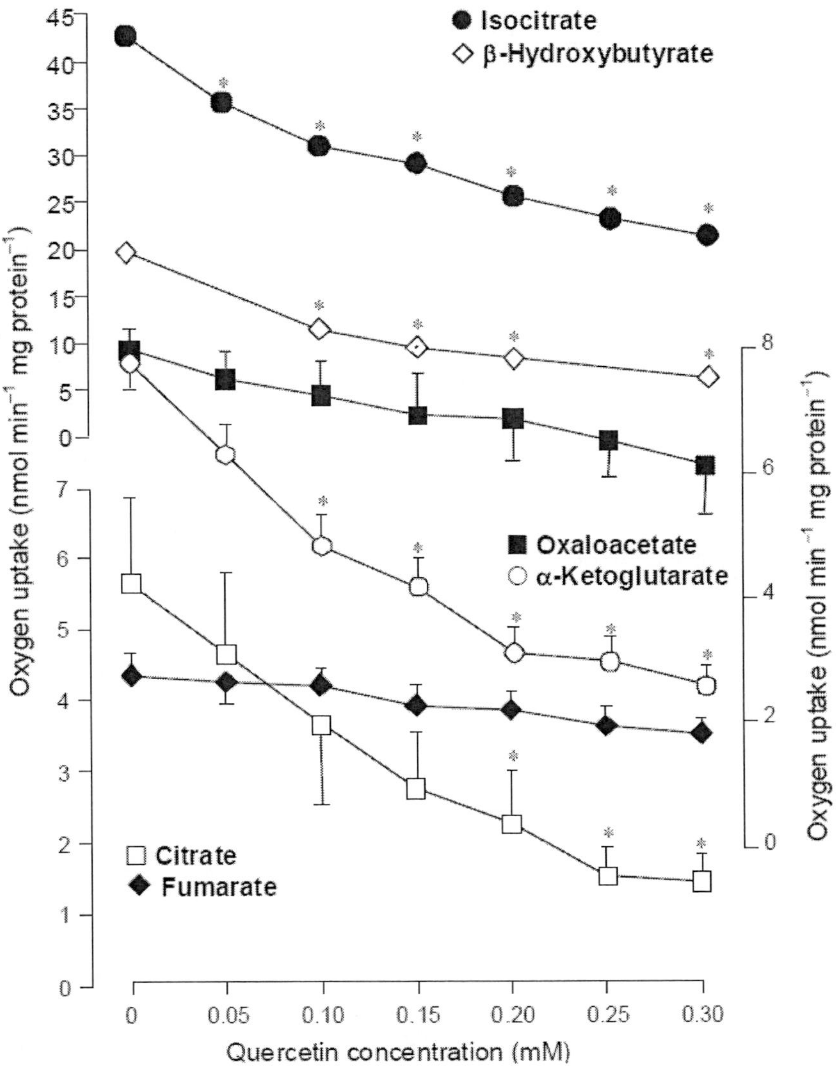

Figure 2. Oxygen uptake by uncoupled rat liver mitochondria in the presence of various substrates that are oxidized by nicotinamide adenine dinucleotide dehydrogenases. The reaction medium described in Materials and Methods (containing 100 μM 2,4-dinitrophenol) was added to the oxygraph chamber. The following additions were: (1) isolated rat liver mitochondria (2 mg protein/ml), (2) quercetin at various concentrations and (3) the corresponding substrate. The oxygen concentration in the closed chamber was recorded polarographically and the rates of oxygen uptake were computed from the slopes of the recorder tracings. Values are means of 3-4 experiments ± mean standard errors. Values obtained in the presence of quercetin which differ statistically from the corresponding controls ($p \leq 0.05$; Student-Newman-Keuls test) are labeled with an asterisk.

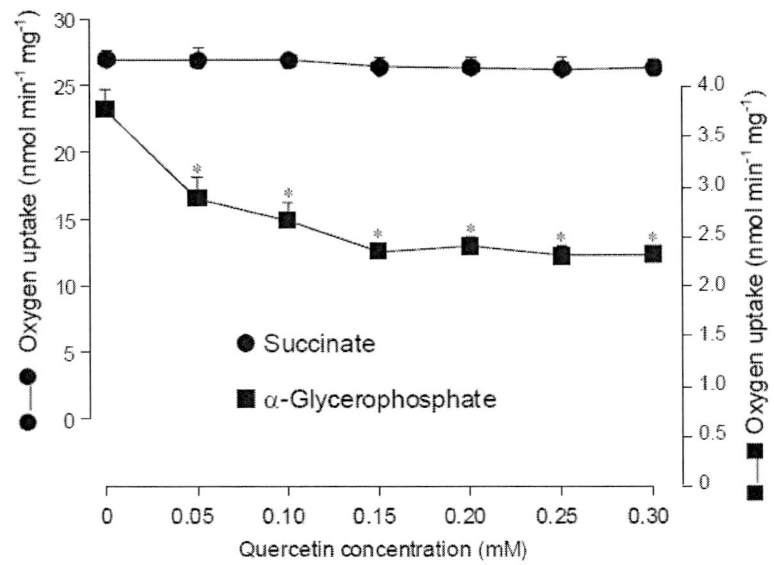

Figure 3. Oxygen uptake by uncoupled rat liver mitochondria in the presence of various substrates that are oxidized by flavin adenine nucleotide dehydrogenases. The reaction medium described in Materials and Methods (containing 100 µM 2,4-dinitrophenol) was added to the oxygraph chamber. The following additions were: (1) isolated rat liver mitochondria (2 mg protein/ml), (2) quercetin at various concentrations and (3) the corresponding substrate. The oxygen concentration in the closed chamber was recorded polarographically and the rates of oxygen uptake were computed from the slopes of the recorder tracings. Values are means of 3-4 experiments ± mean standard errors. Values obtained in the presence of quercetin which differ statistically from the corresponding controls ($p \leq 0.05$; Student-Newman-Keuls test) are labeled with an asterisk.

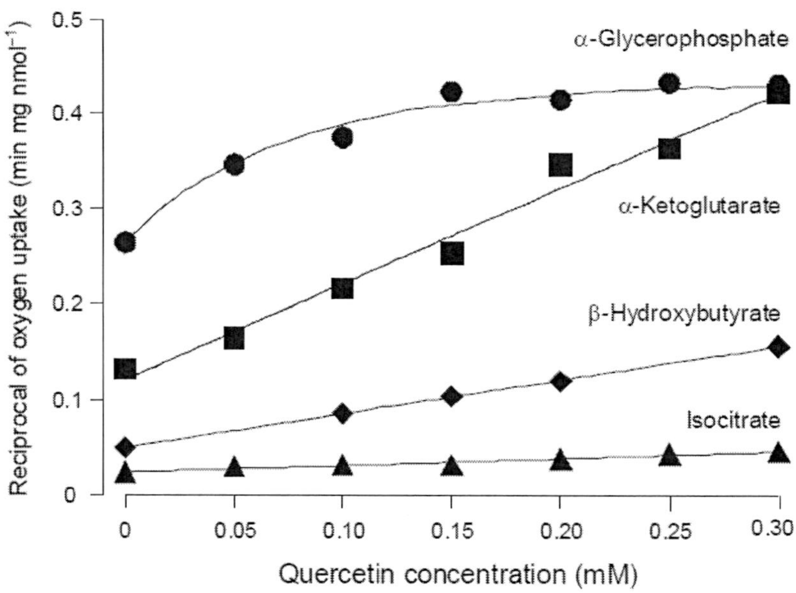

Figure 4. Reciprocals of oxygen uptake with several substrates versus quercetin concentration. The data in reciprocal form are the same already shown in Figures 1 and 2 for the indicated substrates. The straight lines were calculated after a performing linear regression fitting by means of the Scientist® program (*MicroMath Scientific Software Inc.*).

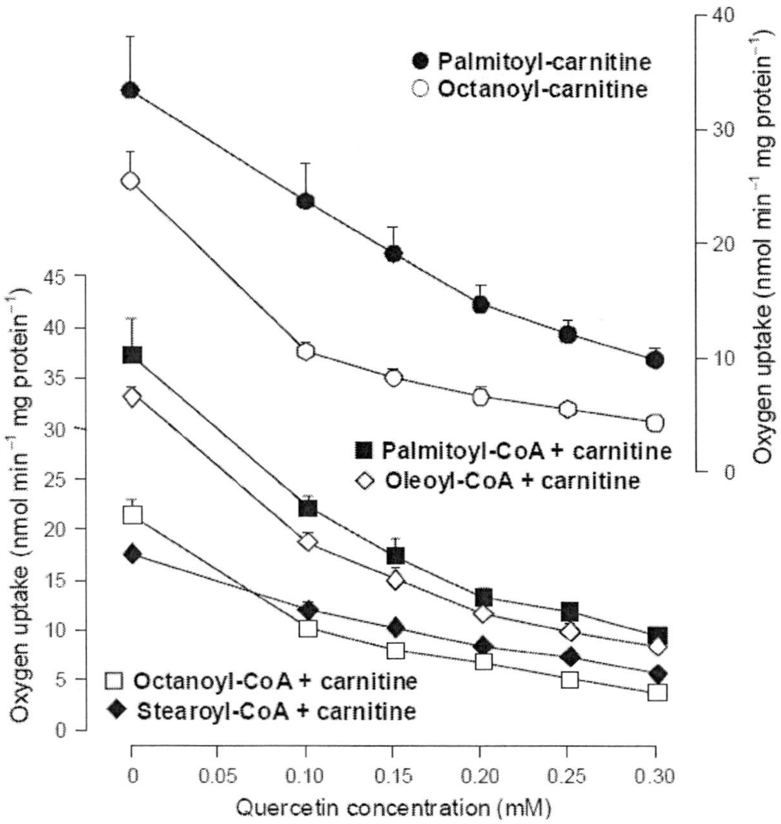

Figure 5. Oxygen uptake by uncoupled rat liver mitochondria in the presence of various activated fatty acids. The reaction medium described in Materials and Methods (containing 100 μM 2,4-dinitrophenol) was added to the oxygraph chamber. The following additions were: (1) isolated rat liver mitochondria (2 mg/ml), (2) quercetin at various concentrations and (3) the corresponding activated fatty acid. The oxygen concentration in the closed chamber was recorded polaro-graphically and the rates of oxygen uptake were computed from the slopes of the recorder tracings. Each value represents the mean of four experiments ± the corresponding mean standard error. All values obtained in the presence of quercetin differed statistically from the corresponding control, according to the Student-Newman-Keuls test ($p \leq 0.05$).

Figure 3 shows the experiments that were done with FAD-dependent substrates, namely succinate and α-glycerophosphate. However no inhibition at all was found with succinate. With α-glycerophosphate as the oxidative substrate inhibition was statistically significant. Maximal inhibition, however, was already achieved at 150 μM quercetin (38%). Inhibition could not be further enhanced by increasing the concentration of quercetin. Inhibition with α-glycerophosphate is different from that found with other substrates as illustrated by Figure 4 where the reciprocals of oxygen uptake rates were represented against the quercetin concentration. With α-ketoglutarate, β-hydroxybutyrate and isocitrate as substrates inhibition was linear, i.e., at least potentially complete. With α-glycerophosphate, however, it was parabolic, i.e., clearly incomplete (Plowman, 1972). In the substrate-free perfused rat liver respiration is mainly dependent on the oxidation of fatty acids. For this reason it is of interest to investigate the action of quercetin on oxygen uptake by mitochondria oxidizing fatty acids. Figure 5 shows the results of a series of measurements in which several activated forms of fatty acids were incubated with uncoupled mitochondria and L-malate (Garland *et al.*, 1969). The latter is readily transformed into oxaloacetate avoiding any limitation in the availability of acceptor molecules for the acetyl-CoA's produced during fatty acid oxidation. As revealed by Figure 5, quercetin inhibited oxygen uptake during the oxidation of all activated fatty acids, with well-defined concentration dependencies. The degrees of inhibition with 300 μM quercetin were: octanoyl-carnitine, 83%; octanoyl-CoA, 82%; palmitoyl-CoA, 74%; oleoyl-CoA, 74%; palmitoyl-carnitine, 70%; and stearoyl-CoA, 67%.

The inhibitory action of quercetin on oxygen uptake observed in isolated rat liver mitochondria as well as in the substrate-free perfused rat liver which has been reported in previous works (Gasparin *et al.*, 2003a; Gasparin *et al.*, 2003b, Buss *et al.*, 2005), raises the question whether these effects are dependent on direct action of the flavonoid on the mitochondrial electron flow.

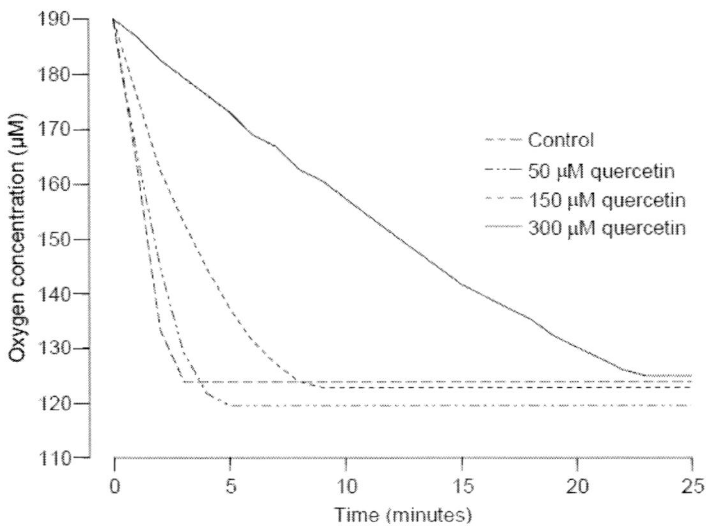

Figure 6. Time courses of oxygen uptake by disrupted rat liver mitochondria in the presence of NADH and quercetin. The reaction medium described in Materials and Methods was added to the oxygraph chamber. The following additions were: (1) isolated disrupted rat liver mitochondria (2 mg protein/ml), (2) quercetin at three concentrations or DMF (control) and (3) NADH. The NADH concentration was equal to 130 μM. Temperature was equal to 37°C. The oxygen concentration in the closed chamber was recorded polarographically and the time courses of oxygen uptake were computed from the slopes of the recorder tracings.

To evaluate this possibility, the effects of several concentrations of quercetin on the NADH-oxidase activity and succinate-oxidase activity were measured in preparations containing freeze-thawing disrupted rat liver mitochondria. Figure 6 shows the time courses of NADH oxidation in the absence (control) and presence of several quercetin concentrations. Considering the stoichiometry of the respiratory chain (NADH/$\frac{1}{2}O_2$), the initial NADH concentration (130 μM) is enough to diminish the initial O_2 concentration (190 μM at 37 °C) to values around 125 μM. Figure 6 reveals that quercetin, in the range between 50 and 300 μM, did not significantly affect the final O_2 concentrationin the reaction medium. This means there was no significant oxidation of NADH by alternative mechanisms in this incubation system (disrupted mitochondria plus reaction medium). It is clear in Figure 6, however, that quercetin diminishes the rate of NADH oxidation. This can be more clearly appreciated in Figure 7, which shows the initial rates of NADH oxidation as a function of the quercetin concentration. The degree of inhibition with 300 μM quercetin was 80%. When succinate was the substrate (succinate-oxidase) a tendency toward inhibition was apparent, but statistical significance was lacking.

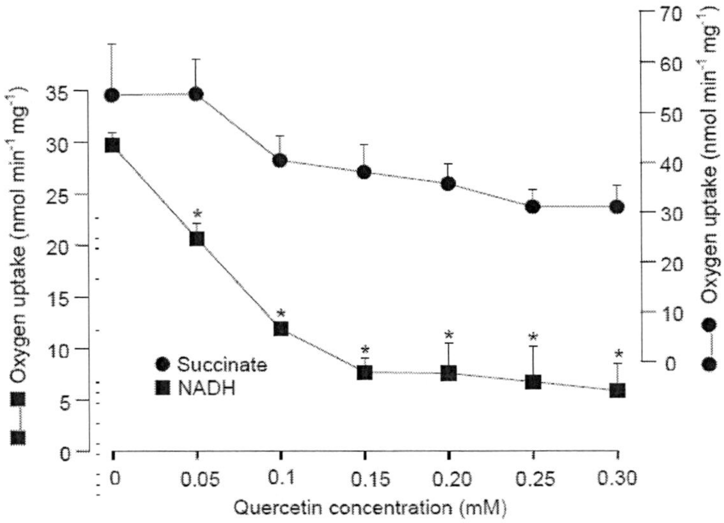

Figure 7. Oxygen uptake by disrupted rat liver mitochondria in the presence of NADH and succinate (NADH-oxidase and succinate-oxidase activities). The reaction medium described in Materials and Methods was added to the oxygraph chamber. The following additions were: (1) isolated disrupted rat liver mitochondria (1 mg protein/ml), (2) quercetin at various concentrations and (3) the corresponding substrate. The oxygen concentration in the closed chamber was recorded polarographically and the rates of oxygen uptake were computed from the slopes of the recorder tracings. Values are means of 3-4 experiments ± mean standard errors. Values obtained in the presence of quercetin which differ statistically from the corresponding controls ($p \leq 0.05$; Student-Newman-Keuls test) are labeled with an asterisk.

Discussion

From the results it becomes clear that quercetin is able to inhibit oxygen uptake by uncoupled rat liver mitochondria oxidizing several substrates and not only when respiration is stimulated by ADP phosphorylation. Inhibition was clear with all fatty acid derivatives that were tested and with all substrates whose oxidation depends on the direct action of NAD^+-dependent dehydrogenases: isocitrate and citrate (isocitrate dehydrogenase), α-ketoglutarate (α-ketoglutarate dehydrogenase) and β-hydroxybutyrate (β-hydroxybutyrate dehydrogenase). Citrate can be included into this group because it is readily isomerized to isocitrate. There was no inhibition with succinate, whose oxidation depends on a flavoprotein (succinate dehydrogenase, FAD-dependent). Inhibition of oxygen uptake dependent on α-glycerophosphate, a compound which is also oxidized by a flavoprotein (α-glycerophosphate dehydrogenase, FAD-dependent), was also observed. This inhibition, however, seems to be of a different kind because it is incomplete and hyperbolic (Plowman, 1972). In addition, in the experiments conducted with disrupted mitochondria, where NADH-oxidase and succinate-oxidase were directly evaluated, inhibition of oxygen uptake dependent on NADH oxidation was found, whereas no significant effect was observed when the substrate was succinate. With substrates that must first undergo reduction or other transformations before effective transfer of electrons to the respiratory chain can occur, such as fumarate and oxaloacetate, no inhibition was found.

The oxidation of fatty acids is under complex control and is dependent on several factors, including NADH reoxidation. When the fatty acid and oxygen availabilies are not limiting, as in the case of the controlled incubations of the experimental conditions, the following factors must be considered: the Krebs cycle activity, fatty acid uptake by mitochondria (carnitine-acyl transferases), and the electron transport chain activity (Lopaschuk *et al.*, 2010; Fromenty and Pessayre, 1995). An inhibitory action of quercetin on the Krebs cycle activity is unlikely if one takes into account the results found in the perfused rat liver, where oxygen uptake inhibition was not accompanied by inhibition of the Krebs cycle. Actually, this metabolic route was clearly stimulated under conditions where oxygen uptake was inhibited, probably due to the decreased NADH/NAD^+ ratio (Buss *et al.*, 2005). The Krebs cycle activity of the liver was measured as $^{14}CO_2$ production after labeling the cellular acetyl-CoA pools with tracer amounts of [1-^{14}C]octanoate. It is also unlikely that inhibition of oxygen uptake when the mitochondria were oxidizing fatty acids was the consequence of an inhibition of the carnitine-acyl transferases by quercetin. It is of general knowledge that octanoyl-CoA permeates the inner mitochondrial membrane as easily as octanoyl-carnitine or long-chain fatty acyl-carnitines (Ishii-Iwamoto *et al.*, 2000). Inhibition of oxygen uptake with octanoyl-CoA, however, was as strong as the one found with octanoyl-carnitine and even somewhat stronger than the one found with the activated long-chain fatty acids. It seems, thus, that inhibition of oxygen uptake when the substrates were fatty acids could be related to the same step (or steps) in the oxidation process of these compounds. The same can be said about the inhibition of the NAD^+-dependent substrates like α-ketoglutarate and isocitrate. This step could be the reoxidation of NADH in the respiratory chain, as suggested by the fact that quercetin was able to inhibit the NADH-oxidase when preparations containing freeze-thawing disrupted rat liver mitochondria were assayed. Since succinate-oxidase was not inhibited, it is reasonable to assume that quercetin inhibited electron flow at the complex I level. It is usually accepted that severe impairment of the respiratory chain at complex I can lead to secondary inhibition of the oxidation process of the fatty acids derivatives that were assayed as well as of all substrates whose oxidation depends on the direct action of NAD^+-dependent dehydrogenases (Mannaerts *et al.*, 1979; Fromenty *et al.*, 1990b; Watmough *et al.*, 1990). Although little can be said about the inhibitory mechanism of complex I by quercetin, a poorly specific mechanism such as hydrophobic interactions of the flavonoid with polypeptides and/or phospholipids of the inner membrane (preventing NADH oxidation) could be raised, similar to what happens with other drugs (Fromenty *et al.*, 1990a; Deschamps *et al.*, 1994). For example, rotenone, a prototypical inhibitor of complex I of the respiratory chain, secondarily inhibits β-oxidation by preventing the reoxidation of the NADH produced during the β-oxidation process. The resulting depletion of NAD^+ soon interrupts β-oxidation because NAD^+ is required by 3-hydroxyacyl-CoA dehydrogenase (Fromenty and Pessayre, 1995).

Although the inhibition of NADH oxidation in the respiratory chain (NADH-oxidase) seems to be the most prominent determinant of the effects observed in the experiments with uncoupled mitochondria, especially at quercetin concentrations above 100 μM, it could well have a secondary importance in the perfused liver and even in intact isolated mitochondria. There is evidence that in the perfused liver the reported ability of the compound to oxidize NADH when activated to *o*-hemiquinones by peroxidases (Buss *et al.*, 2005; Chan *et al.* 2003) plays an important role. In this system, as previously mentioned, the infusion of quercetin produces a diminution in both the lactate/pyuvate ratio (Gasparin *et al.*, 2003a) and the β-hydroxybutyrate/acetoacetate ratio (Buss *et al.*, 2005). These ratios indicate the cytosolic and mitochondrial $NADH/NAD^+$ ratios, respectively. Moreover, the diminution of mitochondrial $NADH/NAD^+$ ratio was accompanied by an increased activity of the Krebs cycle and an inhibition of oxygen consumption, indicating that, in the presence of quercetin, a sort of competition for NADH is established between the respiratory chain and the quercetin metabolites (Buss *et al.*, 2005). The formation of *o*-hemiquinone forms of quercetin could be occurring in the respiratory chain of isolated mitochondria in a way similar to the formation of *p*-hemiquinone forms of ubiquinone (Rich and Wikström, 1986) or, alternatively, by peroxidases contained within microsomes and other structures that normally contaminate isolated mitochondria (Higuti *et al.*, 1985).

It should be recalled, however, that significant oxidation of NADH via *o*-hemiquinone formation was not detected when disrupted mitochondria were used (see Figure 6) even in the presence of 300 μM quercetin. Thisdoes not necessarily mean that the phenomenon does not occur in intact mitochondria, because disruption of the organelles might also have produced considerable dilution of the indispensable factors for *o*-hemiquinone formation, namely a peroxidase reaction catalyzing enzyme and hydrogen peroxide or any other kind of peroxide.

Conclusion

This chapter gives us additional information about the mechanisms of quercetin actions on energy metabolism in isolated mitochondria and intact cells. In addition to its inhibitory action on the ATP-synthase/ATPase (Gasparin *et al.*, 2003) and to its prooxidant effects which result in NADH oxidation (Chan *et al.*, 2003; Buss *et al.*, 2005), a direct action on the NADH oxidation in the respiratory chain is also a likely phenomenon. These three phenomena take place at different concentrations, so that at low concentrations (under 50 μM) the prooxidant effects will predominate, followed by the inhibitory effects on the ATP-synthase (which become significant at concentrations above 50 μM) and finally by the inhibitory action on the NADH oxidation in the respiratory chain.

References

Aziz, NH; Farag, SE; Mousa, LA; Abo-Zaid, MA. Comparative antibacterial and antifungal effects of some phenolic compounds. *Microbios*, 1998;93, 43-54.

Boers, F; Lemiere, G; Lepoivre, JÁ; De Groot, A; Dommisse, R; De Bruyne, T; Vlietinck, AJ; Vanden Berghe, DA. Synthesis and antiviral activity of 7-O-(omega-substituted)-alkyl-3-O-methylquercetin derivatives. *Die Pharmazie*, 1998;53, 512-517.

Bracht, A; Ishii-Iwamoto, EL; Salgueiro-Pagadigorria, CL. O estudo do metabolismo energético em mitocôndrias isoladas de tecido animal. In: Brach A, Ishii-Iwamoto EL editors. *Métodos de Laboratório em Bioquímica*. São Paulo: Manole; 2003; 227-247.

Brouillard, R; Cheminant, A. Flavonoids and plant color. In: Cody V, Middleton E, Harborne JB editors. *Plant Flavonoids in Biology and Medicine: Biochemical, Cellular and Medicinal Properties*. New York: Alan R. Liss, Inc; 1988; 93-106.

Buss, GD; Constantin, J; de Lima, LC; Teodoro, GR; Comar, JF; Ishii-Iwamoto, EL; Bracht, A. The action of quercetin on the mitochondrial NADH to NAD(+) ratio in the isolated perfused rat liver. *Planta* Medica, 2005;71, 1118-1122.

Chan, TS; Galati, G; Pannala, AS; Rice-Evans, C; O'Brien, PJ. Simultaneous detection of the antioxidant and pro-oxidant activity of dietary polyphenolics in a peroxidase system. *Free radical research*, 2003;37, 787-794.

Chan, T; Galati, G; O'Brien, PJ. Oxygen activation during peroxidase catalysed metabolism of flavones or flavanones. *Chemico-biological* interactions, 1999;122, 15-25.

Clark, LC. Monitoring and control of blood O_2 tension. *Transactions of the American Society of Artificial Internal Organs*, 1956;2, 41-49.

Constantin, J; Bracht, A. Quercetin, mechanisms of antiand prooxidant activities. In: Sing K, Govil JN editors. *Recent progress in medicinal plants, volume 21: Phytopharmacology and therapeutic values III*. Houston: TX Studium Press; 2008; 39-61.

Day, AJ; DuPont, MS; Ridley, S; Rhodes, M; Rhodes, MJ; Morgan, MR; Williamson, G. Deglycosylation of flavonoid and isoflavonoid glycosides by human small intestine and liver beta-glucosidase activity. *FEBS* letters, 1998;436, 71-75.

de Vries, JH; Janssen, PL; Hollman, PC; van Staveren, WA; Katan, MB. Consumption of quercetin and kaempferol in free-living subjects eating a variety of diets. *Cancer letters*, 1997;114, 141-144.

Deschamps, D; DeBeco, V; Fisch, C; Fromenty, B; Guillouzo, A; Pessayre, D. Inhibition by perhexiline of oxidative phosphorylation and the beta-oxidation of fatty acids: possible role in pseudoalcoholic liver lesions. *Hepatology*, 1994;19, 948-961.

ElAttar, TM; Virji, AS. Modulating effect of resveratrol and quercetin on oral cancer cell growth and proliferation. *Anti-cancer drugs*, 1999;10, 187-193.

Ferry, DR; Smith, A; Malkhandi, J; Fyfe, DW; deTakats, PG; Anderson, D; Baker, J; Kerr, DJ. Phase I clinical trial of the flavonoid quercetin: pharmacokinetics and evidence for in vivo tyrosine kinase inhibition. *Clinical cancer research: an official journal of the American Association for Cancer Research*, 1996;2, 659-668.

Friesenecker, B; Tsai, AG; Intaglietta, M. Cellular basis of inflammation, edema and the activity of Daflon 500 mg. *International journal of microcirculation, clinical and experimental / sponsored by the European Society for Microcirculation*, 1995;15, 17-21.

Fromenty, B; Pessayre, D. Inhibition of mitochondrial beta-oxidation as a mechanism of hepatotoxicity. *Pharmacology and therapeutics*, 1995;67, 101-154.

Fromenty, B; Fisch, C; Berson, A; Letteron, P; Larrey, D; Pessayre, D. Dual effect of amiodarone on mitochondrial respiration. Initial protonophoric uncoupling effect followed by inhibition of the respiratory chain at the levels of complex I and complex II. *The Journal of pharmacology and experimental therapeutics*, 1990a;255, 1377-1384.

Fromenty, B; Fisch, C; Labbe, G; Degott, C; Deschamps, D; Berson, A; Letteron, P; Pessayre, D. Amiodarone inhibits the mitochondrial beta-oxidation of fatty acids and produces microvesicularsteatosis of the liver in mice. *The Journal of pharmacology and experimental therapeutics*, 1990b;255, 1371-1376.

Garland, PB; Shepherd, D; Nicholls, DG; Yates, DW; Light, PA. Interactions between fatty acid oxidation and the tricarboxylic acid cycle. In: Lowestein JM editor. *Citric Acid Cycle*. New York: Dekker; 1969; 163-212.

Gasparin, FR; Salgueiro-Pagadigorria, CL; Bracht, L; Ishii-Iwamoto, EL; Bracht, A; Constantin, J. Action of quercetin on glycogen catabolism in the rat liver. *Xenobiotica*, 2003a;33, 587-602.

Gasparin, FR; Spitzner, FL; Ishii-Iwamoto, EL; Bracht, A; Constantin, J. Actions of quercetin on gluconeogenesis and glycolysis in rat liver. *Xenobiotica*, 2003b;33, 903-911.

Haenen, GR; Bast, A. Nitric oxide radical scavenging of flavonoids. *Methods in enzymology*, 1999;301, 490-503.

Harborne, JB. Nature, distribution, and function of plant flavonoids. In: Cody V, Middleton E, Harborne JB editors. *Plant Flavonoids in Biology and Medicine: Biochemical, Pharmacological, and Structure- Activity Relationships*. New York: Alan R. Liss, Inc; 1986; 15-24.

Harborne, JB. *The Flavonoids: Advances in Research Since 1986*. New York: Chapman and Hall; 1988a.

Harborne, JB. Flavonoids in the environment: Structure-activity relationships. In: Cody V, Middleton E, Harborne JB, Beretz A editors. *Plant Flavonoids in Biology and Medicine II: BiochemicaL Cellular andMedicinal Properties*. New York: Alan R. Liss, Inc; 1988b; 17-28.

Herrmann, K. Flavonols and flavones in food plants: a review. *International Journal of Food Science and Technology*, 1976;11, 433-448.

Hertog, MG; Hollman, PC; Katan, MB; Kromhout, D. Intake of potentially anticarcinogenic flavonoids and their determinants in adults in The Netherlands. *Nutrition and cancer*, 1993;20, 21-29.

Hertog, MG; Kromhout, D; Aravanis, C; Blackburn, H; Buzina, R; Fidanza, F; Giampaoli, S; Jansen, A; Menotti, A; Nedeljkovic, S. Flavonoid intake and long-term risk of coronary heart disease and cancer in the seven countries study. *Archives of internal medicine*, 1995;155, 381-386.

Higuti, IH; Murata, LY; Stencel, M; De PaivaCampello, A; Do Nascimento, AJ. Studies on rat liver mitochondria. 6. The effect of contaminating particles in mitochondria stored at 0-4 degrees C. *Cell Biochemistry and Function*, 1985;3, 283-288.

Hollman, PC; Katan, MB. Absorption, metabolism and health effects of dietary flavonoids in man. *Biomedicine and pharmacotherapy*, 1997;51, 305-310.

Hollman, PC; Bijsman, MN; van Gameren, Y; Cnossen, EP; de Vries, JH; Katan, MB. The sugar moiety is a major determinant of the absorption of dietary flavonoid glycosides in man. *Free radical research*, 1999;31, 569-573.

Ishii-Iwamoto, EL; Ferrarese, ML; Constantin, J; Salgueiro-Pagadigorria, C; Bracht, A. Effects of norepinephrine on the metabolism of fatty acids with different chain lengths in the perfused rat liver. *Molecular and Cellular Biochemistry*, 2000;205, 13-23.

Kawaii, S; Tomono, Y; Katase, E; Ogawa, K; Yano, M. Antiproliferative activity of flavonoids on several cancer cell lines. *Bioscience, biotechnology, and biochemistry*, 1999;63, 896-899.

Kefford, JF; Chandler, BV. *The Chemical Constituents of Citrus Fruits*. New York: Academic Press;1970.

Kim, HP; Mani, I; Iversen, L; Ziboh, VA. Effects of naturally-occurring flavonoids and biflavonoids on epidermal cyclooxygenase and lipoxygenase from guinea-pigs. *Prostaglandins, leukotrienes, and essential fatty acids*, 1998;58, 17-24.

Knekt, P; Järvinen, R; Seppänen, R; Hellövaara, M; Teppo, L; Pukkala, E; Aromaa, A. Dietary flavonoids and the risk of lung cancer and other malignant neoplasms. *American journal of epidemiology*, 1997;146, 223-230.

Lopaschuk, GD; Ussher, JR; Folmes, CD; Jaswal, JS; Stanley, WC. Myocardial fatty acid metabolism in health and disease. *Physiological reviews,*2010;90, 207-258.

Lowry, OH; Rosebrough, NJ; Farr, AC; Randall, RJ. Protein measurement with the Folin phenol reagent. *The Journal of biological chemistry*, 1951;193, 265-275.

Mannaerts, GP; Debeer, LJ; Thomas, J; De Schepper, PJ. Mitochondrial and peroxisomal fatty acid oxidation in liver homogenates and isolated hepatocytes from control and clofibrate-treated rats. *The Journal of biological chemistry*, 1979;254, 4585-4595.

Nijveldt, RJ; van Nood, E; van Hoorn, DE; Boelens, PG; van Norren, K; van Leeuwen, PA. Flavonoids: a review of probable mechanisms of action and potential applications. *The American journal of clinical nutrition*, 2001;74, 418-425.

Peterson, J; Dwyer, J. Flavonoids: dietary occurrence and biochemical activity. *Nutrition Research*, 1998;18, 1995-2018.

Plowman, KM. *Enzyme Kinetics*. New York: McGraw-Hill Book Company; 1972.

Rich, PR; Wikström, M. Evidence for a mobile semiquinone in the redox cycle of the mammalian cytochrome bc1 complex. *FEBS letters*, 1986;194, 176-182.

Ross, JA; Kasum, CM. Dietary flavonoids: bioavailability, metabolic effects, and safety. *Annual review of nutrition*, 2002;22, 19-34.

Skibola, CF; Smith, MT. Potential health impacts of excessive flavonoid intake. *Free radical biology and medicine*, 2000;29, 375-383.

Strack, D. Phenolic Metabolism. In: Det PM and Harbone JB editors. *Plant Biochemistry*. New York: Academic Press, Inc.; 1997; 387-416.

Singer, TP. Determination of the activity of succinate, NADH, choline, and alpha-glycerophosphate dehydrogenases. *Methods of biochemical analysis*, 1974;22, 123-175.

Timberlake, CF; Henry, BS. Plant pigments as natural food colours. *Endeavour*, 1986;10, 31-36.

Voss, DO; Campello, AP; Bacila, M. The respiratory chain and the oxidative phosphorylation of rat brain mitochondria. *Biochemical and biophysical research communications*, 1961;4, 48-51.

Watmough, NJ; Bindoff, LA; Birch-Machin, MA; Jackson, S; Bartlett, K; Ragan, CI; Poulton, J; Gardiner, RM; Sherratt, HS; Turnbull, DM. Impaired mitochondrial beta-oxidation in a patient with an abnormality of the respiratory chain. Studies in skeletal muscle mitochondria. *The Journal of clinical investigation*, 1990;85, 177-184.

In: Quercetin
Editors: Taiki Chikamatsu and Yuudai Hida
ISBN: 978-1 61942- 057-1

Chapter 11

ORAL HEALTH BENEFITS OF QUERCETIN

***M. Y. Li*[1]*, G. Y. Lai*[2] *and J. Wang*[1]**
[1]Shanghai Key Laboratory of Stomatology, Shanghai Research Institute of Stomatology,
Ninth People's Hospital, Medical College, P. R. China
Shanghai Jiao Tong University, Shanghai, P. R. China
[2]Department of Restorative Dentistry and Periodontology,
Dental School of the Ludwig-Maximilians-University, Munich, Germany

ABSTRACT

Herbs are naturally occurring gifts of nature. Flavonoids are present in fruits, vegetables and beverages derived from plants (tea, red wine), and in many dietary supplements or herbal remedies including Ginkgo Biloba, Soy Isoflavones, and Milk Thistle. Flavonoids have been described as health-promoting, disease-preventing dietary supplements, and have activity as cancer preventive agents. Additionally, they are extremely safe and associated with low toxicity, making them excellent candidates for chemopreventive agents. [1]

Quercetin, one of the most common natural flavonoids, has been reported to possess various excellent activities both in vitro and in vivo. This chapter gives brief survey of current study on quercetin that is commonly used in cosmetic and therapeutic application in oral health care. For cosmetic application it may temporarily control or reduce malodor. For cosmetic application it may reduce plaque, caries, gingivitis, periodontal disease, oral mucosal ulceration or oral cancer. The etiology of malodor involves many factors such as gingivitis, periodontitis, nasal inflammation, chronic sinusitis and diabetes. Plaque is the major etiology of dental caries, gingivitis and periodontal diseases. Antibacterial activities of quercetin could explain how it can help to prevent these diseases. The oral mucosal ulceration or oral cancer is related both on the internal factors, immunological, microbiological, saliva, with digestive, lubricating and other protective properties, and external factors such as nutrition, habits and lifestyle, including stress and coping. Quercetin may be useful in accelerating the healing process of minor aphthous ulcers and inhibiting the cellular grow of human oral cancer cells. Quercetin may be a better candidate material for maintaining perfect oral health at home.

1. Reduce Malodor by Quercetin

Halitosis (oral malodor, bad breath) is defined as an offensive odor arising from the oral cavity or air-filled cavities such as the nose, sinuses, and pharynx. Halitosis can often be a source of embarrassment, can interfere in social situations and marriages, and can create psychological barriers. Primarily, halitosis is often simply a result of poor oral hygiene. Frequently, the cause is heavy accumulation of organisms and resultant plaque on the back third of the top of the tongue. The production of halitosis is multi-factorial and may involve both oral and non-oral sources. [2-3] Non-oral sources of bad breath are generally related to systemic problems and/or medications. Conditions such as diabetes, liver and kidney disorders, and pulmonary disease may contribute to offensive breath odor. This is also true of some medications, especially those that reduce salivary flow such as antidepressants, antipsychotics, narcotics, decongestants, antihistamines, and anti-hypertensives. [4] However, while systemic conditions and medications can contribute to breath problems, most authorities seem to agree the majority of bad breath originates in the oral cavity. It is estimated by many experts in the field that 85% to 90% of the bad breath conditions come from sources in the mouth. Gram-negative organisms (mostly anaerobes) are the specific bacteria responsible for halitosis. [5] particularly those residing on the posterior dorsum of the tongue, utilize sulfur containing amino acids, primarily cysteine and methionine [6] to produce volatile sulfur compounds. Although other organic components (e.g., organic acids, indole/skatole, putrescine, cadaverine) may be involved in the production of halitosis,12 hydrogen sulfide (H_2S), methyl-mercaptan (CH_3SH), and dimethyl sulfide [$(CH_3)_2S$] have been identified as the predominate VSCs responsible for oral malodor. [6]

Primarily, halitosis was prevented by tooth brushing and mouth rinse. But, never before have there been effective method for it until now, which only temporarily treat the problem. Most people will notice the advertising media is saturated with products promoted to help with this condition. Most, if not all of them, really do not work very long and some make the problem worse. Alcohol based mouthwashes can, for example, dry out the tissues in the mouth and cause the tissues to secrete plasma proteins which worsen the condition over time.

The usual treatments of halitosis include the use of compounds containing some kind of chlorine dioxide or combination of chlorine dioxide and chemically altered forms of oxychlorine species and also zinc compounds. The VSCs are then chemically changed into harmless compounds with no odor by the use of toothpastes and mouth rinses containing those oxchloride species. Treatment should also include tongue scrapping with specific instruments to remove the coating of white plaque. This not only removes the odor causing agents but lowers the overall bacteria count in the mouth which can have positive effects on the health of the gum tissues.

A paper has reported a screening study of Chinese herbs on volatile sulfur compounds associated with halitosis. [7] In this study, saliva samples from volunteers were used as the source for the evaluation of bacterial activity and VSC inhibition. Extracted substances from Chinese herbs were identified by VSC inhibition tests with a Halimeter and microbial sensitivity testing. The results of the investigation show that: Of the 40 herbs tested, 14 extracts had percent inhibition rates of VSCs >50%. The 14 herbs that showed inhibition of VSCs from 50.39% to 70.69% included the following: acanthopanax root, chrysanthemum flower, cirsium root, coptis rhizome, eupatorium, gallnut of Chinese sumac, honeysuckle flower, isatis root, moutan root bark, phellodendron bark, stemona root, schisandra fruit, winter jasmine flower, and wintermelon peel. In this 14 herbs, acanthopanax root [8], chrysanthemum flower [9], eupatorium [10], honeysuckle flower [11], and wintermelon peel contain a chemical constituent compound of quercetin which may be responsible for the biological activity to control or reduce malodor. cirsium root [13], coptis rhizome [14], phellodendron bark [15], and schisandra fruit [16] contain a chemical compound of flavonoids. It was also found that agrimony, chrysanthemum flower, cirsium root, clover flower, coptis rhizome, gallnut of Chinese sumac, honeysuckle flower, houtuynia, isatis root, and moutan root bark had a greater effect on microorganisms, with percent inhibition >70%. A weak positive correlation was found between bacteriostasis and the anti-VSC activity of all herbs with a correlation coefficient of 0.2579 (Pearson).

There are many special-purpose care products, such as a dentifrice containing mint, designed to eliminate halitosis that do so with aromaticity. The aromaticity dentifrice covers the halitosis, depending on the aromatic compound. Some products with bacteriostatic function contain certain chemical agents such as a dentifrice containing chlorhexidine acetate. Although these agents may extinguish the bacterium in the oral cavity, they have been found to cause some destruction of the oral microbial ecology. [17] Home-care products designed to reduce tartar and plaque build up (and, subsequently, oral malodor) are intended as an adjunct to professional dental care. The benefits of home-care can be maximized by using better products. In this case, natural plant extract may be one of the choices for use in a dentifrice for reducing halitosis.

The potential of natural plant extract, especially polyphenols, flavonoids or quercetin, may be benefit for their numerous hydroxide ions (OH–) and other groups. [18] The hydroxyl of these extract substances may combine with thiol, amine, ammonia and other groups of malodorous substances. These substances may also combine with thiol-containing proteins of foul smell substances, so the peptide chain amino acids of the proteins are not to be degraded, inhibiting the volatilization of sulfhydryl-containing gases. Quercetin may suspend the fatty acid oxidation of odor by its electrophilic effects. Meanwhile, Quercetin and other flavonoids exhibit a stronger inhibitory effect on the glucosyltransferase activity and bacteria (description below will be on the thematic focus). Quercetin may serve as a good candidate of anti-bad breath in future studies for such potential mechanisms. The application has been processed in some patent of deodorant composition (United States Patent Application 20100158840). Using herbal products in oral health care may have a broad application prospect. However, further in vivo studies are needed to better evaluate the potential effectiveness of these compounds as an antihalitosis agent.

2. Reduce Plaque and Caries by Quercetin

A national oral health survey for school children in China demonstrated that dmft increased during the period 1980 - 1986, from 4.15 to 5.5 in pre-school children aged 1 - 6 years in Beijing and dmft for the same age group increased from 2.6 to 4.7 during 1981 to 1990 in Shanghai. It was pointed out that caries was rapidly increasing in developing urban areas of China and as a developing nation China appeared destined to repeat the experience of an epidemic increase in caries incidence unless effective preventive measures were undertaken. In China, using traditional medicinal herb extracts to prevent dental caries and periodontal disease is a well-known practice. In the Chinese market, 60% of the dentifrice products contain herbs. Investigators and manufactures pay much attention to the research and development of herbs for oral health. Reports on the isolation and identification of natural plaque-inhibiting substances from herbs generate many interests in developing various mouthrinses and dentifrices containing these ingredients. [19.]

Dental caries is a transmissible and poly-microbial ecological disease, in which mutans streptococci (MS), mainly Streptococcus mutans and Streptococcus sobrinus play the major role. Dental caries development and progression ascribe mainly to the bacterial dental plaque. So prevention and treatment of the disease are focused on suppression of the pathogenic dental plaque. The use of antimicrobial agents to control plaque has been advocated for a number of years. Different compounds have been delivered through mouthrinses or toothpastes. Some chemical agents have proven to be helpful against plaque accumulation and caries. One agent widely used to reduce the bacterial load in the mouth is chlorhexidine. It can reduce plaque, caries and gingivitis in humans. However at prolonged periods of use, side-effects such as staining of teeth can occur. Glucosyltransferase (GTF) enzymes of mutans streptococci are considered virulence factors due to their ability to synthesize adhesive glucans, which facilitate cell-to-cell adherence and accumulation. [20] The polysaccharides would maintain the acid production in plaque for a long period. This contributes significantly to tooth decalcification.

Propolis means a gum that is gathered by bees from various plants. It is known for its biological properties, having antibacterial, antifungal and healing properties. A study has evaluated the antimicrobial activity of four different Anatolian propolis samples on different groups of microorganisms including some oral pathogens and comparison between their chemical compositions. The MIC values of the most effective propolis were 2 microg/ml for Streptococcus sobrinus and Enterococcus faecalis, 4 microg/ml for Micrococcus luteus, Candida albicans and C. krusei, 8 microg/ml for Streptococcus mutans, Staphylococcus aureus, Staphylococcus epidermidis and Enterobacter aerogenes, 16 microg/ml for Escherichia coli and C. tropicalis and 32 microg/ml for Salmonella typhimurium and Pseudomonas aeruginosa. The main compounds of four Anatolian propolis samples were flavonoids such as quercetin, naringenin, galangine and etc. Propolis can prevent dental caries since it demonstrated significant antimicrobial activity against the microorganisms such as Streptococcus mutans, Streptococcus sobrinus and C. albicans, which involves in oral diseases. [21]

To investigate the influence of several phenolic compounds isolated from cranberry fruit on some of the virulence properties of *Streptococcus mutans* associated with glucan synthesis and acidogenicity. Individual phenolic acids, flavonols and proanthocyanidins were isolated by semi-preparative high-performance liquid chromatography from fresh cranberry fruit. Quercetin-3-arabinofuranoside etc displayed the most inhibition of *S. mutans* virulence. The combined effects of specific flavonols and proanthocyanidins from cranberry on GTFs activity, acid production and acid tolerance of *S. mutans* make them attractive compounds to fully explore for their anti-biofilm and cariostatic properties. [22]

A study evaluates the trial of dietary quercetin supplementation on dental caries formation in rats. All rats were fed 40% sucrose. Rats were evaluated for occlusal dental caries only using a Kruskal-Wallis H test and analysis of variance. statistically significant reductions in occlusal caries were observed for quercetin in the maxillary molars compared with the control group (P < .05). Significant associations were observed among the experimental groups and maxillary (P < .05) and mandibular (P < .01) occlusal dental caries. Hence, selected bioflavonoids such as quercetin may show promise as an alternative means of reducing dental caries. [23]

An isolated flavonoid, quercetin inhibited the growth of bacteria with minimum inhibitory concentrations (MICs) ranging from 1 to 4mg/ml and minimum bactericidal concentrations (MBCs) from 4 to 16mg/ml. In addition, quercetin and kaempferol at sub-MIC levels significantly inhibited acidogenicity and aciduric of *S. mutans* cells. [24] Certain bioflavonoids reduce dental caries and cariogenic bacteria incidence.

Dental caries is fundamentally a microbial disease, which involves the hard tissue of tooth. The prevention of dental caries have been extensively studied worldwide, however, none of the existed preventive ways of dental caries is exclusive. There are many theories and prescribes in ancient natural medicine dealing with dental caries, which facilitate the study of preventing dental caries by herbal medicine. Although the plants tested had a lower potency than conventional antibiotics they offer hope against resistant species. These results are a starting point for further testing in the lab and clinic. To further study the mechanism of quercetin on caries for providing an experimental basis, however, other related experiments of cariogenic virulence factors, such as inhibiting bacterial acid production, early production of extracellular polysaccharides and hydroxyapatite adhesion experiments should to be further processed. Also, the inhibition of bacterial adhesion on the surface of hydroxyapatite by biofilm model *in vitro* and the demineralization experiments of dental hard tissue has yet to be verified.

3. Reduce Gingivitis and Periodontal Disease by Quercetin (An Experiment)

Gingivitis is the beginning stage of periodontal disease. The etiology of the disease is multifactorial infection and bacterial deposits play an essential role in its pathogenesis. The aerobic gram-positive microflora was predominant in healthy periodontal tissues (gingival crevice). [25] Healthy gingival sulcus has a normal flora dominated by equal proportions of Gram positive cocci, especially Streptococcus spp (*S. sanguis, S. Mitior, S. mutans*), and Actinomuces sp. Later, plaque "matures" resulting in a flora consisting from facultative anaerobic microorganisms, spirochaetes and motile rods. The proportions of strict anaerobic, Gram negative and motile organisms increase significantly in accordance with increasing severity of disease. Significant differences were observed in microbial morphotypes between healthy and disease sites: cocci 18.71% and 78.90%, motile rods 46.12% and 16.70%, total spirochetes 26.48% and 2.80%, respectively. There were significant differences in the subgingival microflora between healthy and disease sites in patients with moderate and severe periodontitis. [26]

Periodontal disease is a bacterium-induced chronic inflammation that destroys tissues that attach teeth to jaw bone. The breakdown of periodontal connective tissues by bacterial pathogens can initiate destruction of structural proteins including collagens. The degradation of collagen can be mediated directly by bacterial proteases. [27] Trypsin-Like cysteine proteinases are major extracellular cysteine proteinases produced by Porphyromonas gingivalis. [28] Bacterial collagenase and trypsin-Like cysteine proteinases could be as potential targets for the development of novel antibiotics.

This research was undertaken to test the hypothesis that quercetin may take differential effect on Gram-positive and Gram-negative bacteria. Gram-negative bacteria are more susceptible to it than aerobic Gram-negative bacteria. The activity inhibition of specific virulence factors of trypsin-like protease and glycosidic enzyme activity may benefited for its medical application. The microbial ecology of periodontal pathogen site may be reformed by quercetin.

Materials and Methods

Quercetin and Bacteria

Quercetin was purchased from Chinese Food and Drug Administration (CFDA). The herb purified molecular components of herbs were dissolved in ethanol at first and then in distilled water (ethanol to distilled water in 1:10) to a concentration of 40mg/ml (Control also used the solvent). Green tea polyphenol, purchased from Zhong-ke natural plant technology company (Hangzhou, China), 40mg/ml in original concentration, was used as control. 12 strains used in this study, which were *Streptococcus intermedius* ATCC 27335, *Lactobacillus acidophilus* ATCC 4356, *Actinomyces viscosus* ATCC 19246, *Peptostreptococcus micros* ATCC 43055, *Porphyromonas gingivalis* ATCC 33277, *Prevotella nigrescens* ATCC 25261, *Prevotella intermedia* ATCC 25611, *Fusobacterium nucleatum* ATCC 25586, *Veillone disper* ATCC 17748T, *Tannerella forsythensis* ATCC 43037, *Aggregatibacter actinomycetemcomitans* Y4 and *Capnocytophaga ochracea* ATCC 27872. The mixed entire bacterium specimen were incubated anaerobically in Wilkins-Chalgren anaerobe broth (Oxoid, Oxoid LTD., Basingstoke, Hampshire, England) in an anaerobic work station (BUG BOX DUAL, Fuskinn, England) with 80% of N_2, 10% of H_2 and 10% of CO_2 at 37°C for at least 4 days. After incubation, the entire bacteria were ready for bacterial activity test, trypsin-like protease and glycosidic enzyme activity inhibition test.

Microbial Sensitivity Tests

Sensitivity tests of bacteria were carried out by broth micro-dilution tests on 96 microwell plate as described by Petra Luber [29] with partly modified. MIC (minimum inhibitory concentration) was determined. Stored bacteria were restituted, identified and incubated anaerobically or aerobically (for *L. acidophilus*) in trypticase soy broth (TSB) supplemented with 2g/L sucrose (for Streptococcus) in an incubator at 37°C for 18 h. Then the strains were smeared on trypticase soy agar (TSA) plate. Anaerobic bacteria were incubated anaerobically in pre-reduced Wilkins-Chalgren Anaerobe Broth (Oxford, England) in an Anaerobic Work Station (BUG BOX DUAL, Fuskinn, England) in an atmosphere of 90%N_2, 10%CO_2 at 37°C for 48 hours. The bacterial inoculums were prepared by suspending colonies in 5 ml of prereduced anaerobe broth to a density equal to that of a no. 1 McFarland standard. The suspension was further diluted to give a final inoculum size of 10^5 CFU per well (10^6 CFU/ml). For evaluation by bacterial sensitive tests, quercetin and green tea polyphenol were prepared in serial twofold dilutions in broth within a dilution range from 0.0195 to 10 mg/ml. In each well contained 50 μl grade diluted herb extracts and 50 μl bacterial stain suspension. In final two ranks, the rank contained herb agent only is considered as negative control and the rank contained bacteria only is considered as positive controls. Tea polyphenol was set as positive controls. After 24 h incubation of the microwell plate anaerobically, bacterial growth was observed by stereoscope and recorded. The MIC was defined as the lowest concentration of each antimicrobial herb that inhibited the visible growth of the test isolate. The tests were carried out by quadruplicating and the result was showed by mean.

Inhibition of Trypsin-Like Protease and Glycosidic Enzyme Activity of Porphyromona Gingivalis by Quercetin

Trypsin-like protease and glycosidic enzyme activities of *Porphyromona gingivalis* were measured using fluorogenic substrates essentially as previously described [30]. Briefly, specific glycosidase activities were determined using 4-MU-linked substrates while trypsin-like protease activities were monitored using N-CBZ-Gly-gly-arg-AMC as model substrates. N-α-benzoyl-L-arginine-AMC and N-CBZ-Gly-gly-arg-AMC (Sigma) for trypsin-like protease and glycosidic enzyme were with a final concentration of 2.5 mM in an assay buffer containing 50% DMSO. Bacterial cells were harvested from plates and ultrasonic extracts (25 W, 10 min at 0°C in 30 s bursts) were prepared. The bacterial inoculums were prepared by suspending colonies in 5 ml of prereduced anaerobe broth to a density equal to that of a no. 1 McFarland standard. The suspension was further diluted to give a final inoculum size of 10^5 CFU per well (10^6 CFU/ml). 500μl bacterial suspension was mixed with 250μl aliquots of quercetin in different concencertion. 500μl bacterial suspension was mixed thoroughly with 250μl aliquots of 50 mmol/ L Tris – HCl as positive control. After preincubated in 37 °C for 15 min, the mixture were added the synthetic chromogenic substrate N-α-benzoyl-L-arginine-AMC and N-CBZ-Gly-gly-arg-AMC in 100μl/ ml 250μl, respectively. The final concentration of the quercetin was from 0.0195 to 10 mg/ml. Quercetin was prepared in serial twofold dilutions in broth within a dilution range from 0.0195 to 10 mg/ml. After incubated in 37 °C for another 15 min, the mixture were checked for fluorescence intensity in RF-5000 spectrofluorophotomer (Shimadzu Co. Japan) in excitation = EX 380 nm, emission = EM 460 nm. The activity was expressed as U · $g_{fw}{}^{-1}$ (=μmol· min^{-1}· $g_{fw}{}^{-1}$) using the extinction coefficient 380=10.21 ·min^{-1}·cm^{-1}. Blanks control values were deducted from the gross value to obtain the test values (test value = actual value –blanks control). Percent inhibition rates of test were calculated with the following formula: (Positive control – test value) / positive control × 100%. The tests were carried out by quadruplicating samples for each and the results provided are a mean value and standard deviation.

Statistical analysis was performed using a statistics package (SPSS 11.0 for Windows). Differences between control and test samples were determined using Student's t-test.

Results and Discussion

The minimal bactericidal concentration (MBC) of quercetin on Gram-negative are 0.0625mg/ml, 0.125mg/ml, 0.125mg/ml, 0.25mg/ml, 0.25mg/ml, 0.5mg/ml, for *Streptococcus intermedius, Peptostreptococcus micros, Propionibacterium acnes, Lactobacillus acidophilus, Actinomyces viscosus* and *Eubacterium lentum* respectively. The minimal bactericidal concentration (MBC) of quercetin on Gram positive bacteria are 0.125mg/ml, 0.25mg/ml, 0.25mg/ml, 0.125mg/ml, 0.125mg/ml, 0.5mg/ml, 0.5mg/ml, 1mg/ml, for *Porphyromonas gingivalis, Prevotella nigrescens, Prevotella intermedia, Fusobacterium nucleatum, Veillonella spp, Tannerella forsythensis, Aggregatibacter actinomycetemcomitans* and Capnocytophaga species, respectively (Table 1). Quercetin showed extensive antibacterial activity against Gram negative bacteria and even more strongly than against Gram positive bacteria. It showed a differential effect of gram-positive versus gram-negative bacteria. The inhibitory effect of quercetin was re-experimented using tea polyphenol as a positive control to confirm the inhibitory effects.

Table 1. Antimicrobial Sensitive tests of quercetin on Caries Pathogenic Bacteria (MIC, mg / ml)

	quercetin	tea polyphenol (control)
Streptococcus intermedius	0.125	0.25
Peptostreptococcus micros	0.125	0.25
Propionibacterium acnes	0.125	0.25
Lactobacillus acidophilus	0.25	0.5
Actinomyces viscosus	0.25	0.5
Eubacterium lentum	0.5	0.5
Porphyromonas gingivalis	0.125	0.25
Prevotella nigrescens	0.25	0.5
Prevotella intermedia	0.25	0.25
Fusobacterium nucleatum	0.125	0.25
Veillonella spp	0.125	0.25
Tannerella forsythensis	0.5	0.5
Aggregatibacter actinomycetemcomitans	0.5	0.5
Capnocytophaga species	1	0.5

The quercetin inhibited both the trypsin-like protease and glycosidic enzyme activity by 82.5% and 94.06% within 2 h. On Figure 1, trypsin-like protease (over 26% of inhibition when quercetin at concentration of 0.078mg/ml, $P<0.05$) and glycosidic enzyme activity (over 73% of inhibition when quercetin at concentration of 0.078mg/ml, $P<0.01$) of *Porphyromona gingivalis* by quercetin, the inhibition of glycosidic enzyme was stronger than that of trypsin-like protease.

In this study, Gram negative bacteria showed overall more sensitivity to quercetin compared to Gram positive ones. Quercetin showed extensive antibacterial activity against Gram negative bacteria and even more strongly than against Gram positive bacteria. The activity inhibition of specific virulence factors may benefit for its medical application. The microbial ecology of periodontal pathogen site may be reformed by quercetin.

In conclusion, quercetin is an efficacious and economical agent in inhibiting bacteria and its trypsin-like protease and glycosidic enzyme activity. These observations suggest that quercetin may be of therapeutic use against periodontal diseases or other oral diseases.

It is likely to be a desirable ideal natural agent for oral care products. The further study of natural antimicrobial agents may allow us to clarify the mechanism of anti-enzyme action *in vitro* and it's toxicological and or other safety issues effects at high doses *in vivo*.

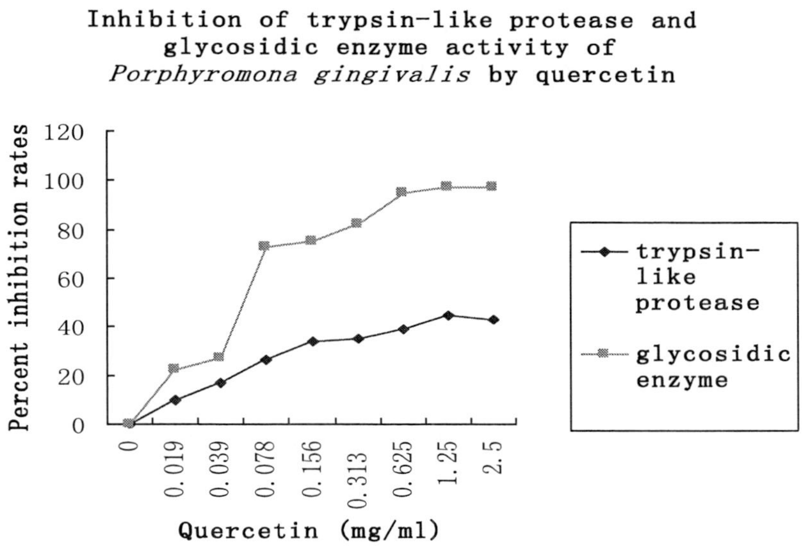

Figure 1. Inhibition of trypsin-like protease and glycosidic enzyme activity of Porphyromona gingivalis by quercetin.

4. ADJUVANT THERAPIES OF RECURRENT ORAL ULCERS BY QUERCETIN

Recurrent aphthous ulceration (RAU) is very common oral disease. Men, women and children may have oral mucosal ulcers throughout the year. It is a characteristic of cyclical by recurrent oral mucosal ulcers limitations of injury, self-healing, can occur in any part of the oral mucosa. There are several factors, such as systemic causes, genetic predisposition, haematinic deficiency, food allergy, sex hormones, psychological illness, immunodeficiency, and other, etc, which contribute to its development. Although it is able to self-healing, but it often repeated attack, in severe case, it could affect eating and language function. The treatments of recurrent oral ulcers are reducing possible causes of local trauma, topical analgesics, topical antimicrobials, topical corticosteroids, topical anti-inflammatories, systemic immuno-suppressives, and others. Natural medicine is an alternative that can be considered to manage recurrent oral ulcers.

Quercetin is a safe, well-tolerated, and highly effective promising new, adjunctive treatment for healing common aphthous ulcers. Although aphthous ulcers typically resolve on their own in one to two weeks, the daily topical application of quercetin may be useful in accelerating the healing process of minor aphthous ulcers. [31] Quercetin, an inhibitor of HSP70 expression, aggravated the infiltration of inflammatory cells and glandular loss in the antrum. [32] Quercetin possesses gastric cytoprotective and gastric ulcer healing-promoting actions. In addition, the free radical-scavenging properties of it may be partly related to its anti-ulcer effects. [33] And the anti-ulcer activity of quercetin could be partly explained by the inhibition of lipid peroxidation, through decrease of reactive oxygen metabolites. [34]

As the etiology and pathogenesis of RAU are unclear, up to the present no entirely satisfactory method for scale prevention has been developed. It is easy to relapse and difficult to control and the long term efficacy of modern medicine therapies is not so satisfactory. Natural medicine, such as quercetin, treatment of RAU focus on the combination of local and systemic has certain advantages.

5. Adjuvant Therapies of Oral Cancers by Quercetin

Cancer is the enemy of human health. It is one of the major killers in human health, therefore, oncology has been the main focus of the study. Cancer treatment, in addition to traditional surgery, radiotherapy and chemotherapy, the treatment by comprehensive regulation of herb medicine is a hot area in recent years. Oral cancer is a subtype of any cancerous tissue growth located in the oral cavity. Oral cancer ranks as the 6th most common cancer in the world. It can occur in tongue, cheek, jaw, any part of the periodontal tissue. The incidence of males is 5 times than that of females. There are several types of oral cancers, but around 90% are squamous cell carcinomas, originating in the tissues that line the mouth and lips.

Many plant polyphenolic compounds have been shown to have cancer-preventing activities in laboratory studies. The polyphenolic or flavone has been shown to inhibit tumorigenesis in a variety of animal models of carcinogenesis. It is suggested that that the mechanisms of cancer preventive of flavonoids include the inhibition of carcinogen-activating cytochrome P450 (CYP) transcription and activities. [35] Quercetin is a flavonoid molecule ubiquitous in nature. A lot of researches have investigated the potency of quercetin against oral cancer risk. Researchers from over the world tested quercetin or extracts containing quercetin from several plants against cells of oral cancer in the lab and clinic. [36-38]

In studies *in vitro*, quercetin has been shown to affect signal transduction pathways, leading to inhibition of cell growth and transformation, enhanced apoptosis [39] modulating enzyme activities resulting in the decreased carcinogenicity of xenobiotics. [40] Quercetin induces necrosis and apoptosis in SCC-9 oral cancer cells. Quercetin initially induces a stress response, resulting in necrosis of these oral epithelial cells. Prolonged exposure of the surviving cells to quercetin causes apoptosis, presumably mediated by inhibition of Thymidylate synthase protein. [41]

Quercetin are also effective inhibitors of oral squamous carcinoma cell (SCC-25) growth and proliferation, and warrant further investigation as cancer chemopreventive agents. [42] Quercetin abrogates chemoresistance in melanoma cells by modulating deltaNp73. [43]

Quercetin induce caspase-3-dependent apoptosis in oral cavity cancer cells. [44] Quercetin would take a function of down-regulating the PI3K/Akt/IKK-alpha/NF-kappaB signaling pathway. [45]

Owing to its potent antioxidant and antiproliferative activities posttreatment, quercetin resulted in a significant hamster tumor growth delay. In addition, quercetin administration induced cell cycle arrest and apoptosis and blocked invasion and angiogenesis. [46]

A large number of clinical practices have shown that for patients with advanced cancer high-dose radiotherapy versus chemotherapy may increase the chances of death. Treating cancer by natural medicine could make up for surgery, radiation therapy and chemotherapy. The treatment of cancer by natural medicine with surgery may prevent postoperative complications and recurrence, accelerate postoperative recovery. The treatment of cancer by natural medicine and chemotherapy was better than the chemotherapy alone, and may also reduce the side effects of chemotherapy.

A number of its actions make quercetin a potential anti-cancer agent. It appears to be associated with little toxicity when administered orally or intravenously.

Much in vitro and some preliminary animal and human data indicate quercetin inhibits tumor growth. More research is needed to elucidate the absorption of oral doses and the magnitude of the anti-cancer effect. [47] More in-depth studies on bioavailability should facilitate correlation of mechanisms determined in vitro with in vivo situations, increase our understanding of dose-response relationships, and facilitate extrapolation of results from animal studies to human situations. [48]

References

[1] Moon, YJ; Wang, X; Morris, ME. Dietary flavonoids: effects on xenobiotic and carcinogen metabolism. *Toxicol In Vitro,* 2006 20, 187-210.

[2] Clark, GT; Nachnani, S; Messadi, DV. Detecting and treating oral and nonoral malodors. *J. Calif. Dent. Assoc.* 1997 25, 133-44.

[3] Scully, C; el-Maaytah, M; Porter, SR; Greenman, J. Breath odor: etiopathogenesis, assessment and management. *Eur. J. Oral. Sci.* 1997 105, 287-93.

[4] Messadi, DV. Oral and nonoral sources of halitosis. *J. Calif. Dent. Assoc.* 1997 25, 127-31.

[5] Kozlovsky, A; Gordon, D; Gelernter, I; Loesche, WJ; Rosenberg, M. Correlation between the BANA test and oral malodor parameters. *J. Dent. Res.* 1994 73, 1036-42.

[6] Kleinberg, I; Westbay, G. Oral malodor. *Critical reviews in oral biology and medicine.* 1990 1, 247-59.

[7] Li, MY; Wang, J; Xu ZT. Effect of a Variety of Chinese Herbs and an Herb-Containing Dentifrice on Volatile Sulfur Compounds Associated With Halitosis: An *In Vitro* Analysis. *Clinical Therapeutics, Current Therapeutic Research.* 2010 71, 129-140.

[8] Lee, S; Jung, SH; Lee, YS; Yamada, M; Kim, BK; Ohuchi, K; Shin, KH. Antiinflammatory activity of hyperin from Acanthopanax chiisanensis roots. *Arch. Pharm. Res.* 2004 27, 628-32.

[9] Wang, YJ; Yang, XW; Guo, QS. Studies on chemical constituents in Huangjuhua (flowers of Chrysanthemum morifolium). *Zhongguo Zhong Yao Za Zhi.* 2008 33, 526-30. Chinese.

[10] Yuan, JQ; Yang, JS; Miao, JH. Studies on flavonoids of *Eupatorium odoratum L. Zhong Yao Cai.* 2007 30, 657-60. Chinese.

[11] Choi, CW; Jung, HA; Kang, SS; Choi, JS. Antioxidant constituents and a new triterpenoid glycoside from *Flos Lonicerae. Arch. Pharm. Res.* 2007 30, 1-7.

[12] Xue, YL; Ahiko, T; Miyakawa, T; Amino, H; Hu, F; Furihata, K; Kita, K; Shirasawa, T; Sawano, Y; Tanokura, M. *J. Agric. Food Chem.* 2011 12. [Epub ahead of print].

[13] Jung, HA; Kim, YS; Choi, JS. Quantitative HPLC analysis of two key flavonoids and inhibitory activities against aldose reductase from different parts of the Korean thistle, *Cirsium. maackii. Food Chem. Toxicol.* 2009 47, 2790-7.

[14] Chen, L; Tang, YP; Chen, MJ; Deng, HS; Yan, XP; Wu, DK. Chemical correlation between Gegen Qinlian dispensing granule and its four raw herbs by LC fingerprint. *Phytomedicine.* 2010 17, 100-7.

[15] Wang, W; Zu, Y; Fu, Y; Reichling, J; Suschke, U; Nokemper, S; Zhang, Y. *In vitro* antioxidant, antimicrobial and anti-herpes simplex virus type 1 activity of *Phellodendron amurense Rupr.* from China. *Am. J. Chin. Med.* 2009 37, 195-203.

[16] Kim, SH; Joo, MH; Yoo, SH. Structural identification and antioxidant properties of major anthocyanin extracted from Omija (*Schizandra chinensis*) fruit. *J. Food Sci.* 2009 74, C134-40.

[17] Marsh, PD. The significance of maintaining the stability of the natural microflora of the mouth. *Br. Dent. J.* 1991 21, 174–177.

[18] Osamu, N. Effect of polyphenol oxidase on deodorizatin. *Biosci. Biotech. Biochem.* 1997 61, 2080-2084.

[19] Zhu, L. Clinical observation of the action of honeysuckle mouth tablets on inhibiting plaque and *Streptococcus mutans* in saliva, *Journal of Guangdong Dental Disease Prevention and Treatments.* 1995 5, 96-97.

[20] Loesche, WJ. Role of Streptococcus mutans in human dental decay. *Microbiol. Rev.* 1986 50, 353-80.

[21] Uzel, A; Sorkun, K; Onçağ, O; Cogŭlu, D; Gençay, O; Salih, B. Chemical compositions and antimicrobial activities of four different Anatolian propolis samples. *Microbiol. Res.* 2005 160, 189-95.

[22] [22] Gregoire, S; Singh, AP; Vorsa, N; Koo, H. Influence of cranberry phenolics on glucan synthesis by glucosyltransferases and *Streptococcus mutans* acidogenicity. *J. Appl. Microbiol.* 2007 103, 1960-8.

[23] Wood, N. The effects of selected dietary bioflavonoid supplementation on dental caries in young rats fed a high-sucrose diet. *J. Med. Food.* 2007 10, 694-701.

[24] Guan, X; Zhou, Y; Liang, X; Xiao, J; He, L; Li, J. Effects of compounds found in *Nidus Vespae* on the growth and cariogenic virulence factors of *Streptococcus mutans. Microbiol. Res.* 2011 16, [Epub ahead of print].

[25] Paolantonio, M; D'ercole, S; Perinetti, G; Tripodi, D; Catamo, G; Serra, E; Bruè, C; Piccolomini, R. Clinical and microbiological effects of different restorative materials on the periodontal tissues adjacent to subgingival class V restorations. *J. Clin. Periodontol.* 2004 31, 200-7.

[26] Nogueira, Moreira, A; Fernández, Canigia, L; Furman, C; Chiappe, V; Marcantoni, M; Bianchini, H. Clinical and microbiological study of adult periodontal disease. *Rev. Argent. Microbiol.* 2001 33, 133-40.

[27] Romanelli, R; Mancini, S; Laschinger, C; Overall, CM; Sodek, J; McCulloch, CA. Activation of neutrophil collagenase in periodontitis. *Infect. Immun.* 1999 67, 2319-26.

[28] Curttis, MA; Kuramitsu, HK; Lanz, M; Macrina, FL; Nakayama, K; Potempa, J; Raynolds, EC and Aduse-Opoku, J. Molecular genetics and nomenclature of proteases of *Porphyromonas gingivalis*. *J. Periodont. Res.* 1999 34, 464–472.

[29] Petra, L; Edda, B; Elke, G; Jutta, W and Helmut, H. Comparison of Broth Microdilution, E Test, and Agar Dilution Methods for Antibiotic Susceptibility Testing of *Campylobacter jejuni* and *Campylobacter coli*. *Journal of Clinical Microbiology*. 2003 41, 1062-1068.

[30] Homer, KA; Beighton, D. Synergistic degradation of transferrin by mutans streptococci in association with other dental plaque bacteria. *Microb. Ecol. Health Dis.* 1992 5, 111-116.

[31] Hamdy, AA; Ibrahem, MA. Management of aphthous ulceration with topical quercetin: a randomized clinical trial. *J. Contemp. Dent. Pract.* 2010 1;11, E009-16.

[32] Liu, WL; Chen, SJ; Chen, Y; Sun, LM; Zhang, W; Zeng, YM; Zhou, TH; Si, JM. Protective effects of heat shock protein 70 induced by geranylgeranylacetone in atrophic gastritis in rats. *Acta. Pharmacol. Sin.* 2007 28, 1001-6.

[33] Suzuki, Y; Ishihara, M; Segami, T; Ito, M. Anti-ulcer effects of antioxidants, quercetin, alpha-tocopherol, nifedipine and tetracycline in rats. *Jpn. J. Pharmacol.* 1998 78, 435-41.

[34] Martín, MJ; La-Casa, C; Alarcón-de-la-Lastra, C; Cabeza, J; Villegas, I; Motilva, V. Anti-oxidant mechanisms involved in gastroprotective effects of quercetin. *Z. Naturforsch C.* 1998 53, 82-8.

[35] Walle, T; Walle, UK. Novel methoxylated flavone inhibitors of cytochrome P450 1B1 in SCC-9 human oral cancer cells. *J. Pharm. Pharmacol.* 2007 59, 857-62.

[36] De, S; Chakraborty, RN; Ghosh, S; Sengupta, A; Das, S. Comparative evaluation of cancer chemopreventive efficacy of alpha-tocopherol and quercetin in a murine model. *J. Exp. Clin. Cancer Res.* 2004 23, 251-8.

[37] Gee, JM; Hara, H; Johnson, IT. Suppression of intestinal crypt cell proliferation and aberrant crypt foci by dietary quercetin in rats. *Nutr Cancer.* 2002 43, 193-201.

[38] Kale, R; Saraf, M; Juvekar, A; Tayade, P. Decreased B16F10 melanoma growth and impaired tumour vascularization in BDF1 mice with quercetin-cyclodextrin binary system. *J. Pharm. Pharmacol.* 2006 58, 1351-8.

[39] Lambert, JD; Hong, J; Yang, GY; Liao, J; Yang, CS. Inhibition of carcinogenesis by polyphenols: evidence from laboratory investigations. *Am. J. Clin. Nutr.* 2005 81(1 Suppl), 284S-291S.

[40] Moon, YJ; Wang, X; Morris, ME. Dietary flavonoids: effects on xenobiotic and carcinogen metabolism. *Toxicol. In. Vitro.* 2006 20, 187-210.

[41] Haghiac, M; Walle, T. Quercetin induces necrosis and apoptosis in SCC-9 oral cancer cells. *Nutr. Cancer.* 2005 53, 220-31.

[42] ElAttar, TM; Virji, AS. Modulating effect of resveratrol and quercetin on oral cancer cell growth and proliferation. *Anticancer. Drugs.* 1999 10, 187-93.

[43] Thangasamy, T; Sittadjody, S; Mitchell, GC; Mendoza, EE; Radhakrishnan, VM; Limesand, KH; Burd, R. Quercetin abrogates chemoresistance in melanoma cells by modulating deltaNp 73. *BMC Cancer,* 2010 11,10, 282.

[44] Kang, JW; Kim, JH; Song, K; Kim, SH; Yoon, JH; Kim, KS. Kaempferol and quercetin, components of Ginkgo biloba extract (EGb 761), induce caspase-3-dependent apoptosis in oral cavity cancer cells. *Phytother. Res.* 2010 24 Suppl 1, S77-82.

[45] Sun, ZJ; Chen, G; Hu, X; Zhang, W; Liu, Y; Zhu, LX; Zhou, Q; Zhao, YF. Activation of PI3K/Akt/IKK-alpha/NF-kappaB signaling pathway is required for the apoptosis-evasion in human salivary adenoid cystic carcinoma: its inhibition by quercetin. *Apoptosis.* 2010 15, 850-63.

[46] Priyadarsini, RV; Vinothini, G; Murugan, RS; Manikandan, P; Nagini, S. The flavonoid quercetin modulates the hallmark capabilities of hamster buccal pouch tumors. *Nutr. Cancer.* 2011 63, 218-26.

[47] Lamson, DW; Brignall, MS. Antioxidants and cancer, part 3: quercetin. *Altern. Med. Rev.* 2000 5, 196-208.

[48] Lambert, JD; Hong, J; Yang, GY; Liao, J; Yang, CS. Inhibition of carcinogenesis by polyphenols: evidence from laboratory investigations. *Am. J. Clin. Nutr.* 2005 81(1 Suppl), 284S-291S.

In: Quercetin
Editors: Taiki Chikamatsu and Yuudai Hida
ISBN: 978-1 61942- 057-1

Chapter 12

REACTIONS OF QUERCETIN AND ITS GLYCOSIDES IN THE ORAL CAVITY AND THE STOMACH

Umeo Takahama[1] and Sachiko Hirota[2]
[1]Department of Bioscience, Kyushu Dental College, Japan
[2]Department of Nutritional Science, Kyushu Women's University, Kitakyushu, Japan

ABSTRACT

After ingestion of foods that contain quercetin glycosides, some of them are hydrolyzed to quercetin in the oral cavity, and quercetin can stay in the cavity for several hours. During its stay in the oral cavity, quercetin can suppress the nitration induced by salivary peroxidase/H_2O_2/nitrite systems by competing with nitrite for peroxidase and/or by scavenging reactive nitrogen oxide species. Accompanying the suppression, quercetin is oxidized and one of the oxidation products is 2-(3,4-dihydroxybenzoyl)-2,4,6-trihydroxy- 3(*2H*)-benzofuranone. In the stomach, quercetin and its glycosides can reduce salivary nitrite to nitric oxide (NO), which has various functions. If quercetin functions as the reductant, quercetin is transformed to the benzofuranone described above, and if a quercetin glycoside such as rutin functions as the reductant, *o*-quinone of rutin is formed, which reacts with salivary component SCN^- to produce an oxathiolone derivative of rutin. In the small intestine, quercetin and rutin may be able to slow down starch digestion by binding to starch. In this chapter, various functions of quercetin and its glycoside in the digestive tract are described, especially from the points of scavenging of reactive nitrogen oxide species and inhibition of its formation.

INTRODUCTION

Quercetin glycosides are present in various foods. It is well known that onion bulbs contain large amounts of quercetin 4'-glucoside and quercetin 3,4'-diglucosides, and that buckwheat flour contains rutin. After ingestion of foods that contain quercetin glycosides, some of them can be hydrolyzed to quercetin in the human oral cavity and quercetin remains in the cavity for several hours (Hirota et al., 2001). Quercetin that remains in the oral cavity can function as an electron donor to salivary peroxidase and myeloperoxidase which is derived from leukocytes migrated into the oral cavity (Al-Essa et al., 1994; Hirota et al., 2002, 2005; Yamamoto et al., 1991). The electron donating activity of quercetin can contribute to the inhibition of oxidation of salivary nitrite, which is induced by salivary peroxidase/H_2O_2 and myeloperoxidase/H_2O_2 systems. Nitrogen dioxide (NO_2) produced by the peroxidase-catalyzed reactions can nitrate salivary components.

Quercetin produced by the hydrolysis of quercetin glycosides in the oral cavity is swallowed into the stomach. In the stomach, salivary nitrite is transformed to nitrous acid that can oxidize quercetin. The redox reactions between nitrous acid and quercetin result in the production of nitric oxide (NO) (Takahama et al., 2002). Because not all of quercetin glycosides are hydrolyzed in the oral cavity, quercetin glycosides in foods can also be oxidized by nitrous acid in the stomach to produce NO. If a catechol group is present in a quercetin glycoside, an *o*-quinone is the oxidation product. Thiocyanate is present in saliva, so that the reaction of SCN^- with the *o*-quinone is possible in the stomach. The reaction product is an oxathiolone derivative of the glycoside (Takahama et al., 2009a). The oxathiolone derivative of a quercetin glycoside is supposed to be hydrolyzed to an oxathiolone derivative of quercetin in the intestine because of the presence of glycosidases.

As described above, quercetin and its glycosides have various functions in the oral cavity and the stomach. This chapter, at first, deals with the antioxidative activity of quercetin in the oral cavity from the points of the scavenging of reactive nitrogen oxide species and inhibition of its production, and then deals with the reduction of nitrous acid to NO by quercetin and its glycosides and the formation of oxathiolones in the stomach. Finally, this chapter deals with the formation of quercetin- and rutin-starch complexes, to discuss the function of these flavonoids from the point of starch digestion.

Functions of Quercetin in the Oral Cavity

Flavonoid glycosides in foods and beverages are mixed with saliva or bound to the tissues in the oral cavity. Because various bacteria, which can secrete glycosidases, are present in the oral cavity (Makinen, 1989; Marsh and Martin, 1999), hydrolysis of flavonoid glycosides to the aglycones is possible in the cavity.

It has been reported that quercetin glucosides in onion soup, which are quercetin 4'-glucoside and quercetin 3,4'-diglucosides, are hydrolyzed to the aglycone in the oral cavity to bind to oral tissues (Hirota et al, 2001). In addition to quercetin glucosides, genistein 7-glucoside and diosmetin 7-rutinoside have also been reported to be able to be hydrolyzed in the oral cavity (Browning et al., 2005; Walle et al., 2005). The flavonoid aglycones including quercetin can inhibit proliferation of oral cancer cells (Browning et al., 2005; Walle et al., 2005).

Polymorphonuclear leukocytes in saliva (SPMN) suspended in a Krebs-Ringer phosphate solution (pH 7.4) consume oxygen and the oxygen consumption is enhanced by phorbol myristate acetate (Al-Essa et al., 1994; Yamamoto et al., 1991). Quercetin inhibits the oxygen consumption in the presence and absence of the phorbol ester (Hirota et al., 2002). During the inhibition of oxygen consumption, absorption spectra of quercetin changes.

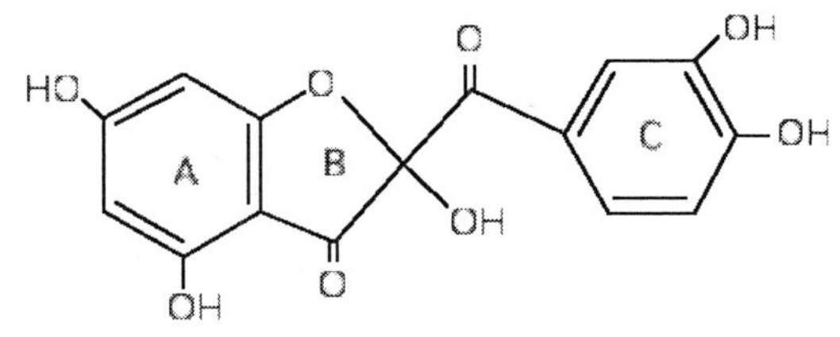

Figure 1. Structure of 2-(3,4-dihydroxybenzoyl)-2,4,6-trihydroxy-3(*2H*)- benzofuranone.

The changes in absorption spectra are enhanced and inhibited by horseradish peroxidase and superoxide dismutase, respectively, suggesting the contribution of H_2O_2 and $O_2^{\bullet-}$ produced by SPMN to the changes in the absorption spectra. The production of $O_2^{\bullet-}$ and H_2O_2 by SPMN has been reported (Al-Essa et al., 1994; Nakahara et al., 1998; Yamamoto et al., 1991). $O_2^{\bullet-}$ can oxidize quercetin by itself to produce H_2O_2, and H_2O_2 can oxidize quercetin by cooperating with myeloperoxidase. In addition to myeloperoxidase, salivary peroxidase also oxidizes quercetin (Hirota et al., 2001). One of the oxidation products of quercetin has been determined to be 2-(3,4-dihydroxybenzoyl)-2,4,6-trihydroxy-3(*2H*)-benzofuranone (Figure 1), which is transformed to 2,4,6-trihydroxyphenylglyoxylic acid and 3,4-dihydroxybenzoic acid (Hirota et al., 2005). Nitrate is present in leafy vegetables such as lettuce and spinach (Tamme et al., 2006). By the ingestion of vegetables, nitrate is absorbed into the human body by the intestine. Part of the absorbed nitrate is secreted into the oral cavity as a component of saliva. Nitrate secreted into the oral cavity is reduced to nitrite by nitrate-reducing bacteria and then NO by nitrite-reducing bacteria (Doel et al., 2004,2005; Palmerini et al., 2003). Because bacteria and SPMN can produce H_2O_2 and salivary peroxidase and myeloperoxidase from SPMN are present in the oral cavity (Tenovuo, 1989), oxidation of nitrite by these peroxidases is possible:

$$\text{Peroxidase} + H_2O_2 \rightarrow \text{Compound I} + H_2O \qquad (1)$$

$$\text{Compound I} + NO_2^- \rightarrow \text{Compound II} + NO_2 \qquad (2)$$

$$\text{Compound II} + NO_2^- + 2H^+ \rightarrow \text{peroxidase} + NO_2 + H_2O \qquad (3)$$

Nitrogen dioxide (NO_2) (NO_2/NO_2^-; $E^{o\prime}$ = 0.99 V at pH 7) (Halliwell and Gutteridge, 1999) produced by the above reactions is an oxidizing and nitrating agent (Burner et al., 2000; Shibata et al., 1995; van der Vliet et al., 1997). 4-Hydroxyphenylacetic acid (HPA) is used to estimate nitration in certain systems, and this component is found in the oral cavity as an intermediate of tyrosine metabolism. SPMN induces nitration of HPA to 4-hydroxy-3-nitrophenylacetic acid in the presence of 1 mM nitrite in Krebs-Ringer phosphate solution (pH 7.4) (Hirota and Takahama, 2003). The following reactions are possibilities as the mechanism of nitration:

$$\text{HPA} + NO_2 \rightarrow \text{HPA radical} + NO_2^- + H^+ \qquad (4)$$

$$\text{2HPA} + H_2O_2 \rightarrow \text{2HPA radical} + 2H_2O \qquad (5)$$

$$\text{HPA radical} + NO_2 \rightarrow \text{Nitrated HPA} \qquad (6)$$

Reaction 5 can be catalyzed by peroxidases. Quercetin inhibited the nitration of HPA induced by SPMN (Hirota and Takahama, 2003) and by salivary peroxidase/H_2O_2/nitrite systems at pH 7 (Hirota et al., 2005), suggesting that phenolic compounds with antioxidative activity can inhibit nitration in the oral cavity. Possible mechanisms of the inhibition are (i) the suppression of peroxidase-catalyzed oxidation of nitrite to NO_2 (reactions 1-3) and HPA to its radical (reaction 5), and (ii) the reduction of NO_2 produced by reactions 1-3 to nitrite. The mechanism (i) is supported by the result that quercetin is oxidized by salivary peroxidase and myeloperoxidase in the presence of H_2O_2 as described above, and the mechanism (ii) is supported by the result that quercetin oxidation induced by salivary peroxidase can be enhanced by nitrite (Hirota et al., 2005; Takahama et al., 2006a). The scavenging of NO_2 by quercetin is also suggested by quercetin-dependent inhibition of the transformation of 4,5-diaminofluorescein (DAF-2) to its triazole form, to which NO plus NO_2 or N_2O_3 may contribute (Takahama et al., 2006b). However, quercetin seems to mainly suppress the nitration by the mechanism (i) at neutral pH, because quercetin is a better electron donor to salivary peroxidase at pH 7 (Hirota et al., 2005).

The nitration of HPA is suppressed by SCN^- at pH 7, a physiological substrate of salivary peroxidase (Tenovuo, 1989), by inhibiting salivary peroxidase-catalyzed oxidation of nitrite and HPA (Takahama et al., 2003a). Uric acid, a major antioxidant in saliva, may also inhibit the nitration by scavenging NO_2 (Prütz et al., 1985; Takahama and Hirota, 2010a). Although the inhibitors of nitration are present in the oral cavity, nitrated HPA is found in saliva from some patients of periodontal diseases (Takahama et al., 2009b). This finding indicates that the nitration reaction can proceed in the human oral cavity under certain conditions.

The pH of dental plaque rapidly decreases to approximately 5 after ingestion of foods with sugars (Marsh and Martin, 1999). Therefore, nitrite-induced transformation of 3-amino-monomethylamino-2',7'-difluorofluorescein (DAF-FM) to its triazole form, which is induced by N_2O_3 and/or NO plus oxidants that can oxidize DAF-FM to its radicals (Espey et al., 2002; Jourd'heuil, 2002; Kojima et al., 1999), is studied at pH 5.3 and pH 7. The transformation is faster at pH 5.3 than pH 7 in bacterial fraction prepared from mixed whole saliva (Takahama et al., 2007a, 2009c). This result implies the faster formation of reactive nitrogen oxide species, which contributes to the transformation of DAF-FM to its triazole form, is faster in acidic than neutral dental plaque. In the paper, it is indicated that the inhibitory effect of 10 μM quercetin on the transformation of DAF-FM is smaller at pH 5.3 than pH 7, whereas 1 μM ascorbic acid equally inhibited the transformation at the two pH values (Takahama et al., 2009c). The result suggests that quercetin [pKa = 6.6 and 9.7 (Zenkevich and Guschina, 2010)] seems to effectively scavenge the reactive nitrogen oxide species, which contributes to the transformation, under the conditions that the phenolic OH groups are partly dissociated. At pH 5.3, about 20% of quercetin is present as the mono-anion, and at pH 7, about 60 and 6% of quercetin is present as the mono-anion and the di-anion, respectively. The faster formation of reactive nitrogen oxide species around pH 5 than pH 7 has also been reported using bacterial fraction prepared from mixed whole saliva by measuring the nitrite-induced oxidation of uric acid (Takahama and Hirota, 2010a). Because NO_2 contributes to the oxidation of uric acid, the result implies that nitrite-induced production of NO_2 in dental plaque can be enhanced by the decrease in pH.

Nitrite-induced transformation of DAF-FM to its triazole form is enhanced by SCN^- at pH 5.3, and suppressed at pH 7 in bacterial fraction prepared from mixed whole saliva

(Takahama et al., 2007a, 2009c). The inhibition at pH 7 can be attributed to the inhibition of peroxidase activity, and the enhancement at pH 5.3 can be attributed to ONSCN produced by the reaction of nitrous acid with SCN^- (see below). ONSCN can dissociate to SCN^- and NO^+ (NO/NO^+; $E^{o'}$ = 1.21 V at pH 7.0) (Licht et al., 1988), which is a strong oxidant (Halliwell and Gutteridge, 1999). At pH 5.3, about 1% of nitrite is present as nitrous acid (pKa = 3.3).

Nitration of HPA by salivary peroxidase/H_2O_2/nitrite systems has been studied in the pH range from 4.5 to 8. The result indicates that the nitration has peaks around pH 5 and pH 7 (Hirota et al., 2005). Quercetin (5 μM) inhibited the nitration about 20 and 90% at pH 5.3 and pH 7.2, respectively. The different degree of inhibition suggests that the mechanism of nitration at pH 7 is different from that at pH 5, in addition to the difference in degree of H^+ dissociation of the phenolic OH groups around pH 5 and pH 7. The oxidation of 5 μM quercetin by salivary peroxidase/H_2O_2 systems has a peak at pH 7.2, and its oxidation is enhanced by nitrite; the degree of the enhancement increases as pH decreases from 8 to 4.5. On the other hand, the oxidation reactions of HPA and nitrite by salivary peroxidase/H_2O_2/nitrite systems have a peak around pH 7 and pH 5, respectively. The faster oxidation of HPA suggests that HPA radicals mainly contributed to the nitration around pH 7. Therefore, if HPA radicals are scavenged and/or its production is inhibited effectively by quercetin, nitration can be effectively suppressed. The faster oxidation of nitrite suggests that NO_2 mainly contributes to the nitration around pH 5. The smaller inhibition of the nitration by quercetin at pH 5 than pH 7 may be due to the less efficient scavenging of NO_2 as opposed to HPA radicals and less efficient inhibition of peroxidase-catalyzed oxidation of nitrite and HPA at pH 5 rather than pH 7 by quercetin.

In addition to NO_2, peroxynitrite ($ONOO^-$/ONOOH) (pKa = 6.8) can be produced in the oral cavity because both NO and $O_2^{\bullet -}$ are formed in the cavity. $ONOO^-$ is stable, but ONOOH decomposes to NO_2 plus OH radicals or rearranges to nitrate (Halliwell and Gutteridge, 1999). The formation of $ONOO^-$/ONOOH in the oral cavity is suggested by the oxidative degradation of aminophenol fluorescein (APF) that is oxidized by strong oxidants such as OH radicals, NO_2, and HOCl, but not $O_2^{\bullet -}$ (Setsukinai et al., 2003). This suggestion is based on the observation that superoxide dismutase inhibited the nitrite-induced oxidation of APF in bacterial fraction prepared from mixed whole saliva filtrate in the pH range from 5.3 to 7.2 (Takahama et al., 2007a).

The contribution of NO^+ formed from ONSCN is discussed for the enhancement of nitrite-induced APF oxidation by SCN^- at pH 5 (Takahama et al., 2007a, 2009c). According to their reduction potentials, quercetin can scavenge NO^+ and $ONOO^-$/ONOOH ($ONOOH/NO_2$; $E^{o'}$ = 2.10 V at pH 7) (Halliwell and Gutteridge, 1999).

Reaction of Quercetin and its Glycosides in the Stomach

As described above, saliva contains nitrite, and the nitrite is mixed with gastric juice, the pH of which is around 2. Therefore, almost all of the salivary nitrite is transformed to nitrous acid in the stomach, which is much more reactive than nitrite ion. Once nitrous acid is formed, it can decompose as the following:

$$NO_2^- + H^+ \rightleftarrows HNO_2 \text{ (pKa = 3.3)} \quad (7)$$

$$HNO_2 + H^+ \rightleftarrows H_2NO_2^+ \rightleftarrows H_2O + NO^+ \quad (8)$$

$$2HNO_2 \rightleftarrows N_2O_3 + H_2O \quad (9)$$

$$N_2O_3 \rightleftarrows NO + NO_2 \quad (10)$$

Ascorbic acid present in gastric juice can reduce nitrous acid,

$$\text{Ascorbic acid} + 2HNO_2 \rightarrow 2NO + \text{Dehydroascorbic acid} + 2H_2O \quad (11)$$

Salivary SCN^- can enhance the ascorbic acid-dependent reduction of nitrous acid (Takahama et al., 2003b):

$$SCN^- + HNO_2 + H^+ \rightarrow ONSCN + H_2O \quad (12)$$

$$\text{Ascorbic acid} + 2ONSCN \rightarrow 2NO + \text{Dehydroascorbic acid} + 2SCN^- + 2H^+ \quad (13)$$

Thus, ascorbic acid/nitrite/SCN^- systems may function as a main NO generation system in the stomach when foods are not ingested. The production of NO results in the lowering of the concentrations of both nitrite and ascorbic acid, but NO can be transformed to N_2O_3 by autoxidation, which can be hydrolyzed to nitrous acid (Halliwell and Gutteridge, 1999).

$$4NO + O_2 \rightarrow 2N_2O_3 \quad (14)$$

$$N_2O_3 + H_2O \rightarrow 2HNO_2 \quad (15)$$

Therefore, no significant decrease in the concentration of nitrite in the stomach will occur as long as the above reactions proceed. If phenolic compounds such as quercetin are supplied as food components, these compounds reduce nitrous acid to NO after almost all of ascorbic acid has been oxidized by nitrous acid in the stomach as follows(Takahama et al., 2003c):

$$PhOH + HNO_2 \rightarrow NO + PhO\ \text{radical} + H_2O \quad (16)$$

PhOH is a phenolic compound and PhO radical is a phenoxyl radical. ONSCN, which may be present in the gastric juice, did not enhance the oxidation of quercetin. The oxidation of quercetin by the above reaction results in absorbance increases at 293 nm (Takahama et al., 2002), and the component is supposed to be 2-(3,4-dihydroxybenzoyl)-2,4,6-trihydroxy-3(*2H*)-benzofuranone (Figure 1). In addition to quercetin, caffeic acid, chlorogenic acid, and rutin can function as efficient reductants for nitrous acid (Peri et al., 2005; Takahama et al., 2007b, 2009a). These compounds are transformed to the *o*-quinones via phenoxyl radicals on oxidation under acidic conditions (Takahama et al., 2007b, 2009a, 2010a). Phenolic compound-dependent reduction of nitrous acid to NO has been suggested after drinking wine (Gago et al., 2007; Takahama et al., 2010a) and eating food prepared from buckwheat flour (Takahama et al., 2010b).

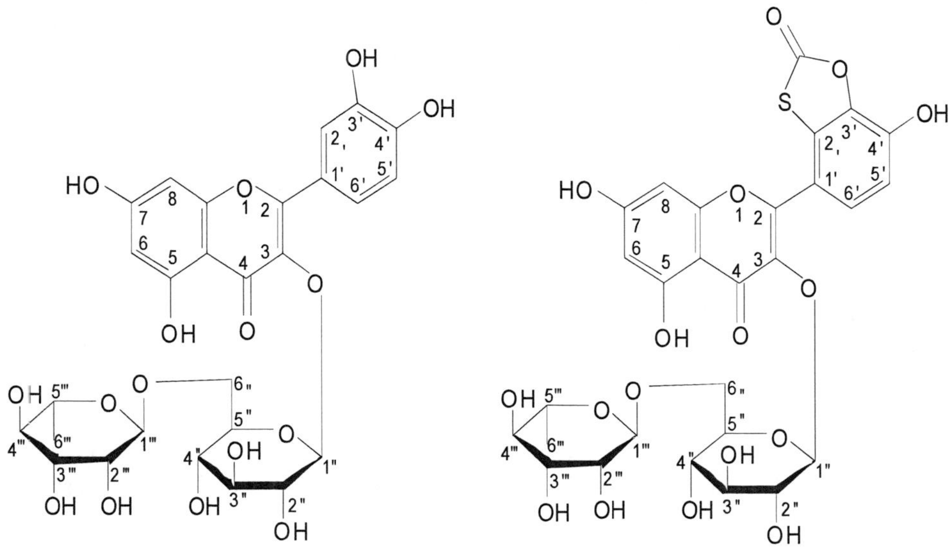

Figure 2. Chemical structures of rutin (left) and an oxathiolone derivative of rutin (right).

It has been reported that NO produced by the reduction of nitrous acid is able to protect against experimentally induced gastric ulcers (Jansson et al., 2007), gastritis (Larauche et al., 2003), and gastric mucosal injury (Miyosh et al., 2003). In addition, as functions of NO, activation of gastric activity (Björne et al., 2004), regulation of gastric acid secretion (Berg et al., 2005; Hasebe et al., 2005; Kato et al., 1998; Tanaka et al., 2001), and antimicrobial activity (Benjamin et al., 1994; Dykhuizen et al., 1996) have been reported. If NO produced in the gastric juice has functions that are beneficial for human health, the ingestion of polyphenol-containing foods and beverages may be recommended from the point of NO production.

Rutin is oxidized by nitrite under acidic conditions to produce the *o*-quinone and NO (Takahama et al., 2009a). The quinone form of rutin can react with SCN^- to produce an oxathiolone derivative of rutin (Figure 2). In addition to the quinone form of rutin, *o*-quinone forms of caffeic and chlorogenic acids can also react with SCN^- producing oxathiolone derivatives of caffeic and chlorogenic acids, respectively (Takahama et al., 2007b, 2010a). Although the above phenolic compounds with a catechol group in each molecule can be transformed to oxathiolone derivatives, quercetin cannot be transformed to its oxathiolone derivative (Takahama et al., 2009a). This may be due to the fact that the quinone intermediate of quercetin is not stable enough to react with SCN^-. An oxathiolone derivative of quercetin has been prepared by acid hydrolysis of the oxathiolone derivative of rutin in Figure 2 (Takahama et al., 2011). Our recent study suggests that an incubation medium of *Escherichia coli* hydrolyzed the oxathiolone derivative of rutin to the oxidation derivative of quercetin, suggesting the occurrence of hydrolysis in the intestine (unpublished result).

Various oxathiolone derivatives have been reported to have various biochemical and biological effects. These include the inhibition of the growth of microorganisms and human cancer cells (Konieczny et al., 2007), the inhibition of carbonic anhydrase (Innocenti et al., 2008), the inactivation of inhibitory kappaB kinase beta (Kim et al., 2008), and the inhibition of xanthine oxidase (Takahama et al., 2011). In our recent study, it is shown that an oxathiolone derivative of quercetin inhibited the growth and the respiration of *Micrococcus luteus* but not *Escherichia coli* and *Staphylococcus aureus*, suggesting that the oxathiolone derivative could suppress the growth of certain bacteria by inhibiting their respiration (unpublished results).

Possible Functions of Quercetin in the Intestine

During the cooking of starch containing foods, phenolic compounds as well as fatty acids can bind to starch, especially amylose, if the foods contain phenolic compounds and/or free fatty acids. The binding of phenolic compounds and/or free fatty acids results in a decrease in the binding of iodine to starch and the inhibition of α-amylase-catalyzed digestion (Takahama and Hirota, 2010b).

Quercetin, rutin, and epicatechin-dimethylgallate isolated from buckwheat flour also bind to starch to inhibit its digestion by α-amylase. Furthermore, a recent study suggests that bile acids also suppress the digestion of starch by α-amylase by making starch-bile acid complexes (Takahama and Hirota, 2011). The above results suggest that not only phenolic compounds but also phytosterols may be able to inhibit starch digestion by binding to starch.

Conclusion

Quercetin glycosides in foods can be hydrolyzed to quercetin in the oral cavity to function as an antioxidant by scavenging O_2^- generated by SPMN and oral bacteria, and NO_2 generated by peroxidase/H_2O_2/nitrite systems. Quercetin can inhibit nitrite oxidation by peroxidase/H_2O_2 systems. When the pH in the oral cavity is decreased to below 5, formation of reactive nitrogen oxide species is increased by self-decomposition of nitrous acid, SCN^-/nitrite systems, and peroxidase/H_2O_2/nitrite systems. Although polyphenols including quercetin can function as scavengers of reactive nitrogen oxide species under acidic conditions, it seems to be important to avoid the frequent or prolonged decrease in pH in dental plaque to keep the oral cavity healthy because the decrease in pH results in the increased production of reactive nitrogen oxide species. In the stomach, quercetin and its glycosides can reduce nitrous acid to NO that has various functions. If compounds with a catechol group such as rutin and chlorogenic acid are oxidized by nitrous acid, oxathiolone derivatives of these components can be produced via their *o*-quinones in the stomach. The functions of oxathiolone derivatives formed in the stomach remain to be elucidated. Finally, quercetin and rutin can bind to starch to slow down its digestion in the intestine to prevent the rapid absorbance of glucose into the human body.

References

Al-Essa, L., Niwa, M., Kohno, K. and Tsurumi, K. (1994) A proposal for purification of salivary polymorphonuclear leukocytes by combination of nylon mesh filtration and density-gradient method: a validation by superoxide- and cyclic AMP-generating responses. *Life Sci.* 55, PL333-PL338.

Benjamin, N., O'Driscoll, F., Dougall, H., Duncan, C., Smith, L., Golden, M. and McKenzie, H. (1994) Stomach NO. *Nature* 368: 502.

Berg, A., Redéen, S., Grenegård, M., Ericson, A.-C. and Sjöstrand, S.E. (2005) Nitric oxide inhibits gastric acid secretion by increasing intraparietal cell levels of cGMP in isolated human gastric glands. *Am. J. Physiol. Gastrointest. Liver Physiol.* 289, G1061-1066.

Björne, H., Petersson, J., Phillipson, M., Weizberg, E., Holm L., and Lundberg, J.O. (2004) Nitrite in saliva increases gastric mucosal blood flow and mucus thickness. *J. Clinc. Invest.* 113, 106-114.

Browning, A.M., Walle, U.K. and Walle, T. (2005) Flavonoid glycosides inhibit oral cancer proliferation – role of cellular uptake and hydrolysis to the aglycones. *J. Pharm. Pharmacol.* 57, 1037-1041.

Burner, U., Furtmuller, P.G., Kettle, A.J., Koppenol, W.H. and Oblinger, C. (2000) Mechanism of reaction of myeloperoxidase with nitrite. *J. Biol. Chem.* 275, 20597-20601.

Doel, J.J., Hector, M.P., Amirtham, C.V., Al-Anzan, L.A., Benjamin, N., Allaker, R.P. (2004) Protective effect of salivary nitrite and microbial nitrate reductase activity against caries. *Eur. J. Oral Sci.* 11, 424-428.

Doel, J.J., Benjamin, N., Hector, M.P., Rogers, M., and Allaker, R.P. (2005) Evaluation of bacterial nitrate reduction in the human oral cavity. *Eur. J. Oral Sci.* 113, 14-19.

Dykhuizen, R.S., Franzer, R., Duncan, C., Smith, C.C., Golden, M., Benjamin, N. and Leifert, C. (1996) Antimicrobial effect of acidified nitrite on gut pathogens: Importance of dietary nitrate in host defense. *Antimicrob. Agents Chemother.* 40, 1422-1425.

Espey, M.G., Thomas, D.D., Miranda, K.M., and Wink, D.A. (2002) Focusing of nitric oxide mediated nitrosation and oxidative nitrosylation as a consequence of reaction with superoxide. *Proc. Natl. Acad. Sci. USA*, 99, 11127-11132.

Gago, B., Lundberg, J.O., Barbosa, R.M. and Laranjinha, J. (2007) Red wine-dependent reduction of nitrite to nitric oxide in the stomach. *Free Radic. Biol. Med.* 43, 1233-1242.

Halliwell, B. and Gutteridge, J.M.C. (1999) Free Radical in Biology and Medicine, Oxford, Oxford University Press.

Hasebe, K., Horie, S., Watanabe, K. and Yano, S. (2005) Stimulatory effects of endogenous and exogenous nitric oxide on gastric acid secretion in anesthetized rats. *Nitric Oxide* 13, 264-271.

Hirota, S., Nishioka, T., Shimoda, T., Miura, K., Ansai, T. and Takahama, U. (2001) Quercetin glucosides are hydrolyzed to quercetin in human oral cavity to participate in peroxidase-dependent scavenging of hydrogen peroxide. *Food Sci. Technol. Res.* 7, 239-245.

Hirota, S., Takahama, U., Ansai, T. and Yoshitama, K. (2002) Oxidation of quercetin by salivary components II. Effects of quercetin on reactive oxygen metabolism by salivary polymorphonuclear leukocytes. *Food Sci. Technol. Res.* 8, 276-280.

Hirota, S. and Takahama, U. (2003) Quercetin and its glucosides inhibit nitration of a salivary component 4-hydroxyphenylactic acid catalyzed by salivary polymorphonuclear leukocytes. *Food Sci. Technol. Res.* 9, 378-382.

Hirota, S., Takahama, U., Ly, T.N. and Yamauchi, R. (2005) Quercetin-dependent inhibition of nitration induced by peroxidase/H_2O_2/nitrite systems in human saliva and characterization of an oxidation product of quercetin formed during the inhibition. *J. Agric. Food Chem.* 53, 3265-3272.

Innocenti, A., Maresca, A., Scozzafava, A. and Supuran, C.T. (2008). Carbonic anhydrase inhibitors; Thioxolone versus sulfonamides for obtaining isozyme-selective inhibitors? *Bioorg. Med. Chem. Lett.* 18, 3938-3941.

Jansson, E.Å., Petersson, J., Reinders, C., Sobko, T., Björne, H., Phillipson, M., Weitzberg, E., Holm, L. and Lundberg, J.O. (2007) Protection from nonsteroidal anti-inflammatory drug (NSAID)-induced gastric ulcers by dietary nitrate. *Free Radic. Biol. Med.* 42, 510-518.

Jourd'heuil, D. (2002). Increased nitric oxide-dependent nitrosylation of 4,5-diaminofluorescein by oxidants: implications for the measurement of intracellular nitric oxide. *Free Radic. Biol. Med.* 33, 676-684.

Kato, S., Kitamura, M., Korolkiewicz, R.P. and Takeuchi, K. (1998) Role of nitric oxide in regulation of gastric acid secretion in rats: effects of NO donors and NO synthase inhibitor. *Br. J. Pharmacol.* 123, 839-846.

Kim, B.H., Roh, E., Lee, H.Y., Lee, I.J., Ahn, B., Jung, S.H., Lee, H., Han, S.B. and Kim, Y. (2008). Benzoxathiole derivative blocks lipopolysaccharide-induced nuclear factor-kappaB activation and nuclear factor-kappaB-regulated gene transcription through inactivating inhibitory kappaB kinase beta. *Molecul. Pharmacol.* 73, 1309-1318.

Kojima, H., Urano, Y., Kikuchi, K., Higuchi, T., Hirata, Y. and Nagano, T. (1999). Fluorecent indicators for imaging nitric oxide production. *Angew. Chem. In*t. Ed. 38, 3209-3212.

Konieczny, M.T., Konieczny, W., Sabisz, M., Skladanowski, A., Wakiec, R., Augustynowicz-Kopec, E. and Zwolska, Z. (2007). Synthesis of isomeric, oxathiolone fused to chalcones, and comparison of their activity toward various microorganisms and human cancer cells line. *Chem. Pharmaceut. Bull.* 55, 817-820.

Larauche, M., Anton, P.M., Gracia-Villar, R., Theodorou, V., Frexinos, J., Buéno, L. and Fioramonti, J. (2003) Protective effect of dietary nitrate on experimental gastritis in rats. *Br. J. Nutr.* 89, 777-786.

Licht, W.R., Tannenbaum, S.R. and Deen, W.M. (1988) Use of ascorbic acid to inhibit nitrosation: kinetic and mass transfer considerations for an in vitro system. *Carcinogenesis* 9, 365-372.

Makinen, K.K. Salivary Enzymes. In: Tenovuo, J.O, editor. Human Saliva: Clinical Chemistry and Microbiology vol. II. Boca Raton, Florida, USA: CRC Press; 1989; pp. 93-119.

Marsh, P. and Martin, M.V. (1999) Oral Microbiology (4th edition). Oxford, UK: Wright.

Miyoshi, M., Kasahara, E., Park, A.-M., Hiramoto, K., Minamiyama, Y., Takemura, S., Sato, E. F. and Inoue, M. (2003) Dietary nitrate inhibits stress-induced gastric mucosal injury in the rat. *Free Radic. Res.* 37, 85-90.

Nakahara, H., Sato, E.F., Ishisaka, R., Kanno, T., Yoshioka, T., Yasuda, T., Inoue, M. and Utsumi, K. (1998) Biochemical properties of human oral polymorphonuclear leukocytes. *Free Radic. Res.* 28, 485-495.

Palmerini, C.A., Palombari, R., Perito, S. and Arienti, G. (2003) NO synthesis in human saliva. *Free Radic. Res.* 37, 29-31.

Peri, L., Pietraforte, D., Scorza, G., Napolitano, A., Fogliano, V. and Minetti, M. (2005) Apples increase nitric oxide production by human saliva at the acidic pH of the stomach: a new biological function for polyphenols with a catechol group? *Free Radic. Biol, Med.* 39, 668-681.

Prütz, W.A., Mönig, H., Butler, J. and Lanf E.J. (1985) Reaction of nitrogen dioxide in aqueous model systems: oxidation of tyrosine units in peptides and proteins. *Arch. Biochem. Biophys*. 43, 125-134.

Setsukinai, K., Urano, Y., Kakinuma, K., Majima, J.J. and Nagano, T. (2003) Development of novel fluorescent probes that can reliably detect reactive oxygen species and distinguish special species. *J. Biol. Chem*. 278, 3170-3175

Shibata, H., Kono, Y., Yamashita, S., Sawa, Y., Ochiai, H. and Tanaka, K. (1995) Degradation of chlorophyll by nitrogen dioxide generated from nitrite by the peroxidase reaction. *Biochim. Biophys. Acta* 1230, 45-50.

Takahama, U., Oniki, T. and Hirota, S. (2002) Oxidation of quercetin by salivary components. Quercetin-dependent reduction of salivary nitrite under acidic conditions producing nitric oxide. *J. Agric. Food Chem*. 50, 4317-4322.

Takahama, U., Hirota, S., Nishiola, T. and Oniki, T. (2003a). Human salivary peroxidase-catalyzed oxidation of nitrite and nitration of salivary components 4-hydroxyphenylacetic acid and proteins. *Arch. Oral Biol*. 48, 679-690.

Takahama, U.; Hirota, S., Yamamoto, A. and Oniki, T. (2003b) Oxygen uptake during the mixing of saliva with ascorbic acid under acidic conditions: possibility of its occurrence in the stomach. *FEBS Lett*. 550: 64-68.

Takahama, U., Yamamoto, A., Hirota, S. and Oniki, T. (2003c) Quercetin-dependent reduction of salivary nitrite to nitric oxide under acidic conditions and interaction between quercetin and ascorbic acid during the reaction. *J. Agric. Food Chem*. 51, 6014-6020.

Takahama, U., Hirota, S. and Oniki, T. (2006a) Thiocyanate cannot inhibit the formation of reactive nitrogen oxide species in the human oral cavity in the presence of high concentrations of nitrite: detection of reactive nitrogen species with 4.5-diaminoflourescein. *Chem. Res. Toxicol*. 19, 1066-1073.

Takahama, U., Hirota, S. and Oniki, T. (2006b) Quercetin-dependent scavenging of reactive nitrogen species derived from nitric oxide and nitrite in the human oral cavity: interactions of quercetin with salivary redox components. *Arch. Oral Biol*. 51, 629-639.

Takahama, U., Ryu, K., Oniki, T. and Hirota, S. (2007a) Dual-function of thiocyanate on nitrite-induced formation of reactive nitrogen oxide species in human oral cavity: inhibition under neutral and enhancement under acidic conditions. *Free Radic. Res*. 41, 1289-1300.

Takahama, U., Tanaka, M., Oniki, T., Hirota, S. and Yamauchi, R. (2007b) Formation of the thiocyanate conjugate of chlorogenic acid in coffee under acidic conditions in the presence of thiocyanate and nitrite. Possible occurrence in the stomach. *J. Agric. Food Chem*. 55, 4169-4176.

Takahama, U., Tanaka, M., Hirota, S. and Yamauchi, R. (2009a) Formation of an oxathiolone compound from rutin in acidic mixture of saliva and buckwheat dough: possibility of its occurrence in the stomach. *Food Chem*. 116, 214-219.

Takahama, U., Imanura, H. and Hirota, S. (2009b) Nitration of the salivary component phenylacetic acid in the human oral cavity: enhancement of nitration under acidic conditions. *Eur. J. Oral Sci*. 117, 555-562.

Takahama, U., Hirota, S. and Kawagishi, S. (2009c) Effects of pH on nitrite-induced formation of reactive nitrogen oxide species and their scavenging by phenolic antioxidants in human oral cavity. *Free Radic. Res*. 43: 250-261.

Takahama, U. and Hirota, S. (2010a) Nitrogen dioxide-dependent oxidation of uric acid in the human oral cavity under acidic conditions: implications for its occurrence in acidic dental plaque. *Chem. Res. Toxicol.* 23, 1067-1075.

Takahama, U. and Hirota, S. (2010b). Fatty acids, epicatechi-dimethylgallate, and rutin interact with buckwheat starch inhibiting its digestion by amylase: implications for the decrease in glycemic index by buckwheat flour. *J. Agric. Food Chem.* 58, 12431-12439.

Takahama, U., Tanaka, M. and Hirota, S. (2010a) Formation of nitric oxide, ethyl nitrite and an oxathiolone derivative of caffeic acid in the mixture of saliva and white wine. *Free Radic. Res.* 44, 293-303.

Takahama, U., Tanaka, M. and Hirota, S. (2010b) Proanthocyanidins in buckwheat flour can reduce salivary nitrite to nitric oxide in the stomach. *Plant Food. Hum. Nutr.* 56, 1-7.

Takahama, U. and Hirota, S. (2011) Inhibition of buckwheat starch digestion by the formation of starch/bile salt complexes: possibility of its occurrence in the intestine. *J. Agric. Food Chem.* 59, 6277-6283.

Takahama, U., Koga, Y. and Hirota, S. (2011) Inhibition of xanthine oxidase activity by an oxathilanone derivative of quercetin. *Food Chem.* 126, 1808-1811.

Tamme, T., Reinik, M.M., Toasto, M., Juhkam, K., Tenno, T. and Kiis, A. (2006) Nitrates and nitrites in vegetables and vegetable-based products and their intakes by the Estonian population. *Food Addit. Contamin.* 23, 355-361.

Tanaka, J., Yuda, Y., Inouye, S. and Yamakawa (2001) The role of nitric oxide in the gastric acid secretion induced by ischemia-reperfusion in the pylous-ligated rat. *Eur. J. Pharmacol.* 424, 69-74.

Tenovuo, J. (1989). Nonimmunologlobin defense factors in human saliva. In: Tenovuo, J.O. and Odont, D. editors. Human Saliva: Clinical Chemistry and Microbiology Vol. 2, pp.55-91, Boca Raton, CRC Press.

van der Vliet, A., Eiserich, J.P., Halliwell, B. and Cross, C.E. (1997) Formation of reactive nitrogen species during peroxidase-catalyzed oxidization of nitrite. A potential additional mechanism of nitric oxide-dependent toxicity. *J. Biol. Chem.* 272, 7617-7625.

Walle, T., Browning, A.M., Steed, L.L., Reed, S.G. and Walle, U.K. (2005) Flavonoid glucosides are hydrolyzed and thus activated in the oral cavity in humans. *J. Nutr.* 135, 48-52.

Yamamoto, M., Saeki, K. and Utsumi, K. (1991) Isolation of human salivary polymorphonuclear leukocytes and their stimulation-coupled responses. *Arch. Biochem. Biophys.* 289, 76-82.

Zenkevich, I.G. and Guschina, S.V. (2010) Determination of dissociation constants of species oxidizable in aqueous solution by air oxygen on an example of quercetin. *J. Anal. Chem.* 65, 371-375.

In: Quercetin
Editors: Taiki Chikamatsu and Yuudai Hida

ISBN: 978-1 61942- 057-1

Chapter 13

Quercetin, Kaempferol, Myricetin, and Fatty Acid Content Among Several Hibiscus Sabdariffa Accession Calyces Based on Maturity in a Greenhouse

J. B. Morris, M. L. Wang and T. Thomas
USDA, ARS, Plant Genetic Resources Conservation Unit, Griffin, GA, US

Abstract

Flavonols including quercetin, kaempferol, myricetin, and fatty acids in plants have many useful health attributes including antioxidants, cholesterol lowering effects, and cancer prevention. Six accessions of roselle, *Hibiscus sabdariffa* calyces were evaluated for quercetin, kaempferol, and myricetin content, while 11 accessions were evaluated for fatty acid content as calyces matured in a greenhouse from late 2009 - early 2010. Variations for all chemical traits were found among the roselle calyces between accessions. The accession, PI 265319 produced the most quercetin (1.134 mg/g) and myricetin (0.972 mg/g). However, PI 286316 produced the most kaempferol (1.882 mg/g). Quercetin, myricetin, and kaempferol declined insignificantly as plants matured. Several fatty acids differed significantly in content among the roselle accessions. The accession, PI 286319 produced the most mono-unsaturated fatty acid, palmitoleic acid (0.046 %) and gadoleic acid (0.213 %), however PI 468409 produced the most oleic acid (5.091 %). The accession, PI 286319 also produced the most omega-6 fatty acid, linoleic acid (6.218 %) while PI 268097 produced the most γ-linolenic acid (0.093 %). The accession, PI 286316 produced the most omega-3 fatty acid, eicosapentaenoic acid (0.038 %), however PI 265319 produced significantly more docsahexaenoic acid (5.296 %) than all other roselle accessions. Stearic, behenic, and docosahexaenoic fatty acids declined significantly over time as roselle plants matured, however gadoleic and arachidonic fatty acid content increased significantly as the calyces matured. Interestingly, the red calyces produced significantly higher amounts of fatty acids overall. Significant correlations were found for many of the flavonol and fatty acid traits tested. Based on these results, sufficient variability exists in these *Hibiscus* accessions for quercetin, kaempferol, myricetin, and fatty acid breeding projects and for use as nutraceutical or functional food plants.

INTRODUCTION

Roselle, (*Hibiscus sabdariffa* L.) is an annual plant in the family Malvaceae and is grown in tropical and subtropical countries for stem fibers, paper pulp and edible calyces, leaves and seeds (Wilson and Menzel, 1964). Most likely, roselle migrated to the western hemisphere by African slaves with its earliest use documented in Jamaica during 1707 (Crane, 1949). However, it is also grown in other sub-tropical countries including Sudan, eastern Taiwan, and Thailand (Chang *et al.*, 2005). Since roselle is an important Jamaican crop, the calyces are used to prepare a Christmas drink (Vaidya, 2000). Roselle calyces are also used in salads, pie filling, sauce, juice, syrup, jam, relish, jelly (Morton, 1987), and as a health tea. The primary import markets for the dried calyx of roselle are the United States and Germany (Agribusiness in Sustainable Natural African Plant Products, 2011).

The flavonols quercetin, kaempferol and myricetin have been shown to contribute to brain tumor chemopreventive properties in children (Labbe *et al.*, 2009). Quercetin can inhibit cancer by inhibiting kinase activity at the cellular level (Boly *et al.*, 2011). A flavonoid rich diet including quercetin and kaempferol may decrease pancreatic cancer risk in male smokers when not consuming alpha-tocopherol and/or beta-carotene (Bobe *et al.*, 2008). Quercetin is considered possibly effective for reducing pain caused by prostatitis (Shoskes *et al.*, 1999).

The omega-3 fatty acid, docosahexaenoic acid has been shown to be possibly effective for age related macular degeneration (Cho *et al.*, 2001), coronary artery disease (Erkkila *et al.*, 2003), and psoriasis (Mayser *et al.*, 1998). Another important omega-3 fatty acid is eicosapentaenoic acid (EPA) with possible effectiveness for coronary artery disease (Erkkila *et al.*, 2003), depression (Peet and Horrobin, 2002), and psoriasis (Mayser *et al.*, 1998). Including EPA in the diet before surgery or after surgery appears to reduce infections and improves wound healing (Daly *et al.*, 1992; Senkal *et al.*, 1995; Kemen *et al.*, 1995; and Tepaske *et al.*, 2001). McKay *et al.*, 2010 found that tea made from roselle calyces lowers blood pressure in pre- and mildly hypertensive adults. The USDA, ARS, Plant Genetic Resources Conservation Unit conserves 140 accessions of roselle from 23 countries. Eighty-four accessions originate from Tanzania, United States, Vietnam and Zambia (National Plant Germplasm System, 2011). The additional 56 accessions originated from Australia, Bangladesh, Brazil, Cuba, Ghana, India, Indonesia, Israel, Japan, Niger, Poland, Rhodesia, Senegal, South Africa, Sudan, Taiwan, Thailand, and Uganda (National Plant Germplasm System, 2011). In temperate areas, roselle requires greenhouse production because the plant is photoperiod sensitive and flowering begins only as the day length shortens and light intensity decreases. In the Griffin, GA area, flower production begins in November and continues through March.

Quercetin and other flavonoids (Maganha *et al.*, 2010) have been identified in roselle, however little is known regarding the variability nor the optimum time of flavonol and fatty acid composition based on maturity. The objectives of this study were to determine quercetin, kaempferol, myricetin, and fatty acid composition in roselle calyces as well as identifying the best time to harvest calyces to maximize quercetin, kaempferol, myricetin, and fatty acid production when grown under greenhouse conditions.

Materials and Methods

Plant Materials

Thirteen randomly chosen roselle accessions were planted in 27.5 cm x 27.5 cm plastic pots containing potting soil grown in a greenhouse from August 1, 2009 – April 1, 2010. Three seedlings per pot were maintained for calyx production. The experimental design was a randomized complete block with 4 replications assigned to roselle accessions, however some of the accessions had poor germination resulting in fewer replications during the experiment. Mean separations were conducted using Duncan's multiple range test ($P < 0.05$, $P<0.01$) and correlations were accomplished using Pearsons correlation in SAS (SAS Institute, Cary, NC). Calyces were harvested between December 9, 2009-March 24, 2010 and were maintained at -20° C until extractions. The country of origins for roselle accessions used in this study are listed.

Table 1. Origin of Hibiscus sabdariffa accessions

PI no.	Origin
265319	Cuba
268097	Nigeria
268100	Nigeria
273388	Taiwan
274245	Nigeria
275413	Senegal
286316	Ghana
286319	Ghana
291128	Ghana
365477	Thailand
468409	U.S.
500696	Zambia
591549	Zambia

Flavonols

Freeze dried roselle calyces from six accessions were ground to a fine powder in a mortar and pestle using liquid nitrogen. Approximately 0.5 g – 1.2 g of calyx tissue from each accession was poured into 5.0 ml test tubes. The test tubes containing roselle calyx tissue were closed and their weights recorded to the nearest 0.001 g. Approximately 5 – 6 ml of 60% methanol in 1.2 M HCL was added to each vial containing the calyces. Each tube containing calyx tissue plus solvent was vortexed and incubated with occasional mixing by inversion in a water bath for 5 hrs at 80° C. An aliquot from each sample was then transferred to a 2 ml test tube and centrifuged at 12000 rpm for 5 min. Afterwards, 1.0 ml of the supernatant was removed from each tube and filtered (0.45 μM pore membrane) into an amber injection vial. Analytes were separated and identified by high performance liquid chromatography (HPLC). The stationary phase consisted of a Zorbax Eclipse XDB-C18 (3.0 x 150 mm, 5 μM particle size) (Agilent Techonologies, Santa Clara, CA) maintained at 40° C. The mobile phase consisted of solvent A (2:1 methanol to acetonitrile) and solvent B (80 % filtered water with 0.1 % formic acid, pH 2.5) with the following gradient: 15 % A for 0-24 min, then 52.5 % A for 25 min, and followed by 95 % A for 25-30 min. The flow rate was 0.8 mL/min and the injection volume was 10 μl. The UV detection was monitored at 340, 370 and 260 nm with a diode array detector. The standards for peak identification and quantification of quercetin, myricetin, and kaempferol were purchased from Sigma Aldrich Chemical Co, St. Louis, MO. Each standard was dissolved in the extraction solvent and diluted to the following concentrations: 5, 20,50,100, 150, and 200 ng/μl.

Fatty Acids

Fatty acid composition was determined by gas chromatography (GC) on an Agilent 7890A GC (Agilent Technologies, Santa Clara, CA) with a split/splitless (S/Sl) inlet and flame ionization detector (FID). Fresh ground roselle calyces from 13 accessions were dried in an oven at 55° C for 2 hrs. The tissue was then transferred to test tubes after the addition of approximately 6 mL of hexane plus isopropanol (3:1). The test tubes containing the calyx tissue were incubated overnight at 65° C. Oil from the ground roselle calyces (~250 mg meal) was extracted in 3 ml heptane and converted to fatty acid methyl esters (FAMEs) with 500 μl of a 0.5 M sodium methoxide in methanol solution were vortexed for 30 sec followed by incubation at 65° C for an additional 2 hrs. The solutions were then cooled at room temperature and the supernatant solutions were washed twice with 3 mL of water with the top layer being transferred to clean test tubes. The solutions were then evaporated by passing nitrogen steam over them. Approximately 2 mL of heptanes/hexane was added to each solution to dissolve the oil sticking to the sides of the test tubes. An aliquot from the heptane layer was transferred to a sample vial for injection into the GC. Peak separation was performed on a DB-225 capillary column (15 m x 250 μm column coated with a 0.25 μm film of 50 % cyanopropyl, 50 % dimethylpolysiloxane) from Agilent Technologies, Santa Clara, CA. One microliter of prepared sample was injected at a 5:1 split ratio into the column with helium as the carrier gas at a flow of 25 mL/min. The initial column temperature was 100° C and later programmed to increase at a rate of 9° min^{-1} to 244° C and was maintained for 18.5 min at 244° C. The carrier gas was helium with an inlet pressure of 12 psi (~39 cm/sec at 195° C). Peaks were identified by retention time comparison to a FAME standard mix RM-3 (Sigma Aldrich, St. Louis, MO).

RESULTS

Flavonols

The results for seed weight and flavonol variation among six roselle accessions are summarized in Table 2. Seed weights for all 6 roselle accessions ranged from 0.2775 – 0.3075 g with no significant differences between accessions. Myricetin, quercetin, and kaempferol ranged from 0.1167 – 0.9727, 0.2624 – 1.1344, and 0.2700 – 1.8826 mg/g, respectively in roselle calyces from all accessions. Both PI 265319 and PI 286316 produced the most myricetin and kaempferol averaging 0.9622 and 1.6749 mg/g of dry weight, respectively, however only PI 265319 produced the most quercetin (1.1344 mg/g). This study showed that roselle calyces contain higher amounts of quercetin (averaging 0.5814 mg/g) than apples with skin (0.0442 mg/g), brussel sprouts (0.0030 mg/g), cranberries (0.1402 mg/g), grapefruit (0.0050 mg/g), raspberries (0.0083 mg/g), black tea (0.0207 mg/g), and green tea (0.0269 mg/g) [USDA, ARS nutrition database, 2003 http://www.nal.usda.gov/fnic/foodcomp].

Fatty Acids

Saturated Fatty Acids

The results for fatty acid variation among thirteen roselle accessions are summarized in Tables 3, 4 and 5. The saturated fatty acids found included myristic (14:0), palmitic (16:0), margaric (17:0), stearic (18:0), arachidic (20:0), behenic (22:0), and cerotic (26:0) acids (Table 3). The percentage of saturated fatty acid content among 13 roselle accessions ranged from 0 to 3.74 % (Table 3). However, only palmitic, stearic, arachidic and behenic acids varied significantly among these 13 roselle accessions.

The accession, PI 468409 from Georgia, U.S.A. produced significantly more palmitic acid than all other accessions. Only the Nigerian, (PI 268097, PI 268100), Cuban (PI 265319), and Ghana accessions (PI 286316) produced significantly more stearic acid than all other accessions. The accessions, PI 268100 and PI 265319 produced significantly more arachidic and behenic acid than all other accessions.

Table 2. Seed weight and flavonol content among 6 Hibiscus sabdariffa accessions

PI no.	Seed wt. (g)	Myricetin (mg/g)	Quercetin (mg/g)	Kaempferol (mg/g)
275413	0.3075a	0.2101ab	0.2624b	0.3230b
268097	0.3000a	0.1167b	0.3017b	0.2700b
500696	0.3000a	0.5767ab	0.3618b	0.4030b
265319	0.2975a	0.9727a	1.1344a	1.4673a
286316	0.2813a	0.9517a	0.8382ab	1.8826a
291128	0.2775a	0.4882ab	0.5902ab	0.9427ab

Table 3. Percent saturated fatty acids in 13 Hibiscus sabdariffa accessions

PI no.	14:0	16:0	17:0	18:0	20:0	22:0	26:0
286319	0.0125a	0.0000b	0.0347a	0.0000b	0.0580b	0.0000b	0.0000a
268097	0.0100a[a]	1.1753b	0.0592a	0.3883a	0.1640b	0.0000b	0.0000a
500696	0.0077a	0.0000b	0.0555a	0.0000b	0.0000b	0.0000b	0.0000a
273388	0.0062a	0.0000b	0.0682a	0.0000b	0.0000b	0.0000b	0.0000a
265319	0.0000a	1.8047b	0.0211a	0.3875a	0.0000b	0.0831a	0.0000a
268100	0.0000a	0.2168b	0.0397a	0.3630a	0.4905a	0.0000b	0.0000a
274245	0.0000a	0.0000b	0.0000a	0.0000b	0.0000b	0.0000b	0.0000a
286316	0.0000a	0.9576b	0.0144a	0.2836a	0.1316b	0.0250b	0.2130a
291128	0.0000a	0.0000b	0.0000a	0.0000b	0.0000b	0.0000b	0.0000a
275413	0.0000a	0.0000b	0.0000a	0.0000b	0.0000b	0.0000b	0.0000a
468409	0.0000a	3.7483a	0.0466a	0.0000b	0.0000b	0.0000b	0.0000a
365477	0.0000a	0.0000b	0.0000a	0.0000b	0.0000b	0.0000b	0.0000a
591549	0.0000a	0.5265b	0.0000a	0.0000b	0.0000b	0.0000b	0.0000a

Table 4. Percent mono-unsaturated fatty acids in 13 Hibiscus sabdariffa accessions

PI no.	16:1	18:1	20:1	22:1
286319	0.0467a	2.8330ab	0.2132a	0.0438a
265319	0.0000b	1.8510b	0.0620b	1.2495a
268100	0.0000b	1.6550b	0.0000b	0.0000a
268097	0.0000b	1.1800b	0.0000b	1.5108a
274245	0.0000b	3.5790ab	0.0000b	0.0000a
275413	0.0000b	2.4310ab	0.0000b	0.0000a
286316	0.0000b	1.6060b	0.0000b	1.4051a
273388	0.0000b	2.4820ab	0.0000b	0.0000a
291128	0.0000b	1.4590b	0.0000b	0.0000a
365477	0.0000b	2.9100ab	0.0000b	0.0278a
468409	0.0000b	5.0910a	0.0000b	0.0000a
500696	0.0000b	2.1030b	0.0000b	0.0000a
591549	0.0000b	2.4100ab	0.0000b	0.0000a

Table 5. Percent poly-unsaturated fatty acids in 13 Hibiscus sabdariffa

PI no.	18:2	18:3α	18:3γ	20:4	20:5	22:6
286319	6.2180a	0.0000c	0.0000b	0.3982a	0.0000a	0.3023b
468409	5.2250ab	4.7720a	0.0000b	0.0000c	0.0000a	0.3710b
591549	5.0590ab	3.7770ab	0.0000b	0.2045b	0.0000a	0.0805b
265319	3.2510abc	1.5130bc	0.0000b	0.0985bc	0.0000a	5.2968a
286316	2.0090bc	1.0940bc	0.0000b	0.1025bc	0.0387a	0.7144b
268097	1.3440bc	0.7970bc	0.0937a	0.0000c	0.0000a	0.0000b
291128	0.7080c	0.3690bc	0.0000b	0.0980bc	0.0000a	0.0000b
268100	0.4270c	1.0120bc	0.0000b	0.0000c	0.0000a	0.0000b
275413	0.0000c	0.0000c	0.0000b	0.0000c	0.0000a	0.0000b
273388	0.0000c	0.0000c	0.0000b	0.2222b	0.0000a	0.0318b
365477	0.0000c	0.0000c	0.0000b	0.1485bc	0.0000a	0.3478b
500696	0.0000c	0.0000c	0.0000b	0.0692bc	0.0000a	0.2025b
274245	0.0000c	0.0000c	0.0000b	0.0000c	0.0000a	0.0000b

Table 6. Correlations for fatty acids and flavonoids from the *Hibiscus sabdariffa* accessions

	14:0	16:0	16:1	17:0	18:0	18:1	18:2	18:3α	18:3γ	20:0	20:1	20:4	20:5	22:0	22:1	22:6	26:0	m	q
16:0	-0.08																		
16:1	0.63***	-0.05																	
17:0	0.41*	-0.01	0.80***																
18:0	0.49**	0.73***	0.31	0.35*															
18:1	0.21	-0.25	0.09	0.15	-0.09														
18:2	0.05	0.39*	0.12	0.007	0.26	0.30													
18:3α	0.99***	-0.07	0.60***	0.42*	0.51**	0.21	0.007												
18:3γ	-0.04	-0.04	0.35*	0.64***	0.08	-0.12	0.08	-0.04											
20:0	0.18	-0.18	-0.09	0.02	0.10	0.07	-0.19	0.19	-0.06										
20:1	0.48**	0.09	0.004	0.16	0.24	0.25	0.15	0.49**	0.21	0.24									
20:4	0.57**	-0.28	0.71***	0.64***	0.09	0.04	0.13	0.55**	0.48**	-0.02	0.43**								
20:5	0.75***	-0.05	0.69***	0.73***	0.50**	0.06	0.08	0.76***	0.60***	0.11	0.51**	0.72***							
22:0	0.95***	-0.04	0.67***	0.57**	0.55**	0.15	0.06	0.96***	0.22	0.17	0.52**	0.65***	0.90***						
22:1	0.35*	0.55**	0.16	0.14	0.63***	-0.05	0.16	0.36*	0.01	-0.02	0.20	0.04	0.28	0.35*					
22:6	0.99***	-0.07	0.60***	0.42*	0.51**	0.21	0.007	1.00***	-0.04	0.19	0.49**	0.55**	0.76***	0.96***	0.36*				
26:0	-0.02	-0.11	0.38*	0.48**	-0.03	-0.09	0.17	-0.07	0.81***	-0.02	0.31	0.54**	0.46**	0.14	-0.05	-0.07			
m	-0.34*	-0.44**	-0.25	-0.31	-0.56**	0.07	0.09	-0.37*	-0.26	0.02	-0.07	-0.04	-0.48**	-0.44**	-0.52**	-0.37*	-0.05		
q	0.03	-0.13	0.16	-0.10	-0.17	0.02	0.17	-0.06	-0.04	0.04	0.22	0.23	-0.08	-0.07	-0.11	-0.06	0.55**	0.29	
k	-0.31	-0.28	-0.32	-0.34*	-0.41*	0.009	-0.18	-0.29	-0.20	-0.12	-0.30	-0.27	-0.35*	-0.33*	-0.58**	-0.29	-0.34*	0.53**	-0.29

Mono-Unsaturated Fatty Acids

Four mono-unsaturated fatty acids were also found including palmitoleic (16:1), oleic (18:1), gadoleic (20:1), and erucic (22:1) acids (Table 4). The percent mono-unsaturated fatty acids ranged significantly from 0 to 5.1 % (Table 4). Only PI 286319 from Ghana produced palmitoleic acid. The majority of the roselle accessions produced more oleic acid (averaging 2.43 %) than any other mono-unsaturated fatty acid. The accession, PI 468409 from the U.S. produced the most oleic acid (5.09 %) while PI 268097 produced the least (1.18 %). Only PI 286319 and PI 265319 produced gadoleic acid averaging 0.1376 %. There were no significant differences for erucic acid production. Five roselle accessions produced erucic acid averaging 0.8474 %.

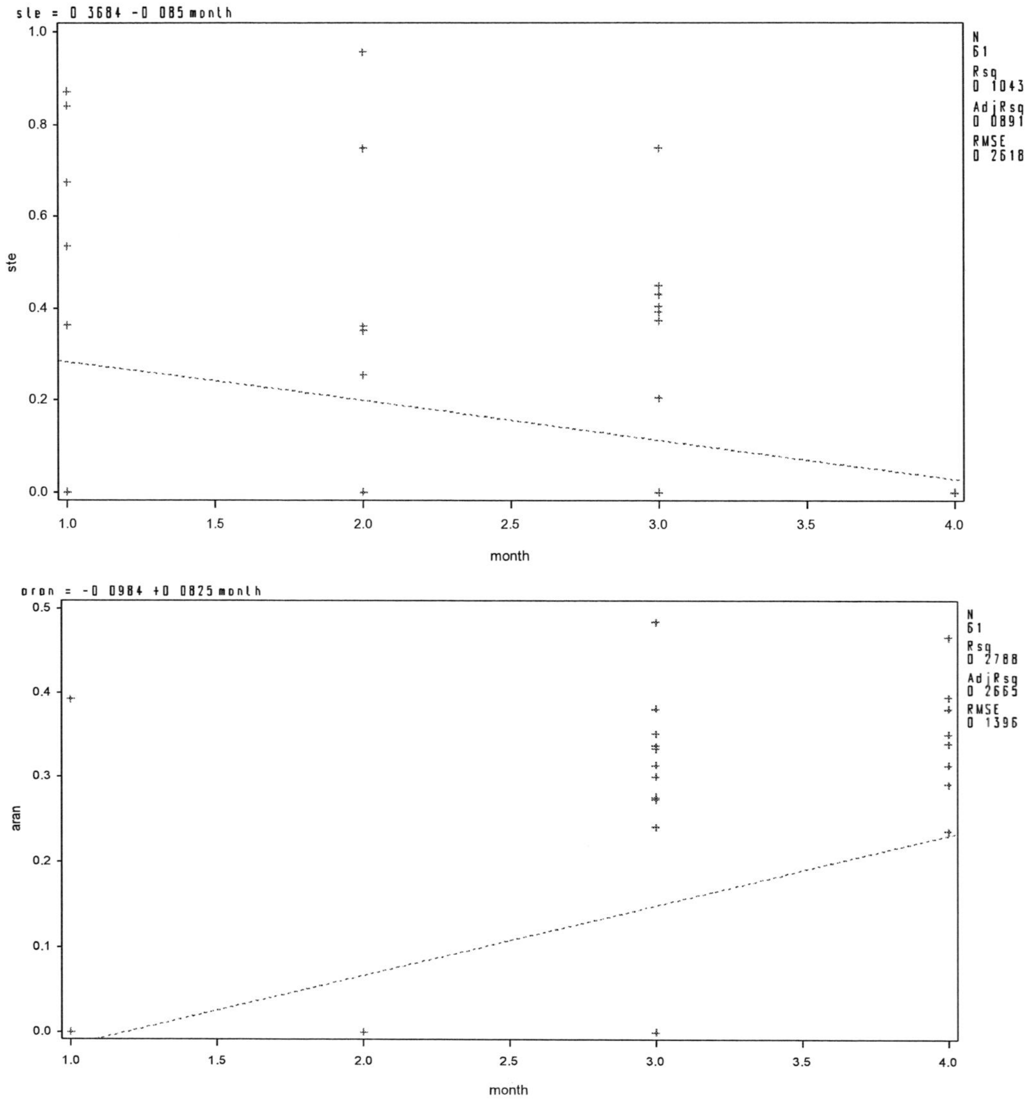

Figure 1. (Continued)

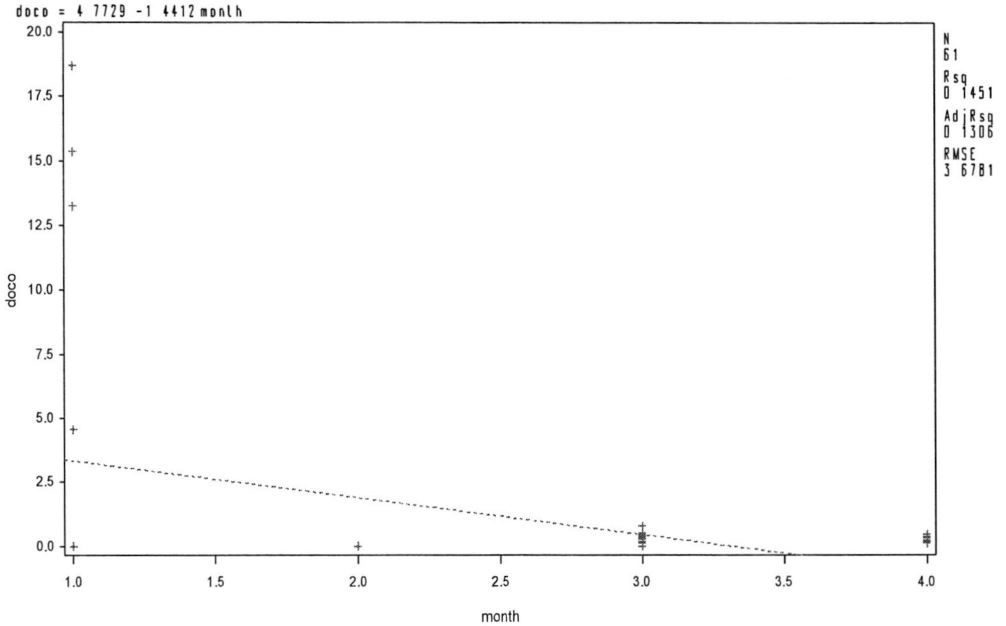

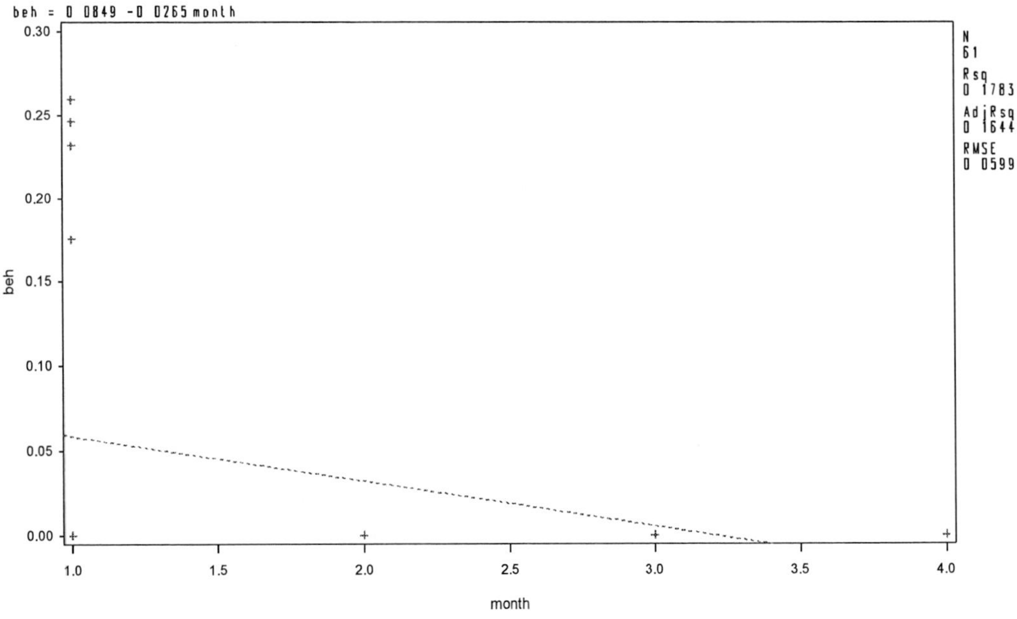

Figure 1. Effect of calyx harvest date on stearic (ste), gadoleic (gad), arachidonic (aran), docosahexaenoic (doco), and behenic (beh) acids.

Poly-Unsaturated Fatty Acids

Six poly-unsaturated fatty acids including linoleic (18:2), α-linolenic (18:3α), γ-linolenic (18:3γ), arachidonic (20:4), eicosapentaenoic (20:5), and docosahexaenoic (22:6) acids (Table 5) were found in these roselle accessions. Several roselle accessions produced variable amounts of all poly-unsaturated fatty acids, except eicosapentaenoic acid (Table 5). The accessions, PI 286319, PI 468409, and PI 591549 from Zambia produced the most linoleic acid, averaging 5.50 % while all other accessions averaged 0.77 %. Both PI 468409 and PI 591549 produced the most α-linolenic acid averaging 4.27 % and all other accessions averaged 0.44 %. Only PI 268097 produced significantly more γ-linolenic (0.0937 %) than all other accessions.

Arachidonic acid varied significantly among accessions as well with PI 286319 and PI 273388 from Taiwan averaging the most (0.3102 %). All other accessions averaged 0.065 % arachidonic acid. Only PI 286316 produced a measureable amount of eicosapentaenoic acid (0.0387 %).

The accession PI 265319 produced significantly more docosahexaenoic acid (5.3 %) than all other roselle accessions, however the other 12 roselle accessions averaged 0.17 %. Several fatty acids and flavonols significantly correlated (Table 6). Myricetin negatively correlated with myristic (r^2 = -0.34*), palmitic (r^2 = -0.44**), stearic (r^2 = -0.56**), α-linolenic (r^2 = -0.37*), eicosapentaenoic (r^2 = -0.48**), behenic (r^2 = -0.44**), erucic (r^2 = -0.52**), and docosahexaenoic (r^2 = -0.37*) acids. Quercetin positively correlated with cerotic acid (r^2 = 0.55**) only, while kaempferol negatively correlated with margaric (r^2 = -0.34*), stearic (r^2 = -0.41*), eicosapentaenoic (r^2 = -0.35*), behenic (r^2 = -0.33*), erucic (r^2 = -0.58**), and cerotic (r^2 = -0.34*) acids. Kaempferol also positively correlated with myricetin (r^2 = 0.53**) (Table 6). All three flavonoids decreased insignificantly as the calyces matured.

Fatty Acid Correlations

Several significant correlations were found for many fatty acids (Table 6) as well. The following are correlations among the most important fatty acids including both mono-unsaturated and poly-unsaturated fatty acids. Among the mono-unsaturated fatty acids, palmitoleic acid positively correlated with myristic acid (r^2 = 0.63***) while gadoleic acid correlated with myristic (r^2 = 0.48**) and α-linolenic (r^2 = 0.49**) acids. Erucic acid correlated with myristic (r^2 = 0.35*), palmitic (r^2 = 0.55**), stearic (r^2 = 0.63***), α-linolenic (r^2 = 0.36*), and behenic (r^2 = 0.35*) acids. Among the poly-unsaturated fatty acids, linoleic acid correlated with palmitic acid (r^2 = 0.39*). α-linolenic acid correlated with myristic (r^2 = 0.99***), palmitoleic (r^2 = 0.60***), margaric (r^2 = 0.42*), and stearic (r^2 = 0.51**) acids while γ-linolenic acid correlated with both palmitoleic (r^2 = 0.35*) and margaric (r^2 = 0.64***) acids. Arachidonic acid correlated with myristic (r^2 = 0.57**), palmitoleic (r^2 = 0.71***), margaric (r^2 = 0.64***), α-linolenic (r^2 = 0.55**), γ-linolenic (r^2 = 0.48**), and gadoleic (r^2 = 0.43**) acids. The omega-3 fatty acid, eicosapentaenoic acid correlated with myristic (r^2 = 0.75***), palmitoleic (r^2 = 0.69***), margaric (r^2 = 0.73***), stearic (r^2 = 0.50**), α-linolenic (r^2 = 0.76***), γ-linolenic (r^2 = 0.60***), gadoleic (r^2 = 0.51**), and arachidonic (r^2 = 0.72***) acids. Another omega-3 fatty acid, docosahexaenoic acid correlated with myristic (r^2 = 0.99***), palmitoleic (r^2 = 0.60***), margaric (r^2 = 0.42*), stearic (r^2 = 0.51**), α-linolenic (r^2 = 1.00***), gadoleic (r^2 = 0.49**), arachidonic (r^2 = 0.55**), eicosapentaenoic (r^2 = 0.76***), behenic (r^2 = 0.96***), and erucic (r^2 = 0.36*) acids.

Regression Analysis

Stearic, docosahexaenoic, and behenic fatty acid content declined significantly as the roselle calyces matured over time (Figure 1).

This indicates that the roselle calyces contain more of these fatty acids soon after initial maturity. However, both gadoleic and arachidonic fatty acid content increased significantly as the calyces matured (Figure 1). Calyces from the roselle accessions should be harvested any time soon after calyx maturity for all other fatty acids and flavonols studied.

Conclusion

Even though relatively small amounts of these various flavonols and fatty acids were found, these roselle accessions showed variability for most of the flavonols and fatty acids when grown in the greenhouse. Quercetin, myricetin, and kaempferol found in roselle calyces may be responsible for contributing antioxidants to the human diet when consumed. Some plants can be used as nutraceuticals and phytochemicals or mixtures of phytochemicals can also be used for nutraceutical products in the form of capsules, tinctures or tablets. Certain phytochemicals or plant extracts with a desirable phytochemical profile are used in the production of many functional foods as bioactives. Since all three flavonols are retained in the calyces for at least three months during maturity in a greenhouse, they can be harvested for use as a nutraceutically herbal tea constituent, functional food, potential cancer preventative, and may be potentially used to lower cholesterol in humans at any time after maturity. Several fatty acids identified in these roselle calyces will provide added health benefits as well. Interestingly, the omega-3 fatty acids, eicosapentaenoic and docosahexaenoic acids were found in the calyces also. According to our study, calyces should be harvested shortly after maturity in a greenhouse to take advantage of their higher poly-unsaturated fatty acid, docosahexaenoic acid. However, we also recommend that greenhouse grown calyces should be harvested later (approximately 3 months after initial calyx maturity) due to the higher amount of both the mono-unsaturated fatty acid, gadoleic acid and the poly-unsaturated fatty acid, arachidonic acid. Calyces from these roselle accessions could be used to develop new products with elevated amounts of flavonols and fatty acids for use as a functional food or nutraceutical.

Those accessions identified to contain superior quantities of both flavonols and fatty acids are likely candidate parents useful in a breeding project for the development of new roselle cultivars or germplasm. Since the fatty acids identified in this research did not add up to 100 %, further research is needed to verify whether or not additional fatty acids exist in roselle calyces. There is also a need to identify and quantitate more flavonoids and additional phytochemicals in roselle accessions due to their health benefits.

ACKNOWLEDGMENTS

We wish to thank Ken Manley for his excellent assistance in maintaining and harvesting of the roselle calyces and Brandon Tonnis for GC and HPLC analysis of fatty acids and flavonols.

REFERENCES

Agribusiness in Sustainable Natural African Plant Products. (2011). Hibiscus Production Manual. Market Survey: *Hibiscus* sabdariffa [http://www.herbs.org/Africa/hibiscus.html]

Bobe, G., Weinstein, S.J., Albanes, D., Hirvonen, T., Ashby, J., Taylor, P.R., Virtamo, J. and Stolzenberg-Solomon, R.Z. Flavonoid intake and risk of pancreatic cancer in male smokers (Finland). *Cancer Epidemiology, Biomarkers and Prevention,* 2008 17:553-562.

Boly, R., Gras, T., Lamkami, T., Guissou, P., Serteyn, D., Kiss, R. and Dubois, J. Quercetin inhibits a large panel of kinases implicated in cancer cell biology. *International Journal of Oncology,* 2011 38:833-842.

Chang, Y.C., Huang, H.P., Hsu, J.D., Yang, S.F. and Wang, C.J. Hibiscus anthocyanins rich extract-induced apoptotic cell death in human promyelocytic leukemia cells. *Toxicology and Applied Pharmacology,* 2005 205:12-201.

Cho, E., Hung, S., Willet, W.C., Spiegelman, D., Rimm, E.B., Seddon, J.M., Colditz, G.A. and Hankinson, S.E. Prospectice study of dietary fat and the risk of age-related macular degeneration. *American Journal of Clinical Nutrition,* 2001 73:209-218.

Crane, J.C. Roselle – a potentially important plant fiber. *Economic Botany,* 1949 3:89-103.

Daly, J.M., Lieberman, M.D., Goldfine, J., Shou, J., Weintraub, F., Rosato, E.F. and Lavin, P. Enteral nutrition with supplemental arginine, RNA, and omega-3 fatty acids in patients after operation: immunologic, metabolic and clinical outcome. *Surgery,* 1992 112:56-67.

Erkkila, A.T., Lehto, S., Pyorala, K. and Uusitupa, M.I. n-3 Fatty acids and 5-y risks of death and cardiovascular disease events in patients with coronary artery disease. *American Journal of Clinical Nutrition,* 2003 78:65-71.

Kemen, M., Senkal, M., Homann, H.H., Mumme, A., Dauphin, A.K., Baier, J., Windeler, J., Neumann, H. and Zumtobel, V. Early postoperative enteral nutrition with arginine-omega-3 fatty acids and ribonucleic acid-supplemented diet versus placebo in cancer patients: an immunologic evaluation of impact. *Critical Care Medicine,* 1995 23:652-659.

Labbe, D., Provencal, M., Lamy, S., Boivin, D., Gingras, D. and Beliveau, R. The flavonols quercetin, keampferol, and myricetin inhibit hepatocyte growth factor-induced medulloblastoma cell migration. *Journal of Nutrition,* 2009 139:646-652.

Maganha, E.G., da Costa Helmenschlager, R., Rosa, R.M., Henriques, J.A.P., de Paula Ramos, A.L.L. and Saffi, J. Pharmacological evidences for the extracts and secondary metabolites from plants of the genus *Hibiscus*. *Food Chemistry,* 2010 118:1-10.

Mayser, P., Mrowietz, U., Arenberger, P., Bartak, P., Buchvald, J., Christophers, E., Jablonska, S., Salmhofer, W., Schill, W.B., Kramer, H.J., Schlotzer, E., Mayer, K., Seeger, W. and Grimminger, F. Omega-3 fatty acid-based lipid infusion in patients with chronic plaque psoriasis: results of a double-blind, randomized, placebo-controlled, multicenter trial. *Journal of the American Academy of Dermatology,* 1998 38:539-547.

McKay, D.L., Oliver Chen, C.Y., Saltzman, E. and Blumbert J.B. *Hibiscus sabdariffa* L. tea (tisane) lowers blood pressure in prehypertensive and mildly hypertensive adults. *Journal of Nutrition,* 2010 140:298-303.

Morton, J. (1987). Roselle. In: Fruits of warm climates. (pp. 281-286). Miami, FL: New Crop Press. National Plant Germplasm System. (2011). Germplasm Resources Information Network (GRIN). Database Management Unit (DBMU), National Plant Germplasm System. US Department of Agriculture, Beltsville, MD.

National Plant Germplasm System. (2011). Germplasm Resources Information Network (GRIN). Database Management Unit (DBMU), National Plant Germplasm System. US Department of Agriculture, Beltsville, MD.

Peet, M. and Horrobin, D.F. A dose-ranging study of the effects of ethyl-eicosapentaenoate in patients with ongoing depression despite apparently adequate treatment with standard drugs. *Archives of General Psychiatry,* 2002 59:913-919.

SAS Institute. (2008). SAS/STAT User's guide SAS Inst., Cary, NC.

Senkal, M., Kemen, M., Homann, H.H., Eickhoff, U., Baier, J. and Zumtobel, V. Modulation of postoperative immune response by enteral nutrition with a diet enriched with arginine, RNA, and omega-3 fatty acids in patients with upper gastrointestinal cancer. *European Journal of Surgery,* 1995 161:115-122.

Shoskes, D.A., Zeitlin, S.I., Shahed, A. and Rajfer, J. Quercetin in men with category III chronic prostatitis: A preliminary prospective, double-blind, placebo-controlled trial. *Urology,* 1999 54:960-963.

Tepaske, R., Velthuis, H., Oudemans-van Straaten, H.M., Heisterkamp, S.H., van Deventer, S.J., Ince, C., Eysman, L. and Kesecioglu, J. Effect of preoperative oral immune-enhancing nutritional supplement on patients at high risk of infection after cardiac surgery: a randomized placebo-controlled trial. *Lancet,* 2001 358:696-701.

USDA, ARS. (2003). USDA database for the flavonoid content of selected foods. *http://www.nal.usda.gov/fnic/foodcomp.*

Vaidya, K.R. Natural cross-pollination in roselle, *Hibiscus sabdariffa* L. (Malvaceae). *Genetics and Molecular Biology,* 2000 23:667-669.

Wilson, F.D. and Menzel, M.M. Kenaf (*Hibiscus cannabinus*), roselle (*Hibiscus sabdariffa*). *Economic Botany,* 1964 18:80-91.

In: Quercetin
Editors: Taiki Chikamatsu and Yuudai Hida
ISBN: 978-1 61942- 057-1

Chapter 14

IN VITRO ANTIBACTERIAL ACTIVITIES AND MURINE STUDIES OF NOVEL QUERCETIN DIACYLGLYCOSYDE ANALOGUES

***Abugafar M. L. Hossion*[1,2,*], *Rafiya K. Kandahary*[1] and *Kenji Sasaki*[1]**

[1]Department of Molecular Design for Medicine, Graduate School of Medicine, Dentistry and Pharmaceutical Science, Okayama University, Kita-Ku, Okayama, Japan
[2]Department of Medical and Bioengineering Sciences, The Graduate School of Natural Science and Technology, Okayama University, Kita-Ku, Okayama, Japan

ABSTRACT

Quercetin is a unique bioflavonoid that has been extensively studied by researchers over past 30 years. Reports of activity in the field of antibacterial flavanoid research are widely conflicting, probably owing to inter- and intra-assay variation in susceptibility testing. However, several high quality investigations have examined the relationship between flavanoid structure and antibacterial activity and these are in close agreement. In addition, numerous research groups have sought to elucidate the antibacterial mechanisms of action of selected flavanoid. The activity of quercetin, for example, has been at least partially attributed to inhibition of bacterial DNA gyrase. In addition, quercetin is one of suitable ligand among flavanoid to fit inside the ATP binding site of DNA gyrase B and Topoisomerase IV ParE. Nevertheless, quercetin can't inhibit the growth of Gram-positive bacterial strains even at high concentrations though it can inhibit the growth of Gram-negative bacterial strains at high concentration.

Keywords: Quercetin, quercetin-3-*O*-glycoside, multidrug-resistant, DNA gyrsae, topoisomerase IV, cell penetration

* Corresponding author. Fax: 81-086-252-8021; E-mail: chem.lokman@gmail.com.

INTRODUCTION

In the past 60 years, antibiotics have been critical in the fight against infectious disease caused by bacteria and other microbes. Antimicrobial chemotherapy has been a leading cause for the dramatic rise of average life expectancy in the Twentieth Century. However, disease-causing microbes that have become resistant to antibiotic drug therapy are an increasing public health problem. Wound infections, gonorrhea, tuberculosis, pneumonia, septicemia and childhood ear infections are just a few of the diseases that have become hard to treat with antibiotics. One part of the problem is that bacteria and other microbes that cause infections are remarkably resilient and have developed several ways to resist antibiotics and other antimicrobial drugs. Another part of the problem is due to increasing use, and misuse, of existing antibiotics in human and veterinary medicine and in agriculture. Animal and agricultural uses of antibiotics are added to human use.

Nowadays, about 70 percent of the bacteria that cause infections in hospitals are resistant to at least one of the drugs most commonly used for treatment. Some organisms e.g., "Super bacteria" are resistant to all approved antibiotics and can only be treated with experimental and potentially toxic drugs. An alarming increase in resistance of bacteria that cause community acquired infections has also been documented, especially in the staphylococci (Methicillin-resistant *Staphylococcus aureus*, MRSA; Methicillin sensitive *S. aureus*, MSSA; Vancomycin resistant enterococci, VRE; Vancomycin-intermediate *S. aureus*, VISA; Vancomycin-resistant *S. aureus*, VRSA) and pneumococci (*Streptococcus pneumoniae)*, which are prevalent causes of disease and mortality. [1−7]

Microbial development of resistance, as well as economic incentives, has resulted in research and development in the search for new antibiotics in order to maintain a pool of effective drugs at all times. While the development of resistant strains is inevitable, the slack ways that we administer and use antibiotics has greatly exacerbated the process. Unless antibiotic resistance problems are detected as they emerge, and actions are taken immediately to contain them, society could be faced with previously treatable diseases that have become again untreatable, as in the days before antibiotics were developed. In other words, while the rate of drug resistance among bacteria is on the rise, there have been very few examples of the development of structurally new classes of antibiotics with truly novel mode of action that can circumvent the prevailing resistance problem. In this chapter, the author is delighted to introduce the quercetin diacylglycoside analogues showing dual inhibition of *E. coli* DNA gyrase and *S. aureus* topoIV as novel and potent antibacterial agents.

BACKGROUNDS AND OBJECTIVES

Flavonoids are well known as herbal medicine, especially, Loquat leaf (known as "Pipaye" in Chinese and "Biwayo" in Japan) is Chinese medicinal herb whose leaves used to apply to resolve phlegm and to stop cough as well as to conduct rebellious *qi* downward and to stop vomiting. A novel kaemferol diacylrhamnoside *1* has recently been isolated from that leaf and reported by Bloor, S. J. (*Phytochemistry*, 1996), Tsuchiya, T. and co. workers (*Biol. Pharm. Bull.* 2008 & 2009) as anti-MRSA agent. [8−10] Respectively, quercetin and quercetin-3-*O*-glycosides are the most abundant flavonoids in the human diet and associated with myriad biological activities, and may contribute to the prevention of human diseases. As quercetin and quercetin-3-*O*-glycoside are widely sold as food supplements and inhibit the growth of Gram-positive and Gram-negative organisms at high concentrations, it is interesting to expand their antibacterial activities. On being encouraged, the author has concerned to develop quercetin derivatives e.g., quercetin diacylglycoside analogues as they strongly inhibit the growth of multidrug-resistant bacterial pathogens.

As shown in Figure 1 the author has explored the discovery, synthesis and biological evaluation of novel as analogues of MRSA strains inhibiting natural lead compound 1, as they inhibit bacterial DNA gyrase and topoisomerase IV and show potent antibacterial activity against a wide spectrum of relevant pathogens responsible for hospital- and community-acquired infections.

1) 3,7-Diacylquercetins (D2)
2) Quercetin 2”,3”-diacylglucosides (D1)
3) Quercetin 6”-acylgalctosides (D3) and
4) Quercetin 2”,6”-diacylgalctosides (D4)

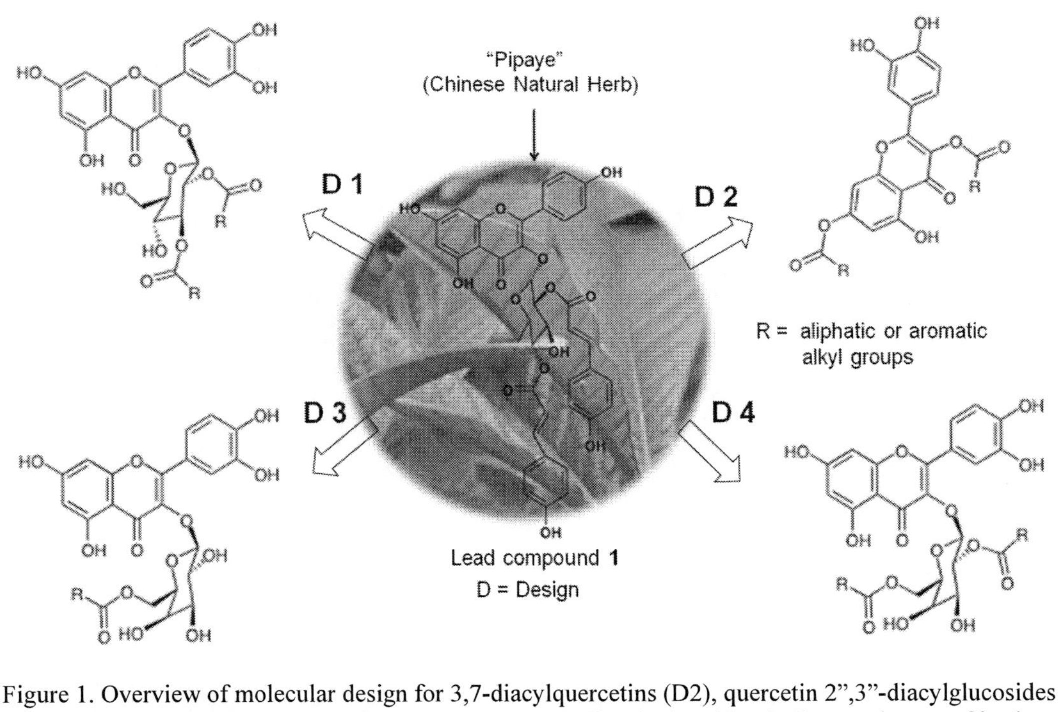

Figure 1. Overview of molecular design for 3,7-diacylquercetins (D2), quercetin 2”,3”-diacylglucosides (D1), quercetin 6”-acylgalctosides (D3), quercetin 2”,6”-diacylgalctosides (D4) as analogues of lead conpound 1.

OUTLINES

The summaries of the author contributions are as follows:

A series of novel quercetin Diacylglucosides [1] (D 1) were designed and synthesized by Steglich esterification [11] on the basis of MRSA strains inhibiting natural compound kaemferol diacylrhamnoside. The *in vitro* inhibition of different multi-drug resistant bacterial strains (MRSA, MSSA, VRE, VISA, K-12, PA01) and *Escherichia coli* DNA gyrase B for these compounds was investigated [12]

In an attempt to clarify the mode of action (MOA) and to explore the extensive Structure Activity Relationships (SARs) of quercetin diacylglycoside analogues (Figure 2); [12] A structure-guided molecular design approach was used to optimize these analogues that inhibit bacterial DNA gyrase and topoisomerase IV and show potent antibacterial activity against a wide spectrum of relevant pathogens responsible for hospital- and community-acquired infections. Such novel 3,7-diacylquercetin (D 2), quercetin 6"-acylgalactoside (D 3) and quercetin 2",6"-diacylgalactoside (D 4) analogues of quercetin 2",3"-diacylglucosides (D 1) as well as lead compound 1 were prepared to assess target specificities and preferences in bacteria. [13] The significant enzymatic inhibition of both *E. coli* DNA gyrase and *S. aureus* topoIV suggest that these compounds are dual inhibitors. Most of the investigated compounds exhibited pronounced inhibition with MIC values ranging from 0.13 to 128 μg/mL towards the growth of multidrug-resistant Gram-positive MRSA, MSSA, VRE, VISA and *Streptococcus pneumoniae* bacterial strains. Structure-activity relationship studies revealed that the acyl moiety was absolutely essential for activity against Gram-positive organisms. The most active compound was minimally 512-fold more potent than vancomycin and 32-fold more potent than 1. It also has realistic *in situ* intestinal absorption in rats, and showed very low acute toxicity in mice. [14]

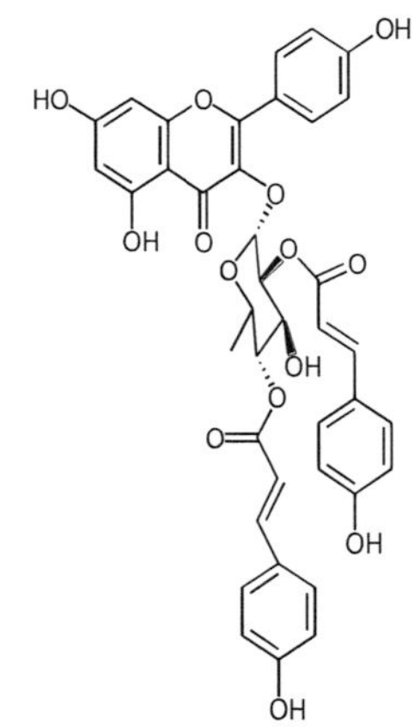

1

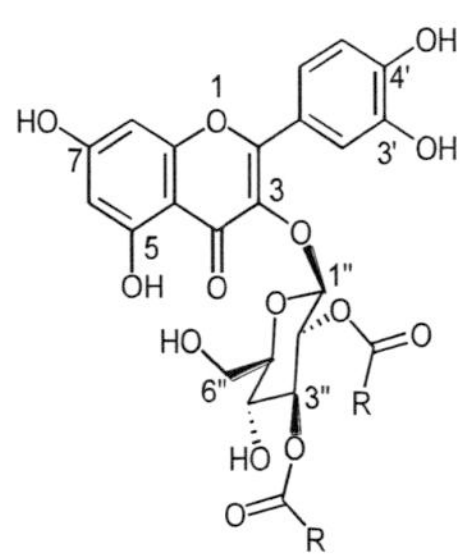

2a–h
D1

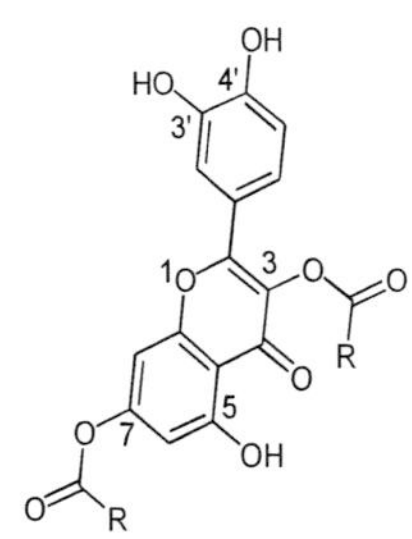

3a,b
D2

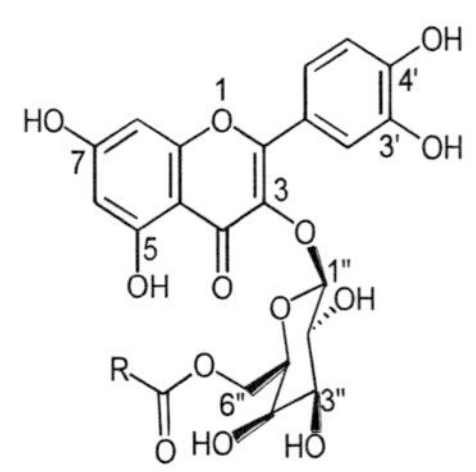

4a,b
D3

Compd	R
2a, 5a	C_6H_4(4-OEt)
2b, 5b	C_6H_4(4-^{n}Pr)
2c, 5c	C_6H_4(4-F)
2d, 5e	$CH_2C_6H_4$(4-F)
2e, 5f	$C_2H_4C_6H_4$(4-OH)
2f, 5g	$C_2H_4C_6H_4$(4-OEt)
2g, 3a, 4a, 5h	$C_2H_4C_6H_4$(4-Me)
2h, 3b, 4b, 5i	$C_2H_4C_6H_4$(4-F)
5d	$CH_2C_6H_4$(4-Me)
5j	$C_3H_6C_6H_4$(4-F)
5k	$C_4H_8C_6H_4$(4-F)

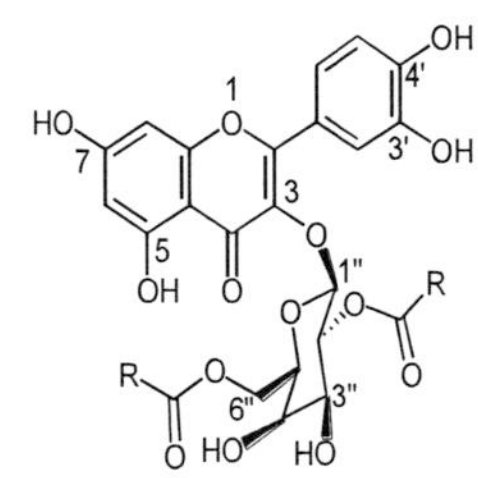

5a–k
D4

Figure 2. Overview of novel quercetin derivatives.

In general, the two factors that contribute to antibacterial potency of quercetin diacylglycoside analogues are the kinetics of drug uptake and the ability to inhibit DNA gyrase or topoIV. For an antibacterial agent to be effective, it must penetrate the bacterial cell first to reach its target enzymes. Ultimately, the antibacterial potency rate for these quercetin derivatives against multidrug-resistant gram-positive bacterial strains is appeared as quercetin 2”,6”-diacylgalactoside (D 4) > quercetin 2”,3”-diacylglucosides (D 1) > 6”-acylglactosides (D 3) > 3,7-diacylquercetins (D 2) > tetraacetyl-quercetin-3-*O*-glycosides > quercetin/ quercetin-3-*O*-glycosides/ quercetin-3,7-di-*O*-glycosides. This potency against gram-negative bacterial strains is appeared to vice versa. The author would like to propose that the primary target of these compounds valued the penetration of bacterial cell even though there is still more desired the investigation to observe the permeability of cell membrane.

THE ROLE OF GRAM-POSITIVE AND GRAM-NEGATIVE ORGANISMS TOWARDS ANTIBIOTICS

Lipinski’s landmark study [15] represented the first systematic attempt to correlate the physicochemical properties of drugs with the predicted successful matriculation of initial hits and subsequent late-stage leads. Major findings from this analysis were the recognition of an ideal property space for orally available drug candidates (MW, lipophilicity, hydrogen bond donors and acceptors), as well as the fact that corporate compound archives had been slowly moving away from an optimal area of this physicochemical space, most likely driven by synthetic convenience rather than by design. This awareness had a major impact on drug discovery, and today it is common to analyze these properties (the “rule of five” or “Lipinski’s rules”) prior to synthesizing novel candidates. Antibacterial compounds, though, have always been considered an exception to these rules primarily because of their higher molecular weight (MW) and polarity. Antibacterial drugs occupy a unique property space that is remarkably different compared to drugs of other therapeutic areas. This fact has been long recognized, and general rules such as Lipinski’s rules of five do not apply to these compounds. The most likely reason for this observed divergence is the different cell architecture of bacteria that, in turn, greatly affects permeability and efflux of compounds. While different groups have addressed the property space of antibacterial drugs as a whole and established algorithms to predict activity, to the best of my knowledge a rigorous distinction between compounds with Gram-positive and Gram-negative activity has to date been lacking. Author proposes that this differentiation is necessary for a significant analysis because of large differences in the cell wall structure of these organisms (Figure 3).

Two major differences between antibacterial and “normal” drugs; Drugs with activity only against Gram-positive bacteria have much less restriction in MW, especially if the target is located in the peptidoglycan matrix or on the outer surface of the underlying lipid bilayer (e.g., glycopeptides such as vancomycin) and permeation through the inner lipid membrane is not required to kill the pathogens. Compounds with activity against Gram-negative organisms must overcome further barriers to function, namely, the penetration of the outer lipid membrane and evasion of efflux pumps. These additional requirements appear to result in even more dissimilar physicochemical properties compared to the reference drug set, with a larger MW (but a quite strict MW) and an increase in polarity, as reflected. Both parameters are partially believed to be driven by the properties of porin proteins that serve as a major entry pathway in Gram-negative bacteria. These proteins form cylinder-shaped openings (*β*-barrels) in the outer membrane with polar amino acid side chains lining the inside of the opening. For a molecule to enter through these hydrophilic channels, the hydration sphere of the channel-lining amino acids has to be removed and replaced temporarily by the drug molecule. [16]

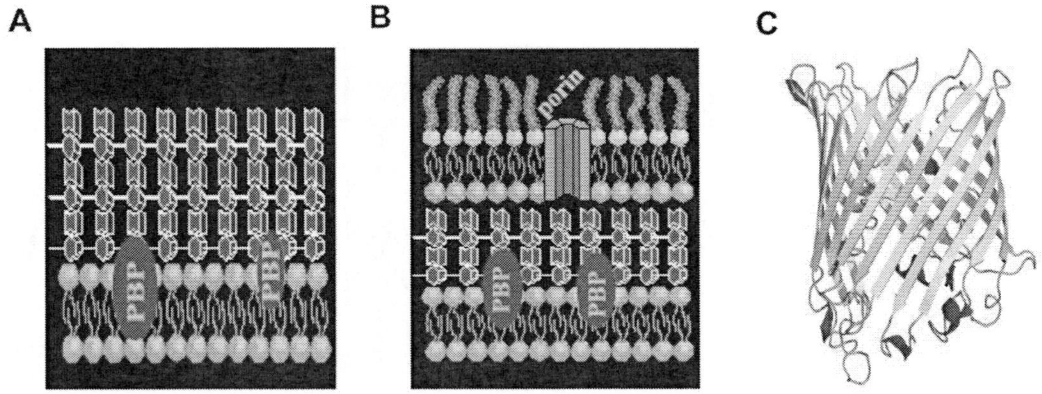

Figure 3. Pictorial view of (A) Gram-positive bacterial cell membrane, (B) Gram-negative bacterial cell membrane and (C) Porin channel.

The regions of physicochemical space required to achieve both Gram-negative activity (high polarity to ensure porin permeability) and oral bioavailability (reasonable level of lipophilicity to guarantee lipid membrane permeability) seem to be largely nonoverlapping.

The unique physicochemical property space required for antibacterially active compounds, and especially Gram-negative antibacterials, must be taken into account during high-throughput screening to identify hits with whole cell activity. A better understanding of the antibacterial property space is one of multiple parameters that are essential to improve the future success rate for the identification of novel antibacterial drugs, especially the badly needed compounds with activity against multi-drug-resistant Gram-positive pathogens that are becoming more prevalent in nosocomial and community based infections.

Methods and Results

As shown in Tables 1 and 2, the minimum inhibitory concentrations (MICs) of quercetin derivatives (2a–h, 3a,b, 4a,b, 5a–k & A, B, C, D) in Figure 2 against a panel of nine selected multidrug-resistant Gram-positive bacterial pathogens [Methicillin-resistant *S. aureus* (MRSA) OM481, OM584, N315, and COL; methicillin-sensitive *S. aureus* (MSSA) 209P; Vancomycin-resistant *S. aureus* (VRE)

FN-1 and NCTC 12201; vancomycin intermediate-resistant *S. aureus* (VISA) Mu50 and *Streptococcus pneumoniae* R6] and two Gram negative bacterial pathogens (*Pseudomonas aeruginosa* PA01 and *Escherichia coli* K-12) were investigated. Furthermore, the effects on *E. coli* supercoiling, *E. coli* topoIV decatenation and *S. aureus* topoIV decatenation activities were evaluated. To observe probable binding conformation of these ligands in the ATP binding pocket, a molecular docking study was performed, and the interaction of these compounds with the 24 KDa fragment of DNA gyrase B and topoIV ParE was explored using the AutoDock 4.0 program (Table 3).

Table 1. Antibacterial activity (MICs) against Gram-positive bacterial strains for 1, 2a–h, 3a,b, 4a,b, 5a–k, Quercetin-3-O-glucose/galactose, Quercetin-3-O-tetraacetateglucose/tetraacetategalactose, Quercetin-3,7-di-O-glucose/glactose, Quercetin-3,7-di-O-tetraacetateglucose/tetraacetategalactose, quercetin, vancomycin, norfloxacin and novobiocin

Compd	MIC[a] (μg/mL, Gram-positive)								
	VRE		VISA	MRSA				MSSA	R6[j]
	FN-1[b]	NCTC 12201[c]	Mu50[d]	OM481[e]	OM584[f]	N315[g]	COL[h]	209P[i]	
3a	64	64	16	32	32	32	32	64	32
3b	64	32	32	16	16	16	32	64	32
4a	32	32	16	16	16	16	32	16	32
4b	16	16	32	16	16	16	32	16	32
5a	8	8	4	4	4	8	16	4	4
5b	8	4	4	4	4	2	16	2	2
5c	4	4	2	2	2	8	8	4	4
5d	8	4	4	2	2	8	16	4	2
5e	0.5	0.5	1	1	1	1	8	1	1
5f	4	4	2	1	1	2	4	2	4
5g	16	16	8	4	4	2	8	8	8
5h	0.5	0.5	0.5	0.25	0.25	0.25	1	0.25	0.25
5i	0.25	0.25	0.5	0.13	0.13	0.13	0.5	0.13	0.13
2h	1	1	1	2	2	0.25	1	0.25	0.50
5j	8	8	4	2	2	4	16	4	4
5k	16	16	16	4	4	2	16	4	8
A	32	32	64	32	32	64	128	64	64
B	>128	>128	>128	>128	>128	>128	>128	>128	>128
C	64	64	128	128	128	128	>128	128	128
D	>128	>128	>128	>128	>128	>128	>128	>128	>128
Qu	>128	>128	>128	>128	>128	>128	>128	>128	>128
Van	>128	>128	8	0.25	0.25	0.25	0.25	0.25	0.25
Norf	>128	4	>128	64	128	2	1	0.5	0.25
Novo	>128	2	8	0.25	0.25	0.13	0.25	0.13	0.25
1	8	4	nt	1	2	1	1	0.5	nt
2a–g	2–16	4–16	1–16	2–32	2–32	1–8	4–16	1–8	1–8

nt, not tested; [a]Microdilution method,[17] MIC determined after 24h; [b]Vancomycin-resistant enterococci FN-1; [c]Vancomycin-resistant enterococci NCTC 12201; [d]Vancomycin intermediate-resistant *S. aureus* Mu50; [e]Methicillin-resistant *S. aureus* OM481; [f]Methicillin-resistant *S. aureus* OM584; [g]Methicillin-resistant *S. aureus* N315; [g]Methicillin-resistant *S. aureus* COL; [i]Methicillin sensitive *S. aureus* 209P; [j]*Streptococcus pneumoniae* R6. Quercetin-3-*O*-glucose/galactose (A), Quercetin-3-*O*-tetraacetateglucose/tetraacetategalactose (B), Quercetin-3,7-di-*O*-glucose/glactose (C), Quercetin-3,7-di-*O*-tetraacetateglucose/tetraacetategalactose (D), Quercetin (Qu), vancomycin (Van), norfloxacin (Norf), and novobiocin (Novo).

Table 2. Antibacterial activity (MICs) against Gram-negative bacterial strains and DNA gyrase supercoiling and topoIV decatenation avtivities for 1, 3a,b, 4a,b, 5a–k, Quercetin-3-*O*-glucose/galactose, Quercetin-3-*O* tetraacetateglucose/ tetraacetategalactose, Quercetin-3,7-di-*O*-glucose/glactose, Quercetin-3,7-di-*O*-tetraacetateglucose/tetraacetategalactose, quercetin, norfloxacin and novobiocin

Compd	MIC[a] (μg/mL, Gram-negative)		Supercoiling inhibition, IC_{50}[d] (μM)	Decatenation inhibition, IC_{50}[d] (μM)	
	PA01[b]	K-12[c]	*E. coli* DNA gyrase	*E. coli* topoIV	*S. aureus* topoIV
3a	64	64	1.66	8.59	0.44
3b	64	64	0.72	6.76	0.29
4a	>128	>128	1.79	11.99	2.57
4b	>128	>128	1.40	11.52	2.99
5a	>128	>128	0.43	11.33	1.78
5b	>128	>128	0.77	10.89	1.93
5c	>128	>128	0.38	11.02	0.52
5d	>128	>128	2.21	10.52	2.69
5e	>128	>128	1.05	10.21	0.46
5f	>128	>128	2.39	10.86	1.59
5g	>128	>128	5.39	>12	2.99
5h	>128	>128	2.09	9.46	1.49
5i	>128	>128	0.78	9.16	0.22
5j	>128	>128	2.98	10.74	2.94
5k	>128	>128	5.02	>12	4.05
A	>128	>128	nt	nt	nt
B	32	16	0.10	3.07	0.07
C	>128	>128	nt	nt	nt
D	32	32	0.26	5.34	0.20
Quercetin	>128	64	0.14	6.42	nt
Norfloxacin	0.25	0.25	0.09	nt	3.50
Novobiocin	8	8	0.05	0.11	nt
1	>128	>128	3.11	nt	2.70

nt, not tested; [a]Microdilution method,[17] MIC determined after 24h; [b]*Pseodomonas aeruginosa* PA01, [c]*E. coli* K-12; IC_{50}[d] the concentration of the drugs that inhibits 50 % of supercoiling (*E. coli* DNA gyrase) and decatenation (*E. coli* and *S. aureus* topoIV) activities,[19,20] Quercetin-3-*O*-glucose/galactose (A), Quercetin-3-*O*-tetraacetateglucose/tetraacetategalactose (B), Quercetin-3,7-di-*O*-glucose/glactose (C), Quercetin-3,7-di-*O*-tetraacetateglucose/tetraacetategalactose (D).

IN SITU ABSORPTION STUDY [18]

The *in situ* absorption was studied in male Wister rats ($n = 4$) weighting from 200 to 300 grams. The rats were fasted with *ad libitum* access to water 18 h, and anesthetized by introperitoneal injection of pentobarbetal at 50 mg/kg 30 min prior to sugery. The *in situ* perfusion technique described in the original publication was used. After the setting up of the cannula and cleaning of the segment under study, 1 mg/mL of 5i was injected into the small intestine. After 1 h, 10 mL saline was pumped through the intestine all the way to the disital cannula and drained back into the intestine to ensure uniform sample concentration throughout the gut segment, and subsquently this 10 mL saline solution along with non-absorbed 5i was collected. The concentration of the collected solution gave amounts of absorption from small intestine by substract from injected cocentration. Thus, the amount of absorption were achieved with following three-step sequence involving initial centrifuging of the intestinal samples at 1500 rpm for 10 min to provide 0.1 mg/mL sample solution, then extraction with chloroform followed by removing the solvent under reduced pressure. Finally the resulting sample was dissolve in 10 mL methanol, and the absorbance of the solution was measured in a UV spectrophotometer at 340 nm.

The most potent compound 5i was selected as a representative compound with which to explore absorption property and acute toxicity of quercetin diacylglycoside analogues in rats and mice, respectively. The required concentration of 5i for *in situ* intestinal absorption and acute toxicity testing, were achieved with 50 % polyoxyethyleneglycol (PEG) in saline. The absorption property was studied by *in situ* prefusion technique in rats (n = 4). The *in situ* intestinal absorption studies in rats demonstrated realistic absorption of 5i from small intestine, 76.6 % ± 0.60.

Acute Toxicity Study

The acute toxicity of 5i was studied in male mice (n = 4) weighting from 15 to 30 grams and animals were purchased from Charles River Co. Ltd.

Table 3. The best docking result on the inhibition constant (K_i) for 3a,b, 4a,b, 5a–k, Quercetin-3-O-galactose, quercetin and novobiocin towards 24 KDa fragment of the DNA Gyrase B and topoisomerase IV ParE from *E. coli*

Compd	K_i^a (μM, *E. coli* DNA gyrase B inhibition constant)	K_i^a (μM, *S. aureus* topoIV ParE inhibition constant)	Compd	K_i^a (μM, *E. coli* DNA gyrase B inhibition constant)	K_i^a (μM, *S. aureus* topoIV ParE inhibition constant)
3a	8.31	2.21	5f	41.96	2.13
3b	3.58	0.93	5g	62.15	29.88
4a	0.46	5.40	5h	19.02	1.88
4b	0.50	8.82	5i	0.91	2.06
5a	2.14	0.70	5j	17.48	3.81
5b	3.83	1.84	5k	394.24	14.23
5c	1.90	1.14	B	0.15	0.32
5d	11.07	14.71	Quercetin	0.18	0.24
5e	0.25	0.43	Novobiocin	0.01	1.00

$^a K_i$ values were calculated by computer aided AutoDock 4.0 soft (AutoDock Tools version 1.5.2 revision 2) [21].

The study was conducted according to internationally accepted principles of laboratory animals. Only water was provided *ad libitum* during the 12 h before experimentation. After intervenous injection of 5i, food and water were provided *ad libitum*. The weight gain of the animals, as well as the mobility and the mortality in animals were observed up to 14 days as an indicator of toxicity. The mortality was zero and the mobility in animals was normal within the period of test.

Intervenous doses of 5i in 50 % PEG via the tail vein were well tolerated by mice (n = 4) at 10 mg/kg/d (for 4 days, total dose was 40 mg/kg, total dose volume was 20 mL/kg) and 50 mg/kg/d (for 4 days, total dose was 200 mg/kg, total dose volume was 20 mL/kg). At 100 mg/kg/d (for 4 days, total dose was 400 mg/kg, total dose volume was 20 mL/kg), the mice showed a transient, seizure-like reaction to fourth injection after ca. 10 min, but all animals appeared normal after 1 day.

Conclusions

Our mechanistic studies revealed that although quercetin diacylglycoside analogues show modest and dual inhibition toward *E. coli* DNA gyrase and *S. aureus* topoIV, their antibacterial activity is not related only to their effect on these enzymes. The two factors that contribute to their antibacterial potency are the ability to penetrate the bacterial cell and their potentiality to inhibit these enzymes. The presence of suitable sizes of liphophilic acyl groups on the sugar moiety of quercetin diacylglycoside is required for activity against multidrug-resistant Gram-positive organisms. Finally, these novel quercetin diacylglycosides represent one of the most exciting recent chemical advances in the antibacterial field.

References

[1] Center for disease control and prevention, public health dispatch: Vancomycin-resistant *Staphylococcus aureus-Pennsylvania. MMWR Morb. Mortal. Wkly. Rep.* 2002, *51*, 902–902.

[2] Levy, S. B.; Marshall, B. Antibacterial resistance worldwide: cause, challenges and responses. *Nat. Med.* 2004, *10*, S122–129.

[3] Aspa, J.; Rajas, O.; Rodriguez de Castro, F.; Blanquer, J.; Zalacain, R.; Fenoll, A.; de Celis, R.; Vargas, A.; Salvanes, F. R.; Espana, P. P.; Rello, J.; Torres, A. Drug-resistant *pneumococcal pneumonia*: clinical relevance and related factors. *Clin. Infect. Dis.* 2004, *38*, 787–798.

[4] Barrett, C. T.; Barrett, J. F. Antibacterials: are the new entries enough to deal with the emerging resistance problems? *Curr. Opin. Biotech.* 2003, *14*, 621–626.

[5] Livermore, D. M. The need for new antibiotics. *Clin. Microbial. Infect.* 2004, *10* (Suppl, 4), 1–9.

[6] Jacobs, M. R. Worlwide trends in antimicrobial resistance among common respiratory tract pathogens in children. *Pediatr. Infect. Dis. J.* 2003, *22*, S109–S119.

[7] Häbich, D.; von Nussbaum, F. Platensimycin, a new antibiotic and "superbug challenger" from nature. *ChemMedChem* 2006, *1*, 951–954.

[8] Bloor, S. J. An antimicrobial kaempferol-diacyl-rhamnoside from *Pentachondra pumila*. *Phytochemistry* 1995, *38*, 1033–1035.

[9] Otsuka, N.; Liu, M. –H.; Shiota, S.; Ogawa, W.; Kuroda, T.; Hatano, T.; Tsuchiya, T. Anti-methicillin resistant *Staphylococcus aureus* (MRSA) compounds isolated from *Laurus nobilis*. *Biol. Pharm. Bull.* 2008, *31*, 1794–1797.

[10] Liu, M, -H.; Otsuka, N.; Noyori, K.; Shiota, S.; Ogawa, W.; Kuroda, T.; Hatano, T.; Tsuchiya, T. Synergistic effect of kaempferol glycosides purified from *Laurus nobilis* and fluloroquinolones on methicillin-resistant *Staphylococcus aureus*. *Biol. Pharm. Bull.* 2009, *32*(3), 489–492.

[11] Neises, B.; Steglich, W. Esterification of carboxylic acids with diacylcyclohexylcarbodiimide/ 4-dimethylaminopyridine: *tert*-butyl ethyl formate. *Org. Synth.* 1990, *Coll. Vol. 7*, 93–93.

[12] Hossion, A. M. L.; Otsuka, N.; Kandahary, R. K.; Tsuchiya, T.; Ogawa, W.; Iwado, A.; Zamami, Y.; Sasaki, K. Design, synthesis and biological evaluation of a novel series of quercetin diacylglucosides as potent anti-MRSA and anti-VRE agents. *Bioorg. Med. Chem. Lett.* 2010, *20*, 5349–5352.

[13] Hossion, A. M. L.; Zamami, Y.; Kandahary, R. K.; Tsuchiya, T.; Iwado, A.; Sasaki, K.; Quercetin Diacylglycoside Analogues Showing Dual Inhibition of DNA Gyrase and Topoisomerase IV as Novel Antibacterial Agents. Submitted to *J. Med. Chem.* 2011, *54*, 3686–3703.

[14] Sasaki, K.; Tsuchiya, T.; Hossion, A. M. L. PCT Int. Pat. Appl. WO 2011013735. Novel flavanone derivative. (National University Corporation Okayama University, Japan) http://www.sumobrain.com/patents/wipo/Novel-flavanone-derivative/WO2011013735.html

[15] Lipinski, C. A.; Lombardo, F.; Dominy, B. W.; Feeney, P. J. Experimental and computational approaches to estimate solubility and permeability in drug discovery and development settings. *Adv. Drug Delivery Rev.* 1997, *23*, 3–25.

[16] O'Shea, R. and Moser, H. E. Physicochemical Properties of Antibacterial Compounds: Implications for Drug Discovery. *J. Med. Chem.* 2008, *51*, 2871–2878.

[17] Clinical and Laboratory Standard Institute (CLSI). *Methods for Dilution Antibacterial Susceptibility Test for Bacteria That Grow Aerobically*; 7th *ed.* Vol. 27; Approved Standard (MA7-A7); Clinical and Laboratory Standard Institute: Wayne, 2007; p133–133.

[18] Doluisio, J. T.; Billups, N. F.; Dittert, L. W.; Sugita, E. T.; Swintosky, J. V. Drug absorption I: an *in situ* rat gut technique yielding realistic absorption rates. *J. Pharm. Sci.* 1969, *58*, 1196–1200.

[19] Hallett, P.; Grimshaw, A. J.; Wigley, D. B.; Maxwell, A. Cloning of the DNA gyrase genes under *tac* promoter control: overproduction of the gyrase A and B proteins. *Gene* 1990, *93*, 139–142.

[20] Peng, H.; Marians, K. J. Overexpression and purification of bacterial topoisomerase IV. *Methods Mol. Biol.* 1999, *94*, 163–169.

[21] Rosenfeld, R. J. Goodsell, D. S.; Musah, R. A.; Morris, G. M.; Goodin, D. B.; Olson, A. J. Automated docking of ligands to an artificial active site: augmenting crystallographic analysis with computer modeling. *J. Comput. -Aided Mol. Des.* 2003, *17*, 525–536.

In: Quercetin
Editors: Taiki Chikamatsu and Yuudai Hida

ISBN: 978-1 61942- 057-1

Chapter 15

SUPPRESSIVE EFFECT OF QUERCETIN ON INTESTINAL TIGHT JUNCTION PERMEABILITY

Takuya Suzuki*

Department of Biofunctional Science and Technology,
Graduate School of Biosphere Science, Hiroshima University, Japan

ABSTRACT

One of the most important functions of gastrointestinal epithelial cells is to provide a physical barrier to the diffusion of pathogens, toxins, and allergens from the external environment into the tissues. Defects in the barrier function play a crucial role in the pathogenesis of various intestinal diseases, such as inflammatory bowel disease, irritative bowel disease, and food allergies. The intestinal barrier function is organized by interactions among several barrier components, including the adhesive mucous gel layer, the mucosal immune system, and intercellular tight junctions (TJ). The TJ is a multi-protein complex, which locates around the apical end of the lateral membrane of polarized epithelial cells, and selectively regulates the paracellular passage of ions, molecules and water. The TJ complex is composed of transmembrane proteins that interact with the perijunctional actin cytoskeleton through intracellular plaque proteins. TJ permeability and assembly are dynamically regulated by various intracellular signaling molecules, such as protein kinase C, mitogen-activated protein kinases, and protein phosphatases. Quercetin is one of the most abundant flavonoids in the human diet and exhibits various biological effects, such as anti-inflammatory and anti-cancer activities. Recent studies have demonstrated that quercetin participates in the regulation of intestinal TJ barrier function. This chapter presents the recent advances in our understanding of the quercetin-mediated suppressive effect on intestinal TJ permeability with a particular focus on intracellular molecular mechanisms.

---

* Address correspondence to: Takuya Suzuki, Ph. D., 1-4-4, Kagamiyama, Higashi-Hiroshima, 739-8528, Japan. TEL: 81-82-424-7984. Fax: 81-82-424-7916; E-mail: takuya@hiroshima-u.ac.jp.

1. Intestinal Barrier Function and Diseases

The gastrointestinal epithelium provides a physical barrier to the diffusion of luminal pro-inflammatory molecules, such as pathogens, toxins, and allergens, into the mucosal tissues and circulation [1]. Defects in intestinal barrier integrity, resulting in the diffusion of these molecules, induce the excessive activation of the mucosal immune system and inflammation. Therefore, intestinal barrier defects are involved in the pathogenesis of various intestinal and systemic inflammatory diseases [1-3]. For example, increased intestinal permeability has received much study in association with inflammatory bowel diseases (IBDs) such as Crohn's disease and ulcerative colitis [4]. Recent studies have suggested that the increased intestinal permeability is the primary cause of IBDs, although IBD pathogenesis is complicated by heredity and life-style factors. This includes the observations that a subset of first-degree relatives of patients with Crohn's disease has increased intestinal permeability despite being completely healthy [5] and that the non-involved segment of the intestines in IBD patients exhibits intestinal hyperpermeability [6]. Furthermore, several reports demonstrate that patients with systemic inflammatory diseases, such as dermatologic and rheumatological disorders, show increased intestinal permeability [7-9]. However, in most instances, it is not evident whether the abnormal intestinal permeability is the primary phenomenon responsible for the activation of systemic immune system or whether it is itself a response to the intestinal inflammation or psychological stress caused by the diseases. Further investigations are required to clarify the contribution of increased intestinal permeability to the pathogenesis of diseases mentioned above; however, maintenance of intestinal barrier integrity may help in preventing the onset of the diseases.

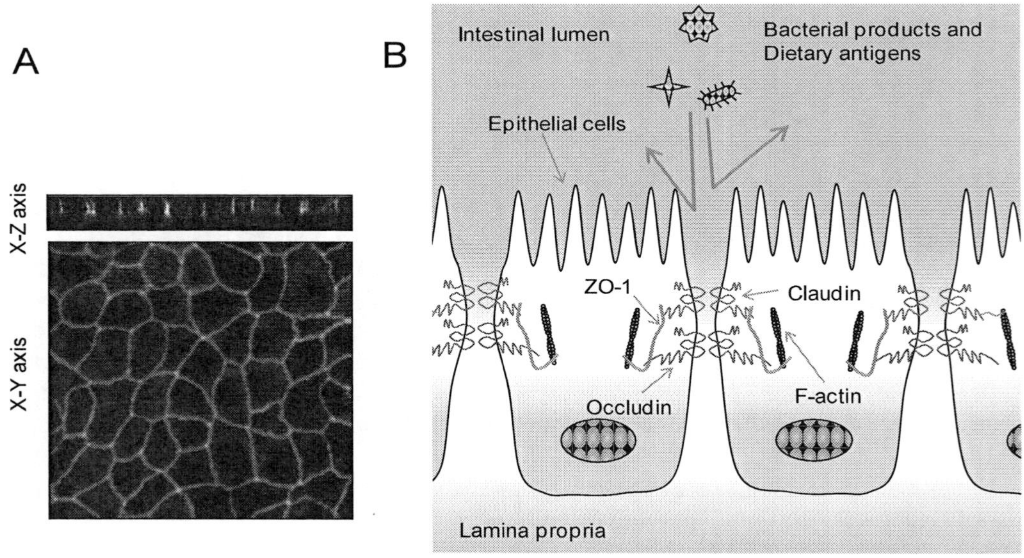

Figure 1. Intestinal tight junctions (TJs) as a physical barrier. (A) Confocal images of an immunolabeled TJ protein, zonula occludens (ZO)-1, collected in human intestinal Caco-2 cells. The TJs are localized at the apical-lateral membrane junction. (B) The TJ is a multiple-protein complex composed of transmembrane and intracellular plaque proteins. The TJs provide a physical barrier to the permeation of pro-inflammatory molecules, such as bacterial endotoxins and dietary antigens, from the luminal environment into the mucosal tissues.

2. Tight Junction Structure

The intestinal barrier is organized by interactions among different components, including the mucus gel layer, antimicrobial peptides, and the tight junctions (TJs). The TJ is a multiple protein complex composed of transmembrane and cytosolic plaque proteins (Figure 1) [2, 10]. It locates on the apical ends of lateral membrane of intestinal epithelial cells and regulates the integrity of paracellular permeability between epithelial cells. Four integral transmembrane proteins, occludin, claudins, tricellulin, and junctional adhesion molecule (JAM), have been identified [11-14]. These transmembrane proteins interact with intracellular plaque proteins, such as zonula occludens (ZO) and cinglin, which in turn anchor the transmembrane proteins to the perijunctional actin cytoskeleton [10]. The interaction of the TJ complex with the actin cytoskeleton is vital for maintaining the integrity of the paracellular pathways [15].

Claudins, occludin, and tricellulin are tetraspanin membrane proteins, which contain 4 transmembrane domains and 2 extracellular loops. The claudin family comprises a multigene family of at least 24 members that exhibit complex tissue-specific expression patterns [10, 13]. Several reports show that claudins play an essential role in determining the size- and charge selectivity of the paracellular pathways [16-18]. In the intestines, claudin-1/3/4/5/8 are known to strengthen TJ integrity (by decreasing paracellular permeability), and claudin-2/7/15 form charge-selective paracellular channels. A number of studies have demonstrated that occludin also plays an important role in the regulation of TJ integrity, although occludin knockout mice show the formation of intact TJs in different epithelia [19]. In human intestinal Caco-2 cells and mouse intestines, occludin knockdown increases the paracellular flux of macromolecules [20]. Interestingly, the phosphorylation status of occludin is implicated with occludin function and barrier integrity. In the intact epithelium, occludin is highly phosphorylated at the threonine and serine residues, and undergoes dephosphorylation at the threonine residues during TJ disassembly under calcium-depleted conditions [21, 22]. Tricellulin is preferentially localized to the tricellular contact points of the epithelium, although it can also be found in the bicellular junctions [11]. A study shows that suppression of tricellulin expression impairs intestinal barrier integrity [11]. The JAMs are single-span transmembrane proteins characterized by a molecular structure composed of 2 extracellular immunoglobulin loops and a cytoplasmic C-terminal domain [14]. Although our knowledge of JAM family proteins remains fragmentary, the accumulating evidence suggests that some members of the family have roles in TJ assembly and barrier function. For example, JAM-1 knockout mice exhibit an impaired intestinal barrier [23].

Several intracellular plaque proteins, such as ZO-1, -2 and -3, have been identified in the TJ complex [10]. The ZO proteins are essentially multi-domain proteins, characterized by 3 PDZ domains, through which they interact with other TJ proteins and the perijunctional actin cytoskeleton [24-26]. Thus, ZO-proteins play a fundamental role as the molecular scaffold in the TJ structure. Further, a recent study has demonstrated that ZO-1 contributes to the assembly of the TJ structure. In ZO-1 deficient cells, the assembly of other TJ proteins into the TJ structure is delayed, although the cells can still form polarized monolayers with a normal TJ structure [27].

3. TJ Regulation

TJ permeability and assembly are regulated by various intracellular signaling pathways, and this regulation is affected by physiological and pathological stimuli, including food factors. Some kinases and phosphatases have been found to directly phosphorylate and dephosphorylate the TJ proteins, resulting in their subsequent assembly and disassembly into the TJ structure.

Protein kinase C (PKC) is one kinase that has been extensively studied in regard to intestinal TJ regulation [28]. PKC, a serine- and threonine-kinase, is classified into 3 subfamilies (conventional, novel and atypical) and includes at least 12 isoenzymes. Interestingly, PKC regulates intestinal paracellular permeability and TJ assembly/disassembly in an isoform-specific manner. Zonula occludens toxin, derived from Vibrio cholerae, increases TJ permeability through activation of PKCα in the rabbit small intestine and rat intestinal IEC-6 cells, and this impairment of the TJs is associated with bacteria-induced diarrhea [29]. PKCδ activity is reported to be essential for the oxidative stress-induced disruption of the microtubule cytoskeleton and the TJ barrier in human intestinal Caco-2 cells [30, 31]. On the other hand, PKCβ/ε/θ/η/ζ have roles in the maintenance, promotion, or protection of intestinal TJ integrity. PKCβ/ε/ζ are reported to be involved in the epidermal growth factor (EGF)-mediated protection of the TJ barrier and structure against oxidative stress, alcohol and acetaldehyde in Caco-2 cells [32, 33]. Meanwhile, knockdowns or inhibitions of PKCθ/η/ζ induce the impairment of the TJ barrier in intestinal and other epithelial cells [34-36]. Further, PKCη and ζ have been found to directly phosphorylate occludin, and this phosphorylation regulates TJ assembly [35, 36].

As the TJ complex is linked with the perijunctional actin cytoskeletal ring in intestinal epithelial cells, TJ permeability is also regulated by the contraction and relaxation of the actin cytoskeleton. The circumferential contraction of the actin-myosin ring is achieved by the phosphorylation of the myosin light chain (MLC) of myosin II by MLC kinase. Several stimuli, such as nutrients and cytokines, are known to influence cytoskeletal contraction and modulate TJ permeability through the activation and expression of MLC kinase [37-39].

4. Effect of Quercetin on Intestinal TJ Permeability

Currently, information on the effect of quercetin on intestinal barrier function is limited; however, a few recent studies have demonstrated that quercetin has a promotive or protective effect on the intestinal barrier. An animal study was performed to examine intestinal TJ permeability in rats fed quercetin-containing diets (~1.0%) for 9 days. Paracellular lucifer yellow (LY) flux (a TJ permeability marker) was found to be dose-dependently decreased in both the small and large intestines of rats fed the quercetin diets (personal observation). In human intestinal Caco-2 cells, treatment with ~100 μmol/L quercetin for 48 hr decreases LY flux and increases transepithelial electrical resistance (TER, a TJ permeability marker) in a dose-dependent manner, indicating the promotion of TJ integrity (Figure 2) [40].

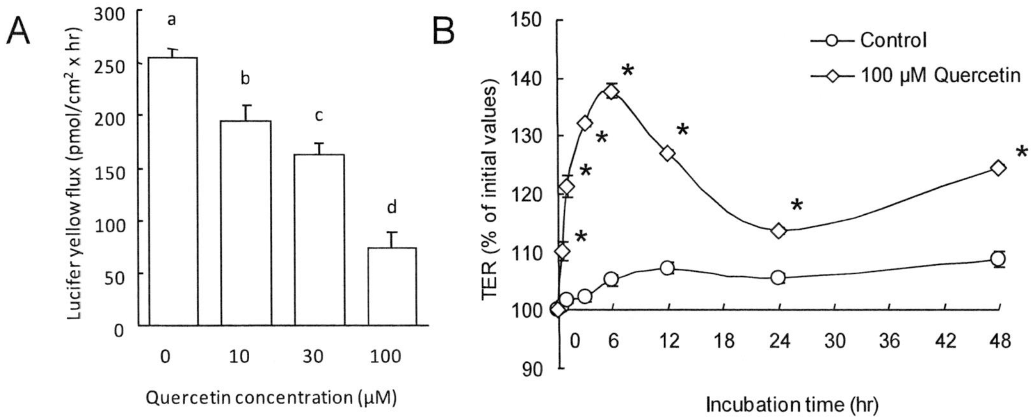

Figure 2. Promotive effect of quercetin on intestinal tight junction (TJ) barrier function. Human intestinal Caco-2 cells were incubated with or without 10-100 μM quercetin for 48 hr in a Transwell culture system. Lucifer yellow flux (A) across the cell monolayers was evaluated for the last 3 hr of incubation, and transepithelial electrical resistance (TER, B) was measured before and at 0.5, 1, 3, 6, 12, 24, and 48 hr. Values are means ± SEM, n = 4. Values not sharing a common letter differ significantly, $P < 0.05$ (A). Asterisks indicate a significant difference from the values before quercetin administration, $P < 0.05$ (B).

In the cells treated with quercetin, the TER rapidly increases over the first 6 hr and then, after a slight decrease, gradually increases again between 24 and 48 hr. Claudin-4 protein expression time-dependently increases from 12 hr after quercetin administration (Figure 3). Another research group has reported, on the basis of a reporter gene assay in Caco-2 cells, that quercetin increases claudin-4 mRNA expression and also induces claudin-4 promoter activity, indicating that quercetin stimulates claduin-4 expression at a transcriptional level [41]. Furthermore, the cytoskeletal association of ZO-2, occludin, and claudin-1 is promoted during the first 6 hr after quercetin administration, although the total expression of the proteins was not influenced (Figure 3) [40]. These findings indicate that the rapid quercetin-mediated increase in TER during the first 6 hr can be attributed to the assembly of ZO-2, occludin, and claudin-1 at the TJs, whereas the promotion of claudin-4 expression results in the increase in TER after 24 hr.

The expression and assembly of TJ proteins are dynamically regulated by various intracellular signaling pathways, including PKC. Treatment of Caco-2 cells with a PKCδ-selective inhibitor produces a promotive effect on TJ integrity in a very similar manner to that of quercetin; the PKCδ inhibitor promotes the assembly of ZO-2, occludin and claudin-1, as well as claudin-4 expression. In fact, quercetin suppresses cellular PKCδ activity, as indicated by the decrease in PKCδ phosphorylation in the cells (Figure 4) [40]. Further, *in vitro* kinase assays using a recombinant PKCδ enzyme has revealed that quercetin directly inhibits PKCδ activity and that the quercetin concentration required for the 50% inhibition of PKCδ is as low as 3.7 μmol/L (Figure 4) [40]. Taken together, these findings indicate that quercetin mediates the promotion of intestinal TJ barrier function through the direct inhibition of the PKCδ isozyme.

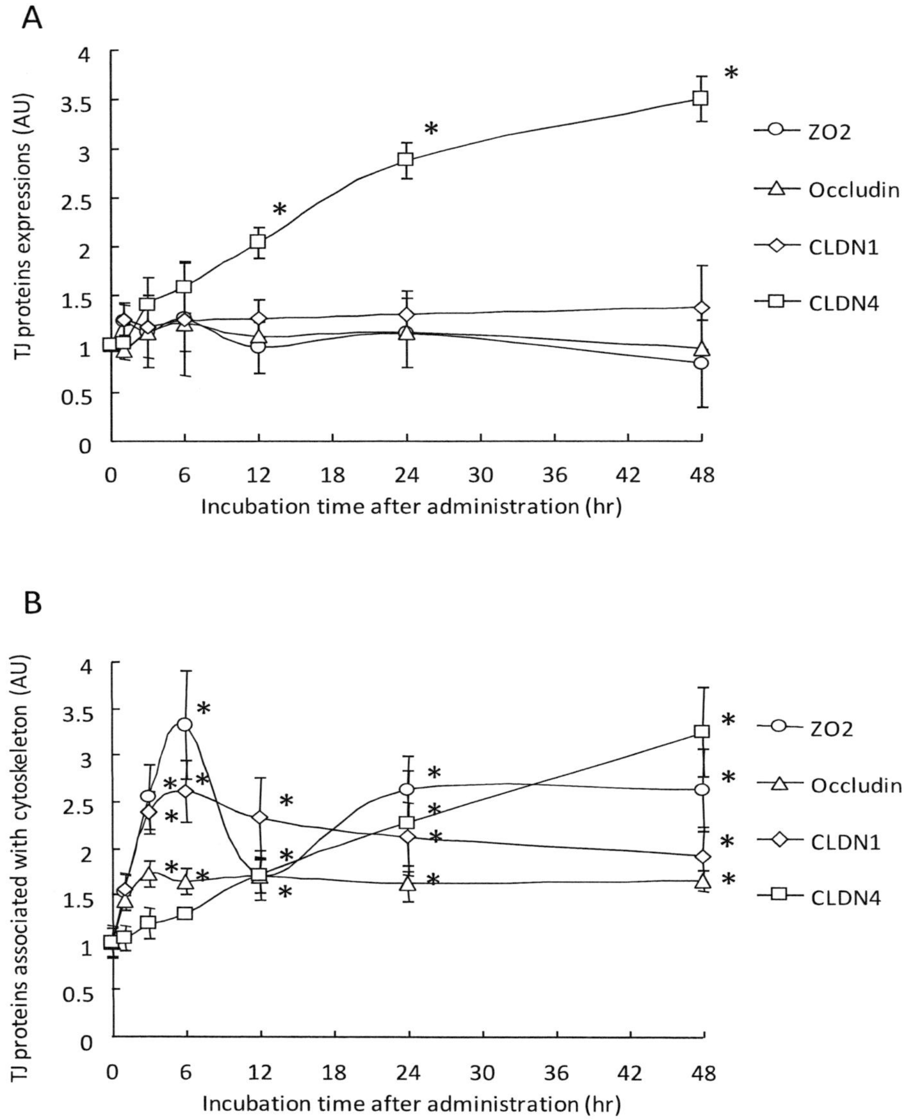

Figure 3. Effect of quercetin on the expression and cytoskeletal association of tight junction (TJ) proteins. Human intestinal Caco-2 cells were incubated with or without 100 μM quercetin for 48 hr in a Transwell culture system. Whole cell extracts (A) and the actin cytoskeleton fraction (detergent-insoluble fraction) (B) were prepared before and at 1, 3, 6, 12, 24 and 48 hr, and immunoblotted for TJ proteins, ZO-1, ZO-2, occludin, JAM-1, claudin-1, claudin-3, and claudin-4. Each specific protein band was quantified by densitometric analysis and the results for ZO-2, occludin, claudin-1 and claudin-4 only are shown, as no differences were found in the other proteins. Values are means ± SEM, n = 4. Asterisks indicate a significant difference from the values before quercetin administration, $P < 0.05$.

Occludin is highly phosphorylated at the Ser and Thr residues in the intact epithelium. TJ assembly and disassembly is associated with the reversible phosphorylation of occludin at these residues, indicating that the Ser/Thr phosphorylation of occludin has a crucial role in the regulation of TJ integrity [21, 22]. Occludin phosphorylation, evaluated by SDS-page migration, increases within 1 hr of quercetin administration, and this increase is closely associated with the actin cytoskeletal association of occludin (Figure 5) [40]. Some protein kinases, such as PKCζ/η and casein kinaseI/II, and phosphatases, such as PP1 and PP2A, have been shown to directly phosphorylate and dephosphorylate occludin [21, 35, 36, 42]. Based on this evidence, it is suggested that quercetin affects the activities of theses kinases or phosphatases via PKCδ inhibition, leading to the promotion of occludin phosphorylation and TJ assembly.

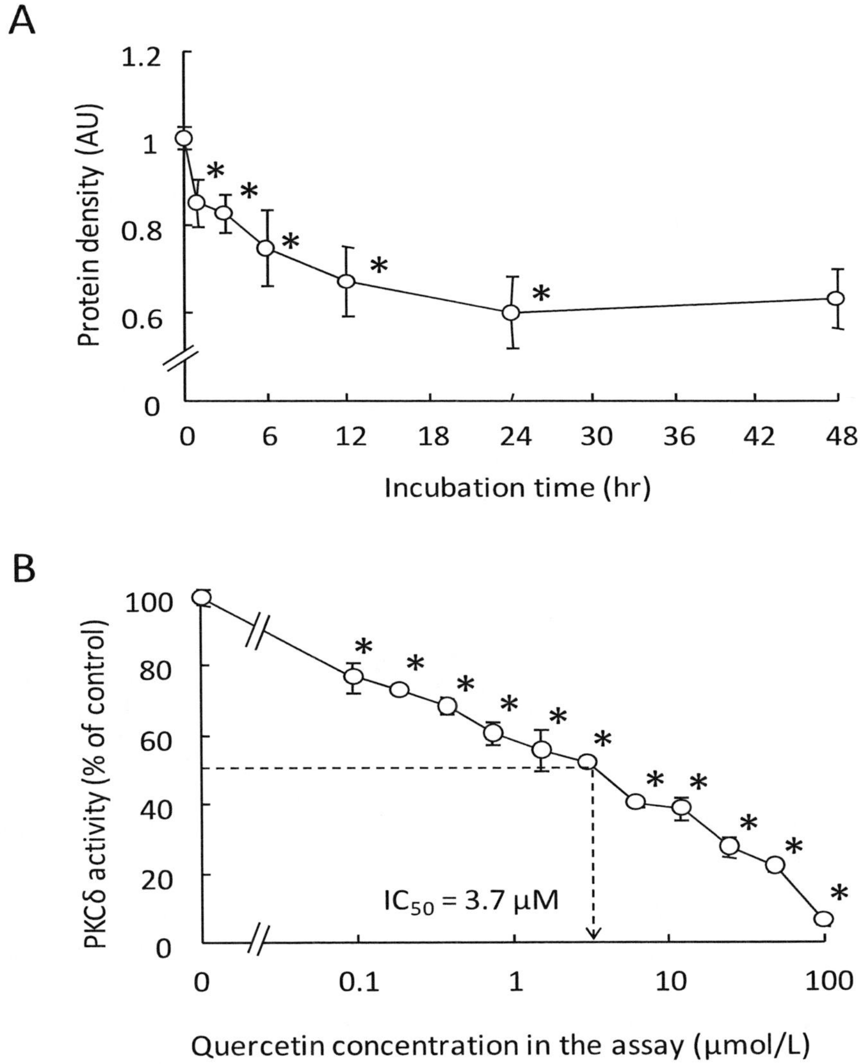

Figure 4. Inhibitory effect of quercetin on protein kinase C δ (PKCδ) activity in Caco-2 cells and in an *in vitro* kinase assay. (A) Human intestinal Caco-2 cells were incubated with or without 100 μM quercetin for 48 hr in a Transwell culture system. Whole cell extracts were prepared before and at 1, 3, 6, 12, 24 and 48 hr, and immunoblotted for phospho- and total PKCδ. Each specific phospho- and total PKCδ band was quantified by densitometric analysis and the ratio of phospho-PKCδ to total PKCδ was calculated. (B) The human recombinant PKCδ enzyme was incubated with the PKC substrate in the absence or presence of quercetin (0 – 100 μM). The activity values were normalized against the control value obtained from the recombinant PKCδ enzyme incubated with the PKC substrate without quercetin. Values are means ± SEM, n = 3. Asterisks indicate a significant difference from the control value, $P < 0.05$.

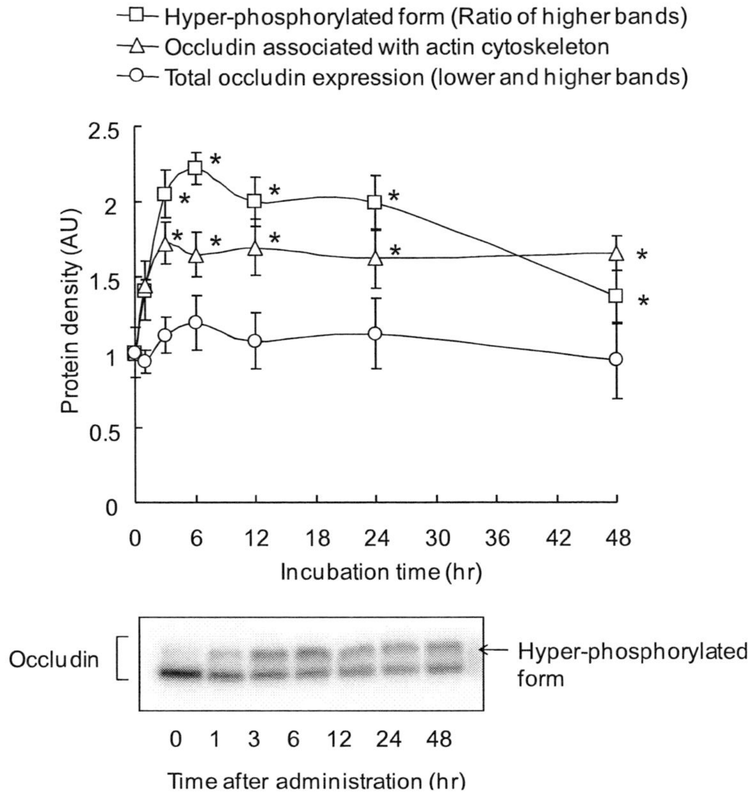

Figure 5. Possible involvement of occludin phosphorylation in the quercetin-induced assembly. Human intestinal Caco-2 cells were incubated with or without 100 μM quercetin for 48 hr in a Transwell culture system. Whole cell extracts and actin cytoskeleton fractions of cells were prepared before and at 1, 3, 6, 12, 24 and 48 hr, and immunoblotted for occludin. Occludin showed double bands in the immunoblots, with the higher band corresponding to the hyper-phosphorylated form of occludin. Each band was quantified by densitometric analysis. The total expression (sum of the lower and higher bands) and the ratio of the hyper-phosphorylated form to total expression were calculated. Values are means ± SEM, n = 4. Asterisks indicate a significant difference from the values before quercetin administration, $P < 0.05$.

A study has shown the protective effect of quercetin on intestinal permeability impaired by ischemic reperfusion injury [43]. The intestinal permeability of sodium fluorescein in the blood-lumen and lumen-blood directions was measured during ischemic reperfusion in anesthetized dogs. They demonstrate that ischemic reperfusion impairs intestinal permeability through increases in mast cell numbers and degranulation. Pretreatment of the intestines with quercetin inhibits the change in permeability, possibly through the stabilization of the mast cells.

Further, there is a report showing that quercetin has a protective effect on oxidative stress-induced TJ disruption in endothelial cells, but not in epithelial cells [44]. However, considering the commonality of TJ structures and regulation between these cells, this finding could be translated to intestinal epithelial cells. Exposure of vascular endothelial ECV304 cells to hydrogen peroxide impaired TJ integrity through decreased expression of TJ proteins, ZO-1 and occludin, *via* ERK1/2 and p38 MAPK activation. Pretreatment of cells with quercetin suppresses the p38 MAPK, but not the ERK1/2, activation, as well as preventing the loss of ZO-1 and occludin, and preserving TJ integrity.

CONCLUSION

Recent studies demonstrate that quercetin has both promotive and protective effects on intestinal barrier integrity. Although the mechanisms underlying the quercetin-mediated effect need to be determined in greater detail, dietary supplementation with quercetin might afford a therapeutic tool for use with diseases associated with intestinal barrier defects.

REFERENCES

[1] Farhadi A, Banan A, Fields J, Keshavarzian A. Intestinal barrier: an interface between health and disease. *J. Gastroenterol. Hepatol.* 2003;18:479-97.

[2] Turner JR. Intestinal mucosal barrier function in health and disease. *Nat. Rev. Immunol.* 2009 Nov;9:799-809.

[3] Groschwitz KR, Hogan SP. Intestinal barrier function: molecular regulation and disease pathogenesis. *J. Allergy Clin. Immunol.* 2009;124:3-20; quiz 1-2.

[4] Wyatt J, Oberhuber G, Pongratz S, Puspok A, Moser G, Novacek G, Lochs H, Vogelsang H. Increased gastric and intestinal permeability in patients with Crohn's disease. *Am. J. Gastroenterol.* 1997 Oct;92:1891-6.

[5] Hollander D, Vadheim CM, Brettholz E, Petersen GM, Delahunty T, Rotter JI. Increased intestinal permeability in patients with Crohn's disease and their relatives. A possible etiologic factor. *Ann. Intern. Med.* 1986 Dec;105:883-5.

[6] Soderholm JD, Peterson KH, Olaison G, Franzen LE, Westrom B, Magnusson KE, Sjodahl R. Epithelial permeability to proteins in the noninflamed ileum of Crohn's disease? *Gastroenterology* 1999;117:65-72.

[7] Hamilton I, Fairris GM, Rothwell J, Cunliffe WJ, Dixon MF, Axon AT. Small intestinal permeability in dermatological disease. *Q. J. Med.* 1985 Sep;56:559-67.

[8] Ukabam SO, Mann RJ, Cooper BT. Small intestinal permeability to sugars in patients with atopic eczema. *Br. J. Dermatol.* 1984 Jun;110:649-52.

[9] Catanoso M, Lo Gullo R, Giofre MR, Pallio S, Tortora A, Lo Presti M, Frisina N, Bagnato G, Fries W. Gastro-intestinal permeability is increased in patients with limited systemic sclerosis. *Scand. J. Rheumatol.* 2001;30:77-81.

[10] Gonzalez-Mariscal L, Betanzos A, Nava P, Jaramillo BE. Tight junction proteins. *Prog. Biophys. Mol. Biol.* 2003 Jan;81:1-44.

[11] Ikenouchi J, Furuse M, Furuse K, Sasaki H, Tsukita S. Tricellulin constitutes a novel barrier at tricellular contacts of epithelial cells. *J. Cell Biol.* 2005 Dec 19;171:939-45.

[12] Furuse M, Hirase T, Itoh M, Nagafuchi A, Yonemura S, Tsukita S. Occludin: a novel integral membrane protein localizing at tight junctions. *J. Cell Biol.* 1993 Dec;123: 1777-88.

[13] Furuse M, Fujita K, Hiiragi T, Fujimoto K, Tsukita S. Claudin-1 and -2: novel integral membrane proteins localizing at tight junctions with no sequence similarity to occludin. *J. Cell Biol.* 1998 Jun 29;141:1539-50.

[14] Martin-Padura I, Lostaglio S, Schneemann M, Williams L, Romano M, Fruscella P, Panzeri C, Stoppacciaro A, Ruco L, et al. Junctional adhesion molecule, a novel member of the immunoglobulin superfamily that distributes at intercellular junctions and modulates monocyte transmigration. *J. Cell Biol.* 1998 Jul 13;142:117-27.

[15] Rao RK, Basuroy S, Rao VU, Karnaky Jr KJ, Gupta A. Tyrosine phosphorylation and dissociation of occludin-ZO-1 and E-cadherin-beta-catenin complexes from the cytoskeleton by oxidative stress. *Biochem. J.* 2002 Dec 1;368:471-81.

[16] Colegio OR, Van Itallie CM, McCrea HJ, Rahner C, Anderson JM. Claudins create charge-selective channels in the paracellular pathway between epithelial cells. *Am. J. Physiol. Cell Physiol.* 2002 Jul;283:C142-7.

[17] Van Itallie CM, Anderson JM. Claudins and epithelial paracellular transport. *Annu. Rev. Physiol.* 2006;68:403-29.

[18] Holmes JL, Van Itallie CM, Rasmussen JE, Anderson JM. Claudin profiling in the mouse during postnatal intestinal development and along the gastrointestinal tract reveals complex expression patterns. *Gene Expr. Patterns.* Netherlands; 2006. p. 581-8.

[19] Saitou M, Furuse M, Sasaki H, Schulzke JD, Fromm M, Takano H, Noda T, Tsukita S. Complex phenotype of mice lacking occludin, a component of tight junction strands. *Mol. Biol. Cell* 2000 Dec;11:4131-42.

[20] Al-Sadi R, Khatib K, Guo S, Ye D, Youssef M, Ma T. Occludin regulates macromolecule flux across the intestinal epithelial tight junction barrier. *Am. J. Physiol. Gastrointest. Liver Physiol.* 2011;300:G1054-64.

[21] Seth A, Sheth P, Elias BC, Rao R. Protein phosphatases 2A and 1 interact with occludin and negatively regulate the assembly of tight junctions in the CACO-2 cell monolayer. *J. Biol. Chem.* 2007 Apr 13;282:11487-98.

[22] Sakakibara A, Furuse M, Saitou M, Ando-Akatsuka Y, Tsukita S. Possible involvement of phosphorylation of occludin in tight junction formation. *J. Cell Biol.* 1997 Jun 16;137:1393-401.

[23] Laukoetter MG, Nava P, Lee WY, Severson EA, Capaldo CT, Babbin BA, Williams IR, Koval M, Peatman E, et al. JAM-A regulates permeability and inflammation in the intestine in vivo. *J. Exp. Med.* 2007;204:3067-76.

[24] Itoh M, Furuse M, Morita K, Kubota K, Saitou M, Tsukita S. Direct binding of three tight junction-associated MAGUKs, ZO-1, ZO-2, and ZO-3, with the COOH termini of claudins. *J. Cell Biol.* 1999 Dec 13;147:1351-63.

[25] Bazzoni G, Martinez-Estrada OM, Orsenigo F, Cordenonsi M, Citi S, Dejana E. Interaction of junctional adhesion molecule with the tight junction components ZO-1, cingulin, and occludin. *J. Biol. Chem.* 2000;275:20520-6.

[26] Furuse M, Itoh M, Hirase T, Nagafuchi A, Yonemura S, Tsukita S. Direct association of occludin with ZO-1 and its possible involvement in the localization of occludin at tight junctions. *J. Cell Biol.* 1994 Dec;127:1617-26.

[27] Umeda K, Matsui T, Nakayama M, Furuse K, Sasaki H, Furuse M, Tsukita S. Establishment and characterization of cultured epithelial cells lacking expression of ZO-1. *J. Biol. Chem.* 2004;279:44785-94.

[28] Farhadi A, Keshavarzian A, Ranjbaran Z, Fields JZ, Banan A. The role of protein kinase C isoforms in modulating injury and repair of the intestinal barrier. *J. Pharmacol. Exp. Ther.* 2006 Jan;316:1-7.

[29] Fasano A, Fiorentini C, Donelli G, Uzzau S, Kaper JB, Margaretten K, Ding X, Guandalini S, Comstock L, Goldblum SE. Zonula occludens toxin modulates tight junctions through protein kinase C-dependent actin reorganization, in vitro. *J. Clin. Invest.* 1995 Aug;96:710-20.

[30] Banan A, Farhadi A, Fields JZ, Zhang LJ, Shaikh M, Keshavarzian A. The delta-isoform of protein kinase C causes inducible nitric-oxide synthase and nitric oxide up-regulation: key mechanism for oxidant-induced carbonylation, nitration, and disassembly of the microtubule cytoskeleton and hyperpermeability of barrier of intestinal epithelia. *J. Pharmacol. Exp. Ther.* 2003 May;305:482-94.

[31] Banan A, Fields JZ, Farhadi A, Talmage DA, Zhang L, Keshavarzian A. Activation of delta-isoform of protein kinase C is required for oxidant-induced disruption of both the microtubule cytoskeleton and permeability barrier of intestinal epithelia. *J. Pharmacol. Exp. Ther.* 2002 Oct;303:17-28.

[32] Suzuki T, Seth A, Rao R. Role of phospholipase Cgamma-induced activation of protein kinase Cepsilon (PKCepsilon) and PKCbetaI in epidermal growth factor-mediated protection of tight junctions from acetaldehyde in Caco-2 cell monolayers. J. *Biol. Chem.* 2008 Feb 8;283:3574-83.

[33] Banan A, Fields JZ, Talmage DA, Zhang L, Keshavarzian A. PKC-zeta is required in EGF protection of microtubules and intestinal barrier integrity against oxidant injury. *Am. J. Physiol. Gastrointest. Liver Physiol.* 2002 May;282:G794-808.

[34] Banan A, Zhang LJ, Shaikh M, Fields JZ, Choudhary S, Forsyth CB, Farhadi A, Keshavarzian A. theta Isoform of protein kinase C alters barrier function in intestinal epithelium through modulation of distinct claudin isotypes: a novel mechanism for regulation of permeability. *J. Pharmacol. Exp. Ther.* 2005 Jun;313:962-82.

[35] Jain S, Suzuki T, Seth A, Samak G, Rao R. Protein kinase Czeta phosphorylates occludin and promotes assembly of epithelial tight junctions. *Biochem. J.* 2011;437: 289-99.

[36] Suzuki T, Elias BC, Seth A, Shen L, Turner JR, Giorgianni F, Desiderio D, Guntaka R, Rao R. PKC eta regulates occludin phosphorylation and epithelial tight junction integrity. *Proc. Natl. Acad. Sci. USA* 2009 Jan 6;106:61-6.

[37] Schwarz BT, Wang F, Shen L, Clayburgh DR, Su L, Wang Y, Fu YX, Turner JR. LIGHT signals directly to intestinal epithelia to cause barrier dysfunction via cytoskeletal and endocytic mechanisms. *Gastroenterology.* 2007 Jun;132:2383-94.

[38] Wang F, Graham WV, Wang Y, Witkowski ED, Schwarz BT, Turner JR. Interferon-gamma and tumor necrosis factor-alpha synergize to induce intestinal epithelial barrier dysfunction by up-regulating myosin light chain kinase expression. *Am. J. Pathol.* 2005 Feb;166:409-19.

[39] Clayburgh DR, Musch MW, Leitges M, Fu YX, Turner JR. Coordinated epithelial NHE3 inhibition and barrier dysfunction are required for TNF-mediated diarrhea in vivo. *J. Clin. Invest.* 2006 Oct;116:2682-94.

[40] Suzuki T, Hara H. Quercetin enhances intestinal barrier function through the assembly of zonula occludens-2, occludin, and claudin-1 and the expression of claudin-4 in Caco-2 cells. *J. Nutr.* 2009 May;139:965-74.

[41] Amasheh M, Schlichter S, Amasheh S, Mankertz J, Zeitz M, Fromm M, Schulzke JD. Quercetin enhances epithelial barrier function and increases claudin-4 expression in Caco-2 cells. *J. Nutr*. 2008 Jun;138:1067-73.
[42] Dorfel MJ, Westphal JK, Huber O. Differential phosphorylation of occludin and tricellulin by CK2 and CK1. *Ann. N. Y. Acad. Sci*. 2009 May;1165:69-73.
[43] Szabo A, Boros M, Kaszaki J, Nagy S. Mucosal permeability changes during intestinal reperfusion injury. The role of mast cells. *Acta Chir Hung*. 1997;36:334-6.
[44] Chuenkitiyanon S, Pengsuparp T, Jianmongkol S. Protective effect of quercetin on hydrogen peroxide-induced tight junction disruption. *Int. J. Toxicol*. 2010;29:418-24.

In: Quercetin
Editors: Taiki Chikamatsu and Yuudai Hida
ISBN: 978-1 61942- 057-1

Chapter 16

THE CHARACTERIZATION AND BIOACTIVITY OF QUERCETIN

Chunhuan He, Hengshan Wang, Yingming Pan**, *Xiaowen Ji and Kai Wang
Key Laboratory for the Chemistry and Molecular Engineering of
Medicinal Resources (Ministry of Education of China),
School of Chemistry and Chemical Engineering of
Guangxi Normal University, Guilin, P. R. China

ABSTRACT

Quercetin is the major representative of the flavonoid subclass of flavonols which mostly present as its glycoside form in onions, olives, tea, beer and red wine. It has a broad range of biological, pharmacological and medical applications which benefit to human health. In present paper, the dietary source, function and health benefits such as antioxidant properties, anticancer properties, anti-inflammatory, anti-aggregatory, vasodilating effects, reverse multidrug resistance and other bioactivity of quercetin and its glycoside form are reviewed.

1. INTRODUCTION

Quercetin (also known as QU, quercetin flavin) and its derivatives are widely distributed in the plant kingdom, with a variety of biological activity of flavonoids. It exists in many plants, flowers, leaves, fruits, mostly in the form of glycosides, such as rutin, quercetin glycosides, hyperin, etc., which acid hydrolysis into quercetin. In recent years, more and more domestic and foreign medical researchers strenghten the study of quercetin, and have found many pharmacological activity of quercetin, such as antioxidant and scavenging oxygen free radicals, anti-aggregatory, anti-tumor effect, vasodilating effects, anti-virus, anti-

* Corresponding author. Tel.: +86-773-5846279; fax: +86-773-5803930; E-mail address: panym2004@yahoo.com.cn (Yingming Pan).

inflammatory, reverse multidrug resistance, pain and diarrhea, etc.. It has been tested in a variety of diseases, and achieved good results. Therefore, we studied the biological activity of quercetin as a review.

2. Chemistry Of Quercetin

The chemical name of quercetin is 2-(3,4-dihydroxyphenyl)-3,5,7-trihydroxy-4*H*-1-Benzopyran-4-one, molecular formula and molecular weight are $C_{15}H_{10}O_7$ and 302.23, and the dihydrate of quercetin is yellow needle-like crystals (dil-ethanol), and in the 95-97 °C become anhydrous, melting point 314 °C (decomposition). 1g dissolved in 290 ml of anhydrous ethanol, 23 ml boiling ethanol, dissolved in glacial acetic acid. Alkaline aqueous solution is yellow, almost insoluble in water, and the ethanol solution tasted bitter.

Quercetin (1) is the prototype antioxidant flavonoid because it exhibits all three structural components necessary for antioxidant activities of this compound class including (a) the presence of a catechol group in ring B, which has electron-donating properties and is a radical target; (b) a 2,3-double bond conjugated with the 4-oxo group, which is responsible for electron delocalization; and (c) the presence of both 3- and 5-hydroxy scavenging groups. These structural characteristics of 1 explain why it has the highest antioxidant activity when compared to other flavonoids. In fact, the most widely recognized biological effects of 1 are related to the antioxidant properties that occur by scavenging oxygen radicals, inhibiting lipid peroxidation as well as protein and DNA oxidation, and chelating metal ions (Valério et al., 2009).

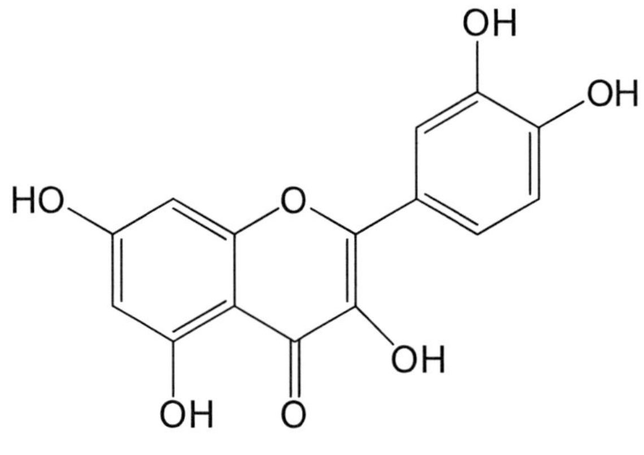

Figure 1. Chemical structure of quercetin.

3. Dietary Sources of Quercetin

Flavonoids, a group of polyphenolic compounds with antioxidant properties, are widely distributed in foods of plant origin such as vegetables, fruit, tea and wine. Within the subgroup of flavonols and flavones the flavonol quercetin is the major compound in foods, especially for onions (Hertog et al., 1992; Vries et al., 1997). It is reported that in onions approximately 90% of the quercetin was localised in the first and second layers of the onion (Ewald et al., 1999). Quercetin is also present in plants in many different glycosidic forms, and quercetin-3-rutinoside (rutin) is one of the most widespread forms. Examples of other dietary quercetin glycosides are quercetin galactosides, quercetin arabinosides, kaempferol, myricetin, and isorhamnetin (Erlund, 2004). They are often found in broccoli, berries, apples and onion.

4. Functions and Health Benefits of Quercetin

4.1. Antioxidant Properties

Previous research show that consumption of fruits and vegetables, which contain high content of antioxidant, can reduce the incidence of cardiovascular diseases and several cancers, whereby especially (cereal) fibers and phenolic compounds play a very important role (Rohn, 2004). Moreover, antioxidant can help preserve food quality because oxidation causes food deterioration. Phenols and flavonoids have gained significant interest among various antioxidants in recent year. Quercetin, one of the most important members in flavonoid family, has been reported to have the greatest antioxidant activity evaluated by B-phycoerythrin fluorimetric method (López et al., 2003). Iacopini et al. (2008) tested the *in vitro* antioxidant activity of quercetin, rutin, catechin, epicatechin and resveratrol in red grape using 2,2-diphenyl-1-picrylhydrazyl (DPPH) free radical and peroxynitrite ($ONOO^-$) scavenging assay and found that quercetin had the lowest IC_{50} value towards both kinds of free radicals, as described by Villaño et al. (2007) and Haenen et al. (1997). The antioxidant activity of quercetin and its protein-phenol derivatives was investigated by Rohn et al. (2004) using a modified TEAC assay. Their results show that the covalent attachment of quercetin to bovine serum albumin decreases the total antioxidant activity in comparison to an equivalent amount of free quercetin depending on the degree of derivatization. The higher amount of covalent bound quercetin, the stronger antioxidant activity of the derivative.

4.2. Anticancer Properties

Quercetin, a lipid-soluble plant pigment, is widely distributed in fruits, vegetables and herbal plants. It's demonstrated to inhibit several types of cancer cells, such as breast and prostrate cells *in vitro* (Kobayashi et al., 2002). It was reported by Choi et al that quercetin induced significant apoptosis in MCF-7 human breast cancer cells through at least two different mechanisms; by inhibiting cell cycle progression through transient M phase accumulation and subsequent G2 arrest, and by inducing apoptosis (Choi et al., 2001). In an animal study, both ellagic acid and quercetin significantly reduced tumor incidence, and ellagic acid can synergistically potentiate the effects of quercetin (at 5 and 10 μM, respectively) (Khanduja et al., 1999). Garcia et al found that higher intake of quercetin can obviously reduce the incidence of stomach cancer (Garcia et al., 1999). Research on human HL-60 leukemia cells showed that quercetin inhibited the growth of HL-60 cells in a concentration-dependent manner and its inhibitory effect on the growth of HL-60 cells may be related to its inhibitory effects on protein kinase C (PKC) and/or tyrosine protein kinase (TPK) *in vitro* and/or on the production of phosphoinositides (Kang and Liang, 1997). Study on hepatic cell suggest that quercetin is a dietary flavonoid that is capable of inducing selective growth inhibition and apoptosis in hepatic tumor cells, but not in normal cells (Son et al., 2004). Similary, Lugli et al found quercetin inhibits lymphocyte activation and proliferation without inducing apoptosis in peripheral mononuclear cells, but it could interfere with effector T cell function (Lugli et al., 2009). The Nagini group found that quercetin suppressed the viability of human cervical cancer (HeLa) cells in a dose-dependent manner by inducing G2/M phase cell cycle arrest and mitochondrial apoptosis through a p53-dependent mechanism (Priyadarsini, et al., 2010). Recently, quercetin-treatment with rats bearing Walker 256 carcinosarcoma show the inhibition of tumor growth, survival increase, decrease of matrix metalloproteinase-2(MMP-2) (related to degradation of extracellular matrix and favoring tumor invasion) and vascular endothelial growth factor (VEGF) levels and reduction of cachexia in animals; these strongly support the anticancer function of this flavonoid. What is more, quercetin can abolishe phospholipase D 1 expression and subsequently inhibits invasion and proliferation of U87 glioma cells (Park et al., 2011).

4.3. Anti-Inflammatory

It is well known that oxidative stress often leads to the accumulation of reactive oxygen species (ROS). And ROS induce the activation of nuclear factor-κB (NF-κB) resulting in the coordinated expression of inflammatory and innate immunity genes and secretion of pro-inflammatory cytokines (Surh and Na, 2008). Quercetin is a potent dietary antioxidant that also displays anti-inflammatory activities. It significantly inhibited mRNA level of inducible nitric oxide synthase (iNOS), cyclooxygenase-2 (COX-2), and reactive C-protein (CRP) and the result may contribute to the anti-inflammatory effects of this flavonoid in Chang Liver cells, *via* mechanisms likely to involve blockade of NF-κB activation and the resultant up-regulation of the pro-inflammatory genes (García-Mediavilla et al., 2007). Previous studies have indicated that quercetin, both added *in vitro* and supplemented *in vivo*, also displays anti-inflammatory effects (Nair et al., 2006; Boots et al., 2008; Boots et al., 2009; Kleemann et al., 2011). It is reported by Boots et al that quercetin is capable of reducing LPS-induced levels of various pro-inflammatory cytokines including TNFa and IL-8, which are known to be elevated in sarcoidosis (Boots et al., 2009; Boots et al., 2011). The effect of quercetin on endoplasmic reticulum (ER) stress, which triggers such disorders as inflammation and cancer, was investigated and found that quercetin suppressed the ER stress caused by calcium dynamics dysregulation by the inhibition of phosphoinositide 3-kinase (Natsume et al., 2009). Another research show that quercetin can not only protect cells from oxidative stress-induced cell death, but also reduced the expression of cytokines interleukin-6 (IL-6) and interleukin-1β (IL-1β) in cells treated with H_2O_2, and increased the expression levels of nuclear factor-erythroid 2-related factor-2 (Nrf2) and heme oxygenase-1 (HO-1) which suggested protective function against oxidative stress (Saviranta et al., 2011). What is more, quercetin exerts anti-oxidative and anti-inflammatory effects in cultured human cells such as endothelial cells and hepatocytes. Meanwhile, it quenched IL-1β-induced C-reactive protein (CRP) expression in human CRP transgenic mice, attenuated atherosclerosis in human ApoE*3Leiden transgenic mice, and also reduced the gene expression of specific factors implicated in local vascular inflammation including IL-1R, Ccl8, IKK, and STAT3.

4.4. Anti-Aggregation

Platelets aggregation is partialy responsible for thromboembolic diseases such as myocardial infarction, unstable angina, stroke and peripheral artery disease (Dogne et al., 2002).

The inhibition of platelet aggregation is a usual way to treat these diseases. Previous study indicate that quercetin inhibits adenosine diphosphate-induced as well as thrombin-induced platelet coagulation, and inhibits the 12-lipoxygenase pathway of arachidonate metabolism, blocking the synthesis of hepoxilins which are mediators of neutrophil activation, calcium mobilisation and vascular permeability (Pace-Asciak, 1993; Pace-Asciak, 1995). Quercetin inhibit platelet aggregation alone, but the combination with α-tocopherol can cause an antiaggregating effect at much lower concentrations than each of these compounds does separately (Kobzar et al., 2005).

The effects of quercetin and dihydroquercetin (DHQ) on hemolysis and platelet aggregation in human blood was compared by Chen and Deuster (2009), and they found lipid-soluble quercetin is more effective for protecting red blood cells against oxidative and enzymatic damages than the water-soluble DHQ, which was more potent than quercetin in inhibiting superoxide but could not inhibit the aggregation of platelets by adenosine diphosphate. Spice active principles showed varied inhibitory effect on *in vitro* human platelet aggregation induced by agonist arachidonicacid (AA), ADP, collagen and calcium ionophore.

The order of potency of spice principles in inhibiting AA-induced platelet aggregation is eugenol > capsaicin > curcumin > cinnamaldehyde >piperine > allyl sulphide > quercetin (Raghavendra and Naidu, 2009).

4.5. Vasodilating Effects

Quercetin can lower blood pressure, increase capillary resistance and expansion of coronary artery, increase coronary blood flow and so on. In recent years, scientist found that quercetin can significantly inhibited pulmonary artery smooth muscle cells proliferation which induced by the blood small plate-derivd growth factor, for the prevention and treatment of pulmonary hypertension has an important role (Wang and Zhang, 1999). Quercetin also has certain role on reversal of myocardial hypertrophy (Qin et al., 1999).

Pretreatment of cultured human umbilical vein endothelial cells with quercetin, at 5 or 50 μM, reduces thrombin-induced endothelin-1 release (Zhao et al., 1999). Comparative vasodilating actions of the constituents of Ginkgo biloba extract, terpenoids (bilobalide, ginkgolides A, B and C) and flavonoids (quercetin and rutin), was found that quercetin, which (100 μmol/l) caused a potent vasorelaxation by 49.9 ± 4.8% ($n = 10$, $P < 0.001$), showed the strongest vasorelaxation (Nishida and Satoh, 2004). In addition, Romero et al (2010) reported that quercetin can reduce systolic blood pressure, left ventricular and renal hypertrophy and improve NO-dependent acetylcholine relaxation, but it was unable to improve insulin sensitivity possibly through its specific interference with the insulin signalling pathway.

4.6. Reverse Multidrug Resistance

Intrinsic or acquired multidrug resistance (MDR) is a major impediment to successful chemotherapy. Overexpression of ATP-binding cassette transporters is thought to be one of main mechanism and has received extensive investigation (Litman et al. 2001). Compounds that inhibit the expression and functional activity of P-glycoprotein, the ATP-dependent efflux pump, will increase cellular accumulation of many chemotherapeutic agents and reverse MDR. Quercetin itself exhibit growth inhibitory activity on both drugsensitive and MDR cells, such as K562 (erythroleukemic cells), HL60 (promyelocyte leukemia cells), CCRF-CEM (T-lymphocytic leukemia cells) and their respective drug resistant counterparts K562/adr, HL60/VCR, CEM/ADR5000, CEM/VLB100 and CEM/E1000 (Chen et al., 2010).

It was reported by Chung et al. (2005) that quercetin treatment resulted in an increased daunomycin accumulation in the resistant cell line MCF-7/ADR, which was similar to that of verapamil, a well-known p-glycoprotein inhibitor. In Brisdelli's study (Brisdelli et al., 2007), quercetin (25μM) causes a marked inhibition of K562 cells growth together with a mild cytotoxicity while HSB-2 cells are practically unaffected. These demonstrate that quercetin triggers the onset and progression of caspase-3 and cytochrome c-dependent apoptosis together with a significant accumulation in G2/M phase in K562 cells, while is almost uneffective in HSB-2 cells. Quercetin has also been studied in animal models.

Wang's study showed that the oral coadministration of 40 mg/kg quercetin increased significantly the Cmax and the AUC of digoxin (substrate for p-glycoprotein) in pigs (wang et al., 2004a, 2004b). In adition, the short-term use of quercetin elevated the plasma concentrations of fexofenadine (Kim et al., 2009).

4.7. Other Bioactivity

Quercetin has many biological activities, in addition to the above, such as anti-virus, hypoglycemic, anti-obesity, antidiarrheal, anti-thrombotic, anti-depression and so on. Wang et al. (2009) have investigated the pathological mechanisms of depression and found that quercetin can siginificantly reduce the Beas-2b cells induced by CSE (cigarette smoke extract) death, and inhibit the reduce of cell activity. The mechanisms may be increase cells' OH-1 protein expression which induced by CSE. Quercetin has a certain analgesic effect, can siginificantly improve animal's Pain threshold, and have a dose-effect relationship. Gong et al. used four different analgesic models: hot plate, writhing, electrical stimulation- screaming law and formalin method found quercetin' effective analgetic dose is 60~100mg/kg, and the effect come to the strongest after 0.5 h, and disappear after 1 h (Gong et al., 1996).

Investigation on neointima hyperplasia with quercetin show that quercetin significantly inhibited neointimal hyperplasia in rat abdominal aorta 14 day safter injury in relatively high doses, and this effect might be partially attributed to the suppression of platelet-derived growth factor-BB, b-fibroblast growth factor, and transforming growth factor-β1 expressions (Huang et al., 2009). Amyloid beta- peptide [Aβ(1–42)], elevated in Alzheimer's disease brain, is associated with oxidative stress and neurotoxicity. Ansari et al. (2009) found that pretreatment of primary hippocampal cultures with quercetin significantly attenuated amyloid beta-peptide [Aβ (1–42)]-induced cytotoxicity, protein oxidation, lipid peroxidation and apoptosis. Recently, treatment with quercetin (5-20 mg/kg, p.o., twice daily, 30 days) in streptozotocin- induced diabetic rats prevented the changes in blood glucose, body weight, and performance in Morris water and elevated plus maze tasks (Bhutada et al., 2010). It means that quercetin treatment ameliorated cognitive dysfunction in the diabetic rats. In addition, quercetin modulates the host response during salmonellosis by protecting the host cells from the toxic effects of bacterial infection and also by decreasing programmed cell death (Paolillo et al., 2011).

CONCLUSIONS

In summary, quercetin has a strong biological activity and a wide range of pharmacological effects and harmless to human body. It's important to human cancer, cardiovascular disease, aging treatment and prevention. Because of its wide range of pharmacological activity, quercetin often as types of the active ingredients of Chinese herbal medicines for quality control. We should fully develop and utilize this class of rich natural medicine resources, contribute to human health according to development of the pharmacological.

ACKNOWLEDGMENTS

This study was supported by 973 projects (2011CB512005), The projects of Key Laboratory for the Chemistry and Molecular Engineering of Medicinal Resources (Guangxi Normal University), Ministry of Education of China (CMEMR2011-15), Guangxi Natural Science Foundation of China (2011GXNSFD018010 and 2010GXNSFF013001), Guangxi's Medicine Talented Persons Small Highland Foundation (0808), and the Fund of Guangxi Key Laboratory of Functional Phytochemicals Research and Utilization (No. FPRU2011-1).

REFERENCES

Ansari, MA; Abdul, HM; Joshi, G. et al. Protective effect of quercetin in primary neurons against Aβ(1–42): relevance to Alzheimer's disease. *Journal of Nutritional Biochemistry*, 2009, 20, 269-275.

Bhutada, P; Mundhada, Y; Bansod, K. et al. Ameliorative effect of quercetin on memory dysfunction in streptozotocin-induced diabetic rats. *Neurobiology of Learning and Memory*, 2010, 94, 293-302.

Boots, AW; Drent, M; de Boer, VCJ. et al. Quercetin reduces markers of oxidative stress and inflammation in sarcoidosis. *Clinical Nutrition*, 2011, 30, 506-512.

Boots, AW; Drent, M; Swennen, EL. et al. Antioxidant status associated with inflammation in sarcoidosis: a potential role for antioxidants. *Respiratory Medicine*, 2009, 103, 364-372.

Boots, AW; Wilms, LC; Swennen, EL. et al. *In vitro* and *ex vivo* anti-inflammatory activity of quercetin in healthy volunteers. *Nutrition,* 2008, 24, 703-710.

Brisdelli, F; Coccia, C; Cinque, B. et al. Induction of apoptosis by quercetin: different response of human chronic myeloid (K562) and acute lymphoblastic(HSB-2) leukemia cells. *Mol. Cellular Biochem*, 2007, 296, 137-149.

Chen, C; Zhou, J; Ji, C. Quercetin: A potential drug to reverse multidrug resistance. *Life Sciences*, 2010, 87, 333–338.

Chen, Y; Deuster, P. Comparison of quercetin and dihydroquercetin: Antioxidant-independent actions on erythrocyte and platelet membrane. *Chemico-Biological Interactions*, 2009, 182, 7-12.

Choi, JA; Kim, JY; Lee, JY. et al. Induction of cell cycle arrest and apoptosis in human breast cancer cells by quercetin. *International journal of Oncology*, 2001, 19, 837-844.

Chung, SY; Sung, MK; Kim, NH. et al. Inhibition of P-Glycoprotein by Natural Products in Human Breast Cancer Cells. *Arch. Pharm. Res*, 2005, 28, 823-828.

de Vries, JHM; Janssen, P ; Hollman, PCH. et al. Consumption of quercetin and kaempferol in free-living subjects eating a variety of diets. *Cancer Letters,* 1997, 114, 141-144.

Dogne, JM; Leval, XD; Benoit, P. et al. Recent advances in antiplatelet agents. *Current medicinal Chemistry*, 2002, 9, 577- 589.

Erlund, I. Review of the flavonoids quercetin, hesperetin, and naringenin. Dietary sources, bioactivities, bioavailability, and epidemiology. *Nutrition Research*, 2004, 24, 851-874.

Ewald, C; Fjelkner-Modig, S; Johansson, K. et al. Effect of processing on major flavonoids in processed onions, green beans, and peas. *Food Chemistry*, 1999, 64, 231-235.

Garcia-Closas, R; Gonzalez, CA; Agudo, A. et al. In take of specific carotenoids and flavonoids and the risk of gastric cancer in Spain. *Cancer Causes Control,* 1999, 10 (1), 71-75.

García-Mediavilla, V; Crespo, I; Collado, PS. et al. The anti-inflammatory flavones quercetin and kaempferol cause inhibition of inducible nitric oxide synthase, cyclooxygenase-2 and reactive C-protein, and down-regulation of the nuclear factor kappaB pathway in Chang Liver cells. *European Journal of Pharmacology*, 2007, 557, 221-229.

Gong, S.; Zhang, YY; Yu, GD. et al. The observe of quercetin analgesic effect. *Chinese Herbal Medicine*, 1996, 27(10), 612-613.

Haenen, GRMM. Paquay, JBG; Korthouwer, REM. et al. Peroxynitrite Scavenging by Flavonoids. *Biochemical and Biophysical Research Communications*, 1997, 236, 591-593.

Hertog, MGL; Hollman, PCH; Katan MB. Content of potentially anticarcinogenic flavonoids of 28 vegetables and 9 fruits commonly used in the Netherlands. *Journal Agriculture Food Chemistry*, 1992, 40, 2379-2383.

Huang, B; Wang, W; Fu, Y. et al. The effect of quercetin on neointima formation in a rat artery balloon injury model. *Pathology–Research and Practice,* 2009, 205, 515-523.

Iacopini, P; Baldi, M; Storchi, P. et al. Catechin, epicatechin, quercetin, rutin and resveratrol in red grape: Content, in vitro antioxidant activity and interactions. *Journal of Food Composition and Analysis*, 2008, 21, 589-598.

Kang, T; Liang, N. Studies on the inhibitory effects of quercetin on the growth of HL-60 leukemia cells. *Biochemical Pharmacology*, 1997, 54, 1013-1018.

Khanduja, KL; Gandhi, RK; Pathania, V. et al. Prevention of N-nitrosodiethylamine- induced lung tumorigenesis by ellagic acid and quercetin in mice. *Food and Chemical Toxicology*, 1999, 37, 313-318.

Kim, KA; Park, PW; Park, JY. Short-term effect of quercetin on the pharmacokinetics of fexofenadine, a substrate of P-glycoprotein, in healthy volunteers. *European Journal of Clinical Pharmacology*, 2009, 65 (6), 609-614.

Kleemann, R; Verschuren, L; Morrison, M. et al. Anti-inflammatory, anti-proliferative and anti-atherosclerotic effects of quercetin in human in vitro and in vivo models. *Atherosclerosis*, 2011, 218, 44-52.

Kobayashi, T; Nakata, T; Kuzumaki, T. Effect of flavonoids on cell cycle progression in prostate cancer cells. *Cancer Letters*, 2002, 176, 17-23.

Kobzar, G; Mardla, V; Samel, N. Effects of α-tocopherol, L-arginine, and quercetin on aggregation of human platelets. *Nutrition Research*, 2005, 25, 569-575.

Litman, T ; Druley, TE ; Stein, WD. et al. From MDR to MXR: new understanding of multidrug resistance systems, their properties and clinical significance. *Cellular and Molecular Life Sciences*, 2001, 58 (7), 931–959.

López, M; Martínez, F ; Del Valle, C.D. et al. Study of phenolic compounds as natural antioxidants by a fluorescence method. *Talanta*, 2003, 60, 609-616.

Lugli, E; Ferraresi, R; Roat, E. et al. Quercetin inhibits lymphocyte activation and proliferation without inducing apoptosis in peripheral mononuclear cells. *Leukemia Research*, 2009, 33, 140-150.

Nair, MP; Mahajan, S; Reynolds, JL et al. The flavonoid quercetin inhibits proinflammatory cytokine (tumor necrosis factor alpha) gene expression in normal peripheral blood mononuclear cells via modulation of the NF-kappabeta system. *Clin. Vaccine Immunol*, 2006, 13, 319-328.

Natsume, Y; Ito, S; Satsu, H. et al. Protective effect of quercetin on ER stress caused by calcium dynamics dysregulation in intestinal epithelial cells. *Toxicology,* 2009, 258, 164-175.

Nishida, S; Satoh, H. Comparative vasodilating actions among terpenoids and flavonoids contained in Ginkgo biloba extract. *Clinica Chimica Acta,* 2004, 339, 129-133.

Pace-Asciak, CR. Hepoxilins. *Gen Pharmacol*, 1993, 24, 805-810.

Pace-Asciak, CR; Hahn, S; Diamandis, EP. et al. The red wine phenolics trans-resveratrol and quercetin block human platelet aggregation and eicosanoid synthesis: Implications for protection against coronary heart disease. *Clinica Chimica Acta*, 1995, 235, 207-219.

Paolillo, R; Carratelli, CR; Rizzo, A. Effect of resveratrol and quercetin in experimental infection by Salmonella enterica serovar Typhimurium. *International Immunopharmacology*, 2011, 11, 149-156.

Park, MH; Min, DS. Quercetin-induced downregulation of phospholipase D1 inhibits proliferation and invasion in U87 glioma cells. *Biochemical and Biophysical Research Communications*, 2011, 412, 710-715.

Priyadarsini, RV; Murugan, RS; Maitreyi S. et al. The flavonoid quercetin induces cell cycle arrest and mitochondria-mediated apoptosis in human cervical cancer (HeLa) cells through p53 induction and NF-κB inhibition. *European Journal of Pharmacology*, 2010, 649, 84-91.

Qin, TC; Gu, ZL; Liu, SZ. The influence of quercetin to rat myocardial hypertrophy caused by overload pressure. *Chinese Herbal Medicine*, 1999, 30(4), 275-277.

Raghavendra, RH; Naidu, KA. Spice active principles as the inhibitors of human platelet aggregation and thromboxane biosynthesis. *Prostaglandins, Leukotrienes and Essential Fatty Acids*, 2009, 81, 73-78.

Rohn, S; Rawel, HM; Kroll, J. Antioxidant Activity of Protein-Bound Quercetin. *Journal Agriculture Food Chemistry*, 2004, 52, 4725-4729.

Romero, M; Jiménez, R; Hurtado, B. et al. Lack of beneficial metabolic effects of quercetin in adult spontaneously hypertensive rats. *European Journal of Pharmacology*, 2010, 627, 242-250.

Saviranta, NMM; Veeroos, L; Granlund, LJ. et al. Plant flavonol quercetin and isoflavone biochanin A differentially induce protection against oxidative stress and inflammation in ARPE-19 cells. *Food Research International*, 2011, 44, 109-113.

Son, Y; Lee, K; Kook, S. et al. Selective effects of quercetin on the cell growth and antioxidant defense system in normal versus transformed mouse hepatic cell lines. *European Journal of Pharmacology*, 2004, 502, 195-204.

Surh, YJ; Na, H K. NF-kappa B and Nrf2 as prime molecular targets for chemoprevention and cytoprotection with anti-inflammatory and antioxidant phytochemicals. *Genes Nutr*, 2008, 2, 313-317.

Valério, DA; Georgetti, SR; Magro DA. et al. Quercetin Reduces Inflammatory Pain: Inhibition of Oxidative Stress and Cytokine Production. *Journal Natural Products,* 2009, 72, 1975-1979.

Villaño, D; Fernández-Pachón, MS; Moyá, ML. et al. Radical scavenging ability of polyphenolic compounds towards DPPH free radical. *Talanta,* 2007, 71, 230-235.

Wang, CM; Zhang, ZX. The influence of quercetin to pulmonary arterial smooth muscle proliferation and pulmonary arterial hypertension of big rat. *China Physical Medicine and Rehabilitation Magazine*, 1999, 21(2), 103-105.

Wang, LJ; Gong, T; Wang, L. et al. The inhibitory effect of quercetin on cigarette smoke extract induced human bronchial epithelial cell death. *Chinese Pharmacology Bulletin*, 2009, 25(7), 960-963.

Wang, Y; Cao, J; Zeng, S. Establishment of a P-glycoprotein substrate screening model and its preliminary application. *World Journal of Gastroenterology,* 2004a, 10 (9), 1365-1368.

Wang, YH; Chao, PD; Hsiu, SL. et al. Lethal quercetin-digoxin interaction in pigs. *Life Sciences*, 2004b, 74 (10), 1191-1197.

Zhao, X; Gu, Z; Attele, AS. et al. Effects of quercetin on the release of endothelin, prostacyclin and tissue plasminogen activator from human endothelial cells in culture. *Journal of ethnopharmacology*, 1999, 67, 279-285.

INDEX

B

C

D

E

F

G

H

I

J

K

L

M

N

O

P

Q

R

S

T

U